Haridimos Kondylakis · Andreas Triantafyllidis
Editors

Pervasive Computing Technologies for Healthcare

18th EAI International Conference, PervasiveHealth 2024
Heraklion, Crete, Greece, September 17–18, 2024
Proceedings, Part II

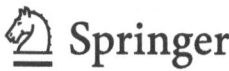 Springer

Editors
Haridimos Kondylakis ⓘ
University of Crete
Heraklion, Greece

Andreas Triantafyllidis ⓘ
Information Technologies Institute Centre
of Research and Technology
Thessaloniki, Greece

ISSN 1867-8211   ISSN 1867-822X (electronic)
Lecture Notes of the Institute for Computer Sciences, Social Informatics
and Telecommunications Engineering
ISBN 978-3-031-85574-0   ISBN 978-3-031-85575-7 (eBook)
https://doi.org/10.1007/978-3-031-85575-7

This Springer imprint is published by the registered company Springer Nature Switzerland AG
The registered company address is: Gewerbestrasse 11, 6330 Cham, Switzerland

If disposing of this product, please recycle the paper.

Lecture Notes of the Institute
for Computer Sciences, Social Informatics
and Telecommunications Engineering

612

The LNICST series publishes ICST's conferences, symposia and workshops.
LNICST reports state-of-the-art results in areas related to the scope of the Institute.
The type of material published includes

- Proceedings (published in time for the respective event)
- Other edited monographs (such as project reports or invited volumes)

LNICST topics span the following areas:

- General Computer Science
- E-Economy
- E-Medicine
- Knowledge Management
- Multimedia
- Operations, Management and Policy
- Social Informatics
- Systems

Preface

We are delighted to introduce the proceedings of the 18th edition of the European Alliance for Innovation (EAI) International Conference on Pervasive Computing Technologies for Healthcare (PervasiveHealth 2024), which took place at Heraklion, Crete, Greece on 17–18 September 2024. This conference brought together researchers, developers, and practitioners around the world who focus on technologies and human factors related to the use of ubiquitous computing for healthcare and wellbeing.

The technical program of PervasiveHealth 2024 consisted of 41 full papers in oral presentation sessions at the main conference tracks. The conference tracks were: Track 1 - Patient Empowerment; Track 2 – Artificial Intelligence; Track 3 – Medical Imaging; Track 4 – Education; and Track 5 – mHealth & Telemonitoring. Aside from the high-quality technical paper presentations, the technical program also featured two keynote speeches and one technical workshop. The two keynote speeches were given by Mary P. Czerwinski from Microsoft, USA and Nicos Maglaveras from Aristotle University of Thessaloniki, Greece. The 3rd IOT-HR workshop: Workshop on Internet of Things in Health Research, which took place in parallel, focused on the challenges and opportunities presented by continuous data acquisition by Internet of Things (IoT) devices, such as smartwatches, fitness trackers, mobile phones, and smart home appliances.

Coordination with the program chairs, Manolis Tsiknakis, Dimitrios Fotiadis, and Guang Yang, was essential for the success of the conference. We sincerely appreciate their constant support and guidance. It was also a great pleasure to work with such an excellent organizing committee team for their hard work in organizing and supporting the conference. We are also grateful to the local chair Kostas Marias for his support, and last but not least, we would like to thank all the authors who submitted and presented their papers at the PervasiveHealth 2024 conference.

We strongly believe that the PervasiveHealth conference provides an excellent forum for all researchers, developers, and practitioners to discuss all science and technology aspects that are relevant to pervasive computing technologies for healthcare. We also expect that the future PervasiveHealth conferences will be as successful and stimulating, as indicated by the contributions presented in this volume.

Haridimos Kondylakis
Andreas Triantafyllidis

Organization

Organizing Committee

General Chair

Haridimos Kondylakis   University of Crete and FORTH-ICS, Greece

General Co-chair

Andreas Triantafyllidis   Centre for Research and Technology Hellas, Greece

Program Chair and Co-chairs

Manolis Tsiknakis   Hellenic Mediterranean University & FORTH-ICS, Greece
Dimitrios Fotiadis   University of Ioannina & FORTH-ICS, Greece
Guang Yang   Imperial College London, UK
Praveen Rao   University of Missouri-Columbia, USA

Local Chair

Kostas Marias   FORTH-ICS, Greece

Workshops Chair

Kostas Stefanidis   Tampere University, Finland

Publicity and Social Media Chair

Sofia Segkouli   Centre for Research and Technology Hellas, Greece

Publications Chair

Vassilis Kilintzis   FORTH-ICS, Greece

Web Chair

Dario Salvi   Malmö University, Sweden

Technical Program Committee

Siddarth Arora   University of Oxford, UK
Karim Lekadir   University of Barcelona, Spain
Stelios Sfakiannakis   FORTH-ICS, Greece
Evangelia Zacharaki   University of Patras, Greece
Manolis Spanakis   FORTH-ICS, Greece
Giuseppe Fico   Universidad Politécnica de Madrid, Spain
Georgios Theodorakopoulos   University of Cardiff, UK
Haodi Zhang   King's College London, UK
Honghan Wu   University College London, UK
Holly Tibble   University of Edinburgh, UK
Tracey Chantler   London School of Hygiene & Tropical Medicine,
                                       UK
Francisco Lupiáñez-Villanueva   Predict By, Spain
Asimina Kiourti   Ohio State University, USA
Ioannis Katakis   University of Nicosia, Cyprus
Gaetano Valenza   University of Pisa, Italy
Iosif Mporas   University of Hertfordshire, UK
Ahmar Shah   University of Edinburgh, UK
Mauro Dragoni   Fondazione Bruno Kessler, Italy
Miriam Kuricova   National Institute of Endocrinology and
                                       Diabetology, Slovakia
Andrea Botikova   Trnava University, Slovakia
Luigi Borzi   Politecnico di Torino, Italy

Contents – Part II

3rd IOT-HR: Workshop on Internet of Things in Health Research

Posters

Contents – Part I

Artificial Intelligence

Medical Imaging

Education

Education

The Virtual Co-design of *Sleep Solved* – A Case Study of an Educational Sleep App Designed with Teens

Anthony Duffy[1,2](✉) (ID), Sarah E. Bennett[2] (ID), Lucy Yardley[2] (ID), and Sylvain Moreno[1] (ID)

[1] School of Interactive Arts and Technology, Simon Fraser University, 250 -13450 102 Avenue, V3T 0A3, Surrey, BC, Canada
anthony.duffy@sfu.ca

[2] School of Life Sciences, Department of Psychological Sciences, University of Bristol, Beacon House, Queens Rd., BS8 1QU, Bristol, UK

Abstract. Background: Sleeplessness is an emerging epidemic amongst young people. Numerous apps exist to mediate sleep problems using a variety of CBT-i workshop design approaches. Virtually crowdsourcing co-design, however, provides the promise of rapid and vastly increased data. The rapid co-design of mHealth apps is an important part of the emerging big data, digital health citizen era.

Objective: This exploratory case study explored the virtual, crowdsourced co-design of Sleep Solved—an educational mHealth sleep app designed with teens, to learn which virtual methods were used to engage teen co-designers and how these methods can be scaled up.

Methods: We conducted an enquiry-based iterative case study utilising the Bayazit 3-stage model. 85 teens participated over 11 months. Data was thematically analysed over several design iterations.

Results: Rapid virtual feedback allowed for quick pivots in a short time frame. Four stages of feedback from teens led to iterative changes to scientific information contextualisation and user experience, from lo-fidelity mock-ups through to a coded app beta.

Conclusion: The co-design of Sleep Solved exemplified the potential of virtually crowdsourcing teens in mHealth. Key to this evolution will be the ability to leverage big data utilising AI and machine learning approaches to data collation and synthesization, such that meaningful and contextual findings can be applied in line with software development timelines.

Keywords: mHealth · digital health citizens · co-design · crowdsourcing · user experience · person-based design · sleep · teens

H. Kondylakis and A. Triantafyllidis (Eds.): PervasiveHealth 2024, LNICST 612, pp. 3–27, 2025.
https://doi.org/10.1007/978-3-031-85575-7_1

1 Background

1.1 Leveraging Mobile Health to Improve Sleep Hygiene in Teens

A worldwide epidemic of sleeplessness is rapidly emerging amongst teens [1]. With one in four young people reporting sleep problems and 4% of all adolescents reporting patterns of sleep disturbance [2], there is great concern that poor sleep habits are fuelling a rise in neurodevelopmental disorders [3] and a variety of mental health challenges[4] in young adults. More specifically, long-term adverse effects include metabolic issues, chemical imbalances, obesity, and chronic disease [4]. It is estimated that this phenomenon is costing the healthcare systems worldwide US $16B annually, with loss in work productivity costs exceeding US $50B annually [5]. These socioeconomic challenges are driving sleep research towards more rapid, instantaneous mobile health (mHealth) solutions that can help teens solve sleep problems into adulthood.

The emergence of mHealth is positively disrupting traditional health approaches on a scale not seen since the emergence of antibiotics [6] mHealth apps provide ubiquitous, instantaneous access to support digital health diagnostics, self-help, preventive behaviour change and various other intervention types [7]. With investments reaching US $410 billion in 2022, [8] mHealth investment is expected to grow beyond half a billion by 2027 [9]. Key to the development of mHealth into the mid 21st century is the contextual design [10] with young people [11]. Teens are digital natives who hold the potential to harness the far-reaching impacts of digitally ubiquitous, instantaneous health technologies throughout life. This is especially important seeing that up to 15% of adolescents today have been diagnosed with a chronic illness or disability, [12] and the downstream impact on an already overwhelmed health care system is concerning. Developing strategies that help transition young people from paediatric to adult health care in the mode of personalised mHealth self-care is therefore paramount [10].

1.2 Teenage Years: A Transition in Sleep and Digital Activity

Considering that adolescence is a period of biological shift in circadian rhythms, [13] this is an important time to connect with teens on developing good sleep hygiene for life. From the age of 13 through to the age of 18, teens see a typical decrease in total sleep time of almost 1.5 h [14, 15]. This, coupled with an increased academic workload and greater independence to utilise digital technologies, provides the opportunity for insomnia and other sleep problems to emerge. Insomnia, which can be defined as "a difficulty in falling asleep, difficulty staying asleep, and non-restorative sleep," leads to symptoms of fatigue, impaired concentration and mood disturbance. Poor sleep habits and their resulting comorbidities can often persist and increase into adulthood, [15] contributing to a flow of downstream health and social problems. A recent study (2020) found adolescent sleep problems persisting into adulthood in approximately 50% of teens, [15] additionally, global estimates in youth mental health problems have risen to between 10% to 20% [16]. These alarming trends call for new and innovative approaches to mediate teen sleep problems. In seeking to address these challenges, the opportunity to curate a mHealth app for sleep awareness is a prospective approach, considering today's teens are digital natives living on the cutting edge of tech culture. In support of this, encouraging research has found that 81% of adolescents have used the internet to seek health related guidance [13]. As digital natives, today's teens are the first generation to grow up with the technological ubiquity of smartphones and other internet of things (IoTs).

1.3   Virtual Crowdsourcing with Teens: The Digital Health Citizens of Tomorrow

Co-designing an mHealth based sleep intervention with teens, one that is embedded into their digital ecosystem is a forward-thinking strategic approach to healthcare intervention design [6]. As healthcare shifts towards more accessible, tailored solutions that prioritise individual needs and preferences, the drive to find better ways to co-design with young health users is heightened [10]. An emerging method to improve this is virtual crowdsourcing the co-design ideas of teens. This method leverages the collective brain of participants, promising a wealth of rapidly collected data touchpoints, towards better understanding how to tailor needs to young mHealth users [17]. More robust, data-rich methods to co-design are foundational towards improving scientific discovery, breakthrough treatments and more personalised care. Crowdsourcing virtually bridges time, distance, and affordability in healthcare in ways traditional co-design methods cannot [18]. In this regard, crowdsourcing teen co-design presents a window to the future of mHealth. More broadly, this aligns with the World Health Organization's (WHO) systematic and cultural transformation of health care ecosystems, led by disruptive technologies that position people as digital health citizens; active engaged participants in the process of curating digital health solutions [19]. Digital health citizens are positioned at the intersection of 'bio and techno-sociality'. They are defined as active, responsible partners in the discourse, technologies, and social practices of health care [20]. This shift in strategy is intended to reduce the downstream cost of sickness services, instead promoting better health services throughout life [21]. As an overarching philosophy, the digital health citizen approach can seek to impact the three core mobile health (mHealth) design challenges of: reduced costs (budget), increased data points (validity) and rapid digital product delivery (time constraints) [22]. This all-digital co-design approach resonates well with the technocentric ecosphere of today's teens.

1.4   Related Work: mHealth Sleep App Design

There have been several efforts to utilise mHealth towards improving sleep deficit and to increase sleep hygiene (Table 1).

Table 1. Summary of prominent mHealth sleep interventions

mHealth app	Focus	Description
Doze	CBT-i	A free transdiagnostic, self-management, cognitive behavioural web app that provides personalised feedback on sleep disturbance, the app was designed using an interactive, experience-based co-design process with end users [23]
Calm	Mindfulness meditation	A commercially successful mindfulness meditation mobile app that includes 'sleep disturbance' as part of a group of health behaviour (change) objectives [24]
Sleep Scheduler	CBT-i	A digital sleep diary that can suggest (or intervene) in sleep scheduling using a CBT-i approach [5]
iREST (interactive Resilience Enhancing Sleep Tactics)	Mindfulness meditation	An mHealth platform designed to provide a just-in-time adaptive intervention (JITAI) in the assessment, monitoring, and delivery of evidence-based sleep recommendations in a scalable and personalised manner. The platform includes a mobile phone–based patient app linked to a clinician portal [25]
Sleepio	CBT-i	A multimedia rich iOS and web app that combines the functionality of a sleep diary, CBT-i coach and virtual sleep expert providing components of CBT, as well as other non-drug treatments for insomnia such as Imagery Relief Therapy [5]

(continued)

Table 1. (*continued*)

mHealth app	Focus	Description
Sleep Ninja	CBT-i	A CBT-i that focuses on psychoeducation, stimulus control, sleep hygiene and sleep-related cognitive therapy, this is delivered via training lessons, recommendations and sleep tips; a six-week program that concludes with a black belt in sleep [2]
Better Nights, Better Days – Youth	CBT-i	A CBT-i with strategies that target adolescents (age 14–18) with neurodevelopmental disorders (NDD) and sleep problems [26], the app aims to educate on healthy sleep behaviours towards effective sleep practices. It does this by providing recommendations and a daily sleep diary for sleep tracking [15]
SHUTi (Sleep Healthy Using the Internet™)	CBT-i	A personalised, interactive web app built on predetermined "if-then" algorithms [25], SHUTi is designed to improve the sleep of adults with insomnia. In the form of an online course, users have daily and weekly tasks to monitor and record the subjectivity of their sleep data,[3] as part of the broader Sleep Well project, SHUTi is currently being adapted for teens in the UK

To summarise, where apps like Doze and Calm are focused on self-management, and apps like Sleep Scheduler and Sleepio combine sleep scheduling and CBT-i, and apps like iREST and SHUTi centred on behaviour change, there was a need for a teen-centric educational sleep app that serves to 'on-board' with sleep hygiene education, building towards diary, tracking and CBT-i approaches. In essence, a gap was identified that segues teens towards sleep management and CBT-i; one that is educational, informative, and in the vein of today's teen tech culture.

1.5   Understanding the Motivation Behind Case Studying Sleep Solved: A Teen Sleep Awareness App

The need for a teen-centric educational sleep app is strongly supported by the fact that only 36% [24] of the teenage demographic actively seeks mental health support through traditional methods. With adolescent sleep problems frequently persisting into adulthood, it is essential to address this issue, as it is adding stress to an already strained health system in the UK. A recent study [15] by Toguas et al. cited inaccessibility, cost, time and stigmas as key factors dissuading teens from seeking traditional help. Contrastingly, mHealth offers the potential to increase accessibility, reduce costs, and provide private, instantaneous interventions. mHealth is uniquely positioned as a medium that lives in the "digisphere" of today's teens: the app space.

However, despite there being more than 2000 mHealth apps targeting sleep [27], there is little in the way of evidence-based support for their development. A 2017 study [28] noted that only 13% of sleep apps provided links to evidence-based scientific literature. A recent review by Aji et al. [29] noted that various attempts to incorporate a user-centred design (UCD) in sleep apps was bridging the gap between patients and health professionals. Nonetheless, approximately half of the sleep apps reviewed did not utilise a person-centred design (PCD) approach. In this regard, there is a unique and important opportunity for the co-design of Sleep Solved to culminate in the three design objectives of: person-based, science-focused, and intelligent design.

Given the important potential of virtual crowdsourcing in mHealth research, we endeavoured to case study this online, iterative process to create Sleep Solved. The app was designed by a team of health experts (sleep, psychology) and digital designers (artists and developers). A person-based approach (PBA) [30] was adopted to engage in the co-design with teens. The stages of ideating and testing with teens was conducted entirely by virtual crowdsourcing. Virtual crowdsourcing, which can be defined as an "online, distributed problem-solving and production model that leverages the collective intelligence of online communities for specific purposes" [31] is not a new concept [32]. However, it remains nascent in the digital health design space, providing the potential for a rapid, vast crop of data-points utilising various mixed-method approaches to ideation and testing [33]. Studies have lauded the ability for crowdsourcing to garner feedback from thousands of participants in a matter of hours [17]. As Swan et. al have noted, crowdsourced health research is an emerging contemporary trend that accentuates the emerging "citizen science" approach to Health 2.0, [33] wherein patients become active participants—practitioners of their own good health—utilising the best of web 2.0 technologies that incorporate big data techniques and artificial intelligence (AI), towards providing intuitive, information analytics for "health citizens". The virtual crowdsourcing approach in digital health co-design may represent an important bridge between the challenge to rapidly create digital solutions within a constricted timeline and traditionally slower, safer large data needs in health care research. In essence, virtual crowdsourcing may bridge top-down (health care) and bottom-up (digital design) approaches around faster, richer, user data points.[31] Gaining more data points in a shorter time frame is of mutual interest to digital and health stakeholders alike. With these objectives in mind, our research questions were:

[RQ1]: How were virtual methods used to engage teens in the co-design of a sleep self-help app?

[RQ2]: How can these virtual co-design methods be adapted for large-scale ideation and testing in the emerging digital health citizen ecosystem?

It is hoped that through this virtual crowdsourced project, broad feedback may be collected towards better understanding how to effectively co-design virtually with young mHealth end users at-scale. Considering that 95% of adolescents (aged 13–17) use a smartphone, [4, 16] and with behavioural strategies being considered the frontline in healthcare prevention [3], an educational mHealth sleep app provides a way to engage teens before negative habits form. It is expected that this novel approach to designing a sleep app for teens will uncover more challenges and opportunities, something that should be embraced in the digital health community.

2 Methods

Seeing that our research questions were exploratory in nature, we modelled this enquiry-based iterative case study after Bayazit's 3-stage model: [34, 35].

Model 1: Find out about current design practices (e.g., pursue a design project to help uncover decision-making processes and social responsibilities).

Model 2: Devise improvements in design methods (e.g., help conceive and develop new design procedures, information, priorities, and tools).

Model 3: Make improvements to designed artefacts (e.g., help contribute to how a type of product can or ought to be designed, how it can be improved, and to demonstrate benefits).

The Bayazit methodology culminates in three key outcomes of which we provide our contextual output:

1. **Knowledge elicitation:** This involved the documentation of co-designers' thinking, archived in an unstructured, unanalyzed form, inclusive of all internal project team meetings, online Young Person's Advisory Group (YPAG) workshops (n = 1), think-aloud interviews (n = 20), online surveys, online user testing and feedback focus groups (n = 7). In essence, the raw data from the co-design journey.
2. **Data analysis and interpretation:** This involved thematic analysis of the data, resulting in themes and subthemes reflective of the plus points, pain points and gaps and opportunities derived from the co-design process.
3. **Knowledge synthesis:** This involved the data synthesis of findings relative to the virtual co-design journey with teen collaborators, and the wider validity and implications relative to scaling up methods for larger virtual data collection into the digital health citizen era.

2.1 Settings

The Sleep Solved co-design took place over the course of 15 months (June 2022-August 2023). All participants, including health researchers, designers and developers co-designed virtually, with some internal work and meetings taking place on-site at the University of Bristol. A virtual codesign was selected in order to increase ease of participation amongst teens across the UK.

2.2 Participants

Over the course of 11 months, 85 Participants aged 14–18 were recruited from colleges and schools across England through partnership with two organisations: E-ACT [36] and the Association of Colleges [37]. Wider PPI consultation was achieved in partnership with UK based charities for sleep and mental health: The Sleep Charity, [38] the McPin Foundation, [39] and a Young Person's Advisory Group (YPAG) [40] from Bristol. Sleep Solved co-designers were recruited from college and secondary school students from some of the most deprived neighbourhoods in the UK. In order to recruit young people to PPIE activities within the target age range (14–18), a video and QR poster describing the study was shared with partner schools and colleges.

2.3 Ethics

Ethics was sought and approved by Ethics and Research Governance, University of Bristol. The main feasibility study was approved by the North West-Greater Manchester Central Research Ethics Committee. For PPIE activities, consent was not required from contributors, in line with National Institute for Health and Care Research (NIHR) Centre for Engagement and Dissemination guidance on patient and public involvement in research [41].

2.4 Data Collection and Analysis

Teen participants were engaged in the form of virtual surveys, focus groups and think-aloud interviews (Appendix 1). Fieldnotes were taken throughout the project reflective of internal meetings, discussions, meeting recordings, interviews, think-alouds and surveys. Data was then collectively organised, and coded and themed in a thematic analysis. Following the Braun and Clarke analysis protocol [42], data was carefully scrutinised, line-by-line, resulting in the organic arrival at codes, themes and sub-themes.

3 Results

In this section, we present an analysis of our findings in a narrative format that recollects the virtual co-design experience. The themes and subthemes listed construct the findings of the design project including the advancements and challenges encountered.

3.1 Virtual Co-design

Young Person Advisory Group (YPAG) Brainstorming Session
To kick-off the PPIE sessions, the Bristol YPAG group [40, 43] was consulted to understand the message, medium(s) and design approach. Teen participants agreed with the

core message proposal (i.e. how science can help you sleep better), and noted that an app that was simple, soothing and informative about sleep hygiene would be beneficial, particularly one that provides a format that answers key questions and clears up common misconceptions. They also noted that most of their teen friends may be unaware of the science surrounding sleep.

Branding and Theming

Before venturing into the app design and features, the first design step was to develop an app name, colour palette (theme) and branding approach (Appendix 1). Six names were proposed by the research team to teen co-designers with Sleep Solved being the most popular choice. Three colour palettes were mocked up by a design agency with the most popular responses being the playful and approachable stylised neon pastel iconography and night blue sky backgrounds (resonating with sleep time).

First Iteration: Discovery (low-fidelity PowerPoint)

With conceptual ideas for branding and theming in place, the research team began to refine an approach to bridge pertinent scientific information on sleep hygiene with intelligent design approaches (Appendix 1). As a first step in the app development process, the research team utilised a blue-sky approach by iterating information and design layout concepts in low fidelity PowerPoint mock-ups (Appendix 1). This would allow for rapid testing of both the interpretation of scientific information and the UX, with easy on-the-fly adjustments.

Information was kept concise, led by snippets of information called "micro learning moments", that presented quick engaging copy mediated by soft imagery and icons. This approach was built upon preliminary research pointing to challenges in language comprehension, engagement, and reducing the intimidation surrounding scientific information. The design was refined several times internally before being scaled-up in fidelity for presentation to teen co-designers.

Second Iteration: Visualising the App Design Concept (medium-fidelity Figma prototype)

Through a process of internal co-designing, the challenge to strike a balance between presenting scientific information whilst making it visually simple was explored repeatedly. Since the first iteration mock-up was focused on deciding on scientific information and how to present it, it was not formulated considering the constraints and affordances of mHealth design. The second iteration then focused on co-designing app screen mock-ups that would provide a viable design concept to integrate the scientific information with an intelligent app design. Successful apps like Duolingo and Mercedes-Benz were explored for design approaches to app onboarding, gestures and calls to action, in order to evaluate the intuitiveness of interactions with end users. A UX designer reconceptualised the first iteration mock-ups within an app design framework in Figma considering mobile app gestures and calls to action (Appendix 1).

The initial PPIE feedback pointed to simplicity through visible, relaxing but relative and informative, intelligent design. This began to take form in the second iteration, through app screen mock-ups that utilised soft but bright pastel images and fun, playful iconography that was semiotic. In this vein, two theme concepts were polished and tested with teens. One theme was darker in tone with text on coloured background panels, whereas the other utilised sharper imagery and white panel background sliders. The latter of the two was more popular with teen co-designers with preference given to good contrast (background/foreground), and bright neon colours to draw attention to imagery with less text (Appendix 1).

Key teen co-designer PPIE feedback: *"[It's] simple, doesn't have too much writing and gets to the point, not overwhelming to look at."*

Key Themes from PPIE: Concision, visualising meaning, soft icons (imagery).

Additionally, the research team understood from the preliminary brand research that the app name and logo design would be an important mediator with teens. To this end, four versions of the Sleep Solved logo were tested with teens (Appendix 1).

"The logos are better being colourful I think as they are aimed at younger audiences." (PPI feedback from teen co-designer, 16, F).

Key Themes from PPIE: Colourfulness, legibility, demographically contextual.

Third Iteration: Coded App for Testing (high-fidelity). With feedback on both app and branding mock-ups from teen co-designers, a web developer from the research team began to code the app for user testing. A focus group was formed to use and test the beta version of Sleep Solved for one week. Seven teens with existing sleep challenges gave their feedback. They enjoyed the visual nature of the app experience and found the information relevant and relatable. Teen co-designers identified numerous bugs and design improvements ranging from menu navigation buttons to continuity errors. Of key importance was the desire for more interactive multimedia (i.e. rewards) and retention concerns (i.e. one-and-done experiences). Overall, users found the tips in the app (sleep hacks) useful when put into practice but were curious about related apps in the project that would provide metrics from sleep tracking.

Key Themes from PPIE: Navigability, informativeness, relevance, relatability.

These findings from teen co-designers led to a final beta-launch version that incorporated layers of UX feedback on the scientific information, usability and retention (Fig. 1, Appendix 1).

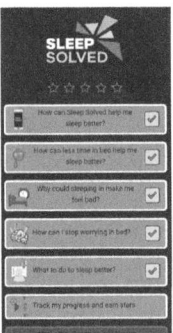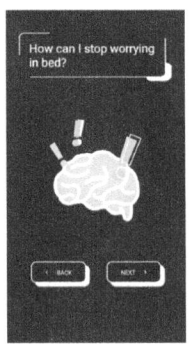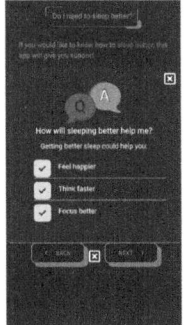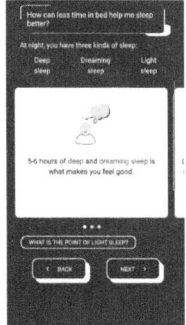

Fig. 1. Sleep Solved coded beta app (high fidelity)

This concluded the co-design phases of the project and the case study. A video walk-through of the project is available in Appendix 3. This final stage of the feasibility trial was to be begin autumn, 2023.

4 Discussion

This exploratory case study sought to investigate methods to rapidly iterate a virtual co-design with teen participants facing sleep challenges, and to understand how these methods could be scaled-up to increase validity and reliability of data in the emerging Health 2.0 era. Our findings illustrate the advancements and challenges to co-design outside of traditional workshop environments. As with any approach, there are pros and cons to its utilisation. Whilst virtual crowdsourcing brings the promise of more data, challenges exist in how to recruit and vet participants, and how to analyse emotional UX data acquired remotely. The virtual co-design of Sleep Solved garnered two key themes (Table 2).

Table 2. Summary of themes and subthemes

Theme	Subtheme
Information Contextualisation	simplicity, informativeness, demographically relative
User Interface and User Experience	visibility, navigability, visualisation

These two themes dominated user feedback such that teen users felt the information presented in the app needed to be scientific yet simple to understand, informative not boring, and demographically relative (i.e. interesting and easy for the teen audience to absorb). Additionally, much of the feedback on the UI and UX was focused on imagery and text being visible yet concise, easy to navigate, and a true visualisation of the scientific message. It was interesting to note that teen users understood the seriousness of a sleep awareness app and the mental health challenges that surround it. A brand affinity survey showed that many of the brands in teen popular culture and their forms of mediation (like TikTok) were deemed unsuitable design references for a sleep self-help app by teen co-designers. This illustrates the astuteness of teen mHealth app users, that they are not in need of mere entertainment for engagement.

A key positive of the design process was the rapid data collection from a wide pool of participants, something that speaks to the need for larger population studies in mHealth co-design (towards improving validity, reliability) [33]. However, one of the key challenges was the lack of digitisation of traditional UX workshop exercises (e.g. sketching, dot-voting etc.) and the rich emotional feedback it garners, data that often speaks beyond statistical feedback. Additionally, some of the design concepts that were popular amongst expert research team members were less popular amongst teen co-designers and quickly dismissed (despite the small subject pool). This gulf of evaluation supports the need for the further involvement of teens alongside designers in the co-design space at-scale, into the Health 2.0 era. Although the themes discovered during this virtual co-design process satisfied the goals of an iterative design process, to envision Créquit et al.'s "citizen science" approach, much larger, richer mixed-method data collection is needed to improve the validity and reliability of data, improving the contextuality of the co-design process[44]. With these general observations in mind, we turn our attention specifically to the research questions.

4.1 The Utilisation of Virtual Methods to Engage Teens in the Co-design of a Sleep App

Data Collection Approaches

The four PPIE events with teen co-designers ranged from 23–40 recruitments with an average participation rate of 32.7%, and a median (n = 7). Participation rates were similar in size to typical in-person workshops. By incorporating national charities, the research team was able to recruit from a larger pool (nationally), making the core demographic more rapidly attainable in this study. The first three PPIE events were surveys which provided the benefit of rapid and blunt assessment of digital assets and copy. The research team was very attentive to teen co-designer feedback and made changes accordingly. However, as with many traditional co-design studies, the number of subjects was limited, such that strong design determinations were built upon limited end-user feedback. This is consistent with recent findings in a 2024 systematic review of Challenges to Incorporate End Users in the Design of DHIs [45] that found 78.3% of studies included less than 20 subjects, with only 7.8% including more than 50 subjects. Although survey feedback is rapid and statistical, it is often brought into question for margin of error (deviation) in small sample sizes. To this end, richer approaches to crowdsource more data could be helpful.

Co-design Approaches

The prototypical on-site co-design workshop which garners mainly emotional, qualitative feedback in a fail-fast agile environment, was not replicated virtually. Instead, traditional research approaches such as surveys and think-alouds were conducted to gain rapid insights. Where co-design may more broadly refer to the involvement of stakeholders in the design process, *how* this takes place is much more subjective. In app design, the process of defining the questions, examining assumptions, exploring personas and mapping user journeys are typically in-person workshop collaborations. During this blue-sky phase, the (research) question may pivot, misconceptions may arise, and challenges often surface. Solutions, be they information or design oriented, are often prioritised and voted on. Sketching exercises wherein the design team (including end-users) flesh together a vision of the solution is common. These approaches would have been beneficial to Sleep Solved but would have added scope and strained delivery timelines. Additionally, these emotionally rich methods are also tagged with the same challenges of reliability and validity due to a similarly limited sample size. Moving forward, the challenge for virtual co-design workshops may lie in how they can be utilised at-scale, in a cost-effective, timely manner. A core challenge exists in digital health on how to utilise proven industry co-design methods: at-scale, with scientific validation, all within the constraints of an mHealth app timeline.

Testing Approaches

The testing phase was conducted with a group of seven teens who used Sleep Solved over the period of one week. Teens were asked open-ended questions like "How did you find using Sleep Solved over the past week?" and about their routines and methods to calm their minds or spend less time lounging in bed. This think-aloud group format allowed teens to scaffold their design feedback as well as stating their misunderstandings or misconceptions about the science of sleep. They were also able to contrast the 'sleep hacks' learned from Sleep Solved with the practical impact (or not) on their sleep-related behaviour. They were then able to suggest better personalisation in the form of more enriching engagement (rewards) and progress markers (checkboxes). Overall, teen co-designers found the app helpful and were intrigued to learn even more about the science of sleep. Nonetheless, virtual ideation and testing approaches that produce large filterable datasets, representing user preferences and tracked usage of the prototype would provide richer more contextual feedback. Attaining this will require novel database-driven co-design interfaces, as we will propose.

To this end, the three iterative design phases built around three surveys, a one-week beta trial, and subsequent focus group, provided rounds of changes that improved Sleep Solved. However, just how effective this co-design process could be with virtual approaches that garner much more data is a question of much intrigue. Concerns regarding reliability and validity may be soothed by methods that generate a larger data pool with a more diverse array of virtual UX workshops. In that regard, our attention shifts to our second research question on the potential methods to scale-up virtual co-design.

4.2   Methods to Scale up Virtual Co-design for Large-Scale Ideation and Testing in the Health 2.0 Era

While Sleep Solved showed that virtual crowdsourcing can be effective, it utilised methods (surveys and think-alouds) that only scratch the surface of virtual co-design data collection. To mediate broader challenges in digital health, new approaches are needed that produce larger datasets rapidly, without losing the richness of emotional feedback or falling into siloed perspectives that can limit the potential of the co-design. Reflecting on the co-design approach in this study, we developed the following five recommendations on how to scale up virtual co-design for large-scale ideation and testing in mHealth:

Recruitment: This study revealed a 32.7% participation rate amongst recruited teens. Researchers can use this marker to consider the scope of outreach needed. Scaled-up, gaining 327 participants from 1000 recruitments would be a much-improved dataset. This underscores—despite any challenges—the potential for virtual crowdsourcing. With the assistance of The Association of Colleges (and other charities), demographically relevant recruitment took place across the country. This process could be further enhanced by utilising teen-centric social media such as TikTok, Snapchat and Instagram for demographically-driven recruitment ad campaigns. This opens the potential for 1000s of responses that form the cornerstone of improved validity and reliability (more data, less margin of error) in digital health co-design studies [46].

Big Data Virtual Co-design: As alluded to previously, traditional workshops are largely qualitative, synchronous and time consuming, with small but rich data pools (typically 5–8 people). Sleep Solved utilised remote surveys and think-alouds for rapidity and reach. However, by digitising workshop UX exercises asynchronously—as our concept exemplifies (Fig. 2)—with a co-design interface that presents mood boards that can be annotated with memes or stickers, by providing lo-fidelity sketches that can be drawn over or highlighted, and logos that can be annotated or doodled over—visual and interactive forms of asynchronous feedback can be obtained en masse. Each section of the co-design could be timeboxed for usage tracking. This of course would require meaningful data that can be filtered and organised in an automated fashion. This is where expanded virtual approaches become very prospective. This approach, deployed on a website or mHealth app may resonate with teens using social cues they enjoy. Additionally, it would allow for some of the best industry practices to be digitised, producing larger datasets. In the Sleep Solved study, financial incentive was provided to teen survey subjects, this approach could also be utilised for a synchronous online design jam, that seeks to utilise industry-styled zero-to-hero design approaches in developing an initial prototype (with teens) in remotely deployed half-day virtual workshops.

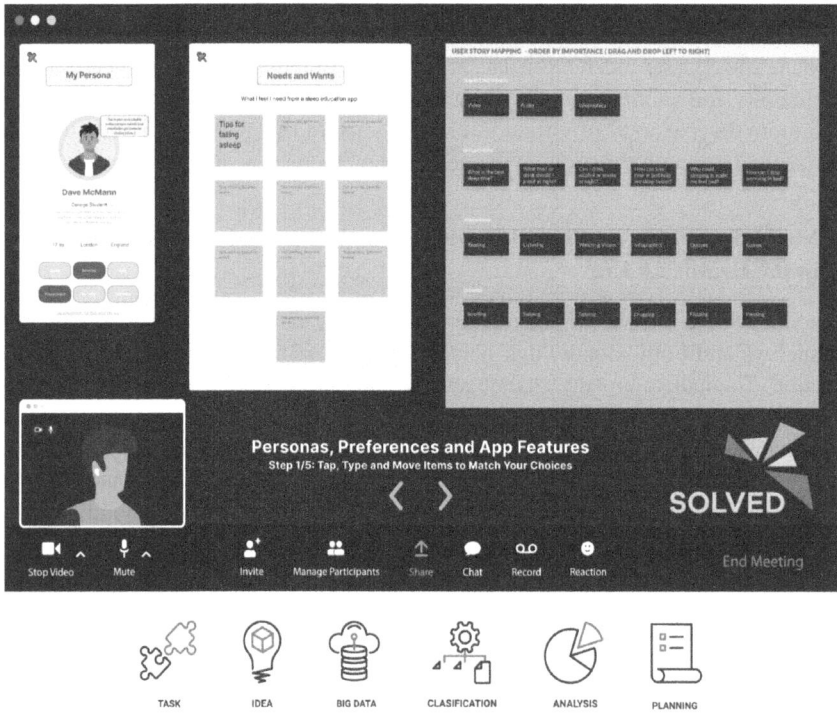

Fig. 2. Prototype for an asynchronous co-design experience jamboard

AI and Machine Learning in Co-design: The aforementioned concepts for digital recruitment and co-design are in need of automated processes that reduce the inundation of uncollated data. It would be an exhaustive process for researchers to comb through extensive online data, one that would negate the gains of digitising feedback. In this regard, there is a need to automate user responses in the forms of stickers, ratings, heat-mapping areas of mockups that gain the most activity, pitch recognition of voice feedback and speech-to-text processing that can generate keyword themes and subthemes auto-matically (automated thematic analysis)— all of this to better understand usage metrics and preferences in co-design. This is a mixed-method approach where qualitative and quantitative approaches can meet, where statistical and emotional feedback can comple-ment one another, a silo-free approach that leverages the best of various sciences in the coproduction of an mHealth app. This is difficult to envision without the smart metrics derived from the automation of workshop data that is collated smartly and instantly.

Observational User Testing: Asynchronous testing that captures both emotional feed-back (vibes) and user actions (metrics) can be obtained by observational user testing. This emotional feedback may include speech (pitch and tone, text-to-speech) and body language (reaction to media or calls to action) which can be linked to the given app screen in view. This data can be automated and mapped to the actionable metrics of the end user. This combination may address the longstanding variance in qualitative and quantitative analysis of an mHealth app that often juxtaposes user feedback with user activity. In this, there is the opportunity to 'draw a line' through trends in the data that better combines the actions and opinions of end users, seeking to vastly improve the challenges of validity and reliability; iterating design based on richer data.

Co-design Vlogging: In addition to leveraging teen social media platforms for recruit-ment, publishing the digital co-design experiences of participants may garner mass feedback in the form of ideation through social commentary. It is also an additional way of gauging broader feedback to design concepts. A popular activity amongst teens nowadays is the publishing of multiplayer online role-playing games (MMORPG) expe-riences to be viewed online, or for young people to publish lived experiences, or their own tutorials (vlogging). The observation of co-design experiences itself may be of intrigue to young people, garnering important secondary feedback at-scale. This data can be mined using algorithmic generative artificial intelligence (AI) software such as AirOps,[47] to collect social media keyword filtering towards thematic trends in social responses.

Key Challenges and Limitations
These concepts, though promising in principle, are untested and would face key chal-lenges. Logistically, the richness of observational analysis is challenged when shifting workshops from in-person to online. Without the value of face-to-face validation, greater challenges exist regarding data integrity. Big data approaches bring data variability and scrutiny into the lens of analysis. There is the danger of obtaining inappropriate data (outside of the target demographic), and falsified tests or designs (junk data), especially when participation may be financially incentivised. This is a longstanding challenge in research that would only be multiplied in larger virtual recruitments. AI and machine

learning is an emerging field that can be manipulated to 'lie with statistics'. Ethics and integrity loom large in the scientific discussion of automating metrics. Researchers will need to account of these challenges.

4.3 Crowdsourcing Digital Health Co-design into the Health 2.0 Era

Whilst tempering the promise of large-scale virtual co-design with the challenges of a domain still very much in its adolescent years, there is an inevitability that digital health co-design must trend in the direction of increasing the scope and uniqueness of data points for mHealth evaluation [33]. It is well-established in the literature that smaller qualitative studies jeopardise validity and reliability and that clinical trials are long and cumbersome, often outliving the life of an mHealth project [48]. The Health 2.0 approach that envision digital health citizens as active participants in their own healthcare necessitates the need for deeper involvement of end users in co-design, an approach that has richer, more plentiful data points that better justify design decisions, reducing the gulf in evaluation amongst stakeholders spread across government, research, industry and consumers. The Sleep Solved study exhibited the potential to rapidly crowdsource with teen co-designers through digital outreach and asynchronous online data collection. However, a mixed methods approach that scales up these data points utilising AI and machine learning to digitise UX workshop data represents a potential step forward, such that from both digital and health perspectives, enough confidence in the data can occur in a reasonable amount of time, in line with project deliverables. This novel idea combines a number of core digital health challenges under one proposed umbrella solution as cited in our introduction: reducing costs (budget), increasing data points (validity) and rapid digital product delivery (time constraints).

5 Conclusion and Acknowledgement

This paper presented the novel virtual co-design process of creating an educational sleep app with teens. Our findings illustrate some of the benefits and challenges encountered in virtual co-designing. This study has led us to several promising suggestions for future experimental research that may increase data points, improve reliability and validity and further involve co-designers. Delivering fast, quantifiable and emotionally rich data in a rapidly synthesizable co-design platform represents a key objective in the diverse arena of digital health. We hope that this exploratory study encourages further experimentation in virtual crowdsourcing in mHealth, leveraging big data approaches into the Health 2.0 era.

We gratefully acknowledge the funding support for this project from: Simon Fraser University Community Trust Endowment Fund, Graduate Dean's Entrance Scholarship at the School of Interactive Arts & Technology at Simon Fraser University, The Prudence Trust (UK) and University of Bristol.

Appendix 1

Summary of co-design events

Event	Method	Participants and Objectives
Young People's Advisory Group (2022/09/08)	Focus group	Ideation. 6 young people, 3 young women, 3 young men, aged 14–17
PPIE feedback (2022/11/22)	Qualtrics survey	App names, colour palette, logo, themes, poster, information sheet. 5 respondents: 4 young women, 1 'prefer not to say', age range 14–17, half from 10% most deprived areas of the UK
PPIE feedback (2022/12/02)	Qualtrics survey	App themes, ranking Theme 1 vs Theme 2. 7 respondents: 5 young women, 2 young men, 6 of White British ethnicity, 1 Sri-Lankan/Sinhalese. All aged 16. From the 30–40% least deprived areas of the UK
Virtual Meetings (2023/01/19 - 2023/07/14)	Think-aloud interviews	20 participants: 8 young men, 10 young women, 1 non-binary, 1 genderfluid. 13 White British, 1 Arab, 1 African 1 White and Black Caribbean, 1 Pakistani, 1 South Asian, 1 Middle Eastern. Age range 16–18 (average age: 17 years). 10 of the 20 from the 10–50% most deprived areas of the UK
PPIE feedback (2023/14/02)	Qualtrics survey	4 logo options. 9 respondents: all young women, 7 of White British ethnicity, 1 White and Black African. Aged 16–17. 6 of the 9 from the 20–50% most deprived areas of the UK

(continued)

(continued)

Event	Method	Participants and Objectives
Sleep Solved app trial Feedback (2023/04/12)	Focus group	Recruited from McPin. 7 users tested the prototype app; six young women and one non-binary person, aged between 16 and 18 years old (average age: 17.12 years). Six were of White British ethnicity, and one user was of Middle Eastern ethnicity. Levels of deprivation ranged from the 40% most deprived, to the 20% least deprived.39 The majority had self-identified sleep problems ranging from 2–3 times per week, to more than 4 times per week
PPIE feedback (2023/05/16)	Qualtrics survey	Recruited from McPin. 7 users tested the prototype app; six young women and one non-binary person, aged between 16 and 18 years old (average age: 17.12 years). Six were of White British ethnicity, and one user was of Middle Eastern ethnicity. Levels of deprivation ranged from the 40% most deprived, to the 20% least deprived.39 The majority had self-identified sleep problems ranging from 2–3 times per week, to more than 4 times per week

Appendix 2

Pre-iteration: Ideation

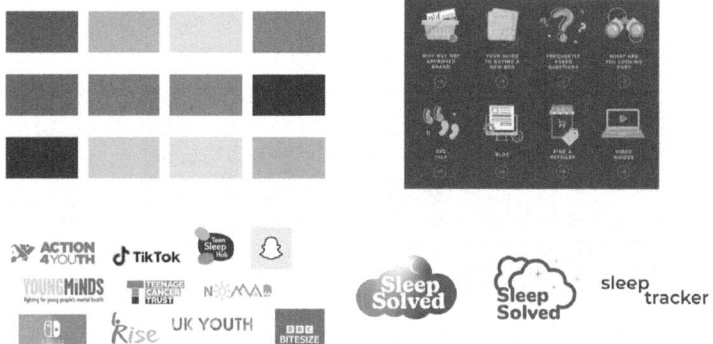

Pre-ideation: mood boards, colour palettes and branding

Branding and theming co-design resolutions

Problem	Resolution
App name	Sleep Solved
App theme	stylised neon pastel with night sky
Design themes	simple, visible, relative, relaxing, informative, intelligent design

"Style is clear...colours are visible...easy to find" (PPIE feedback from teen co-designer).

First Iteration: Discovery (low-fidelity PowerPoint)

App interactions and engagement objectives.

Interaction Type	Objective
Micro (learning) moment	quick bites of scientific information
Pop-ups	optional supplementary information
Enlightenments	pivotal questions that are often misunderstood

Second Iteration: Visualising the app design concept (medium-fidelity Figma prototype)

Figma mock-up (porting the scientific information into a prototype with constraints, affordances and calls to action):

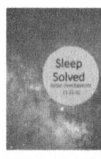

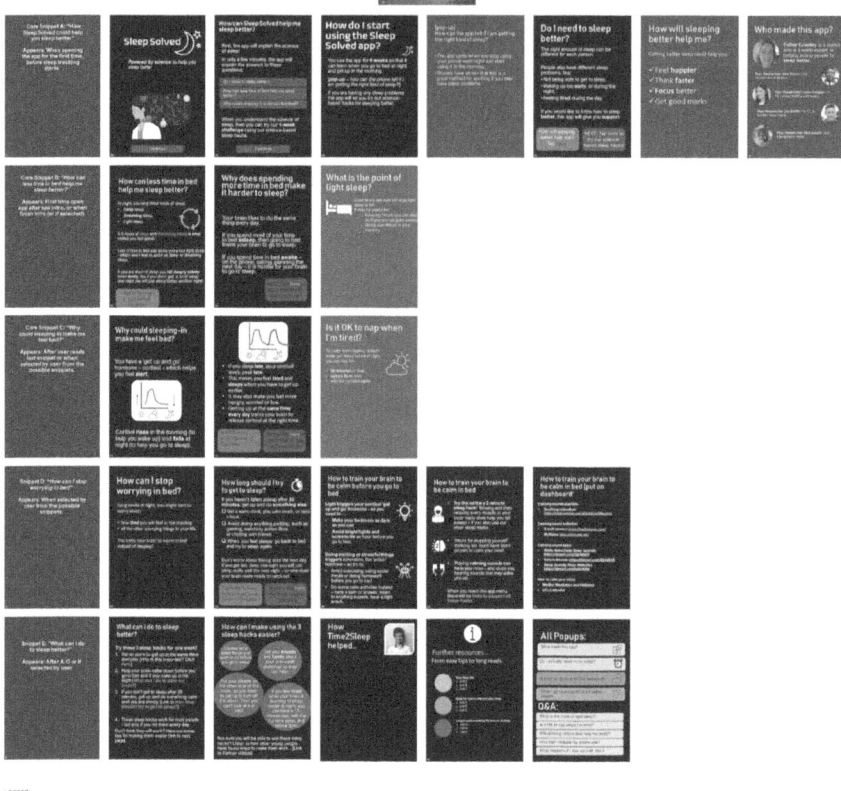

Fig. 3. Sleep Solved low fidelity mock-up mapping with micro-moment snippets of scientific information

First coded concept for testing:

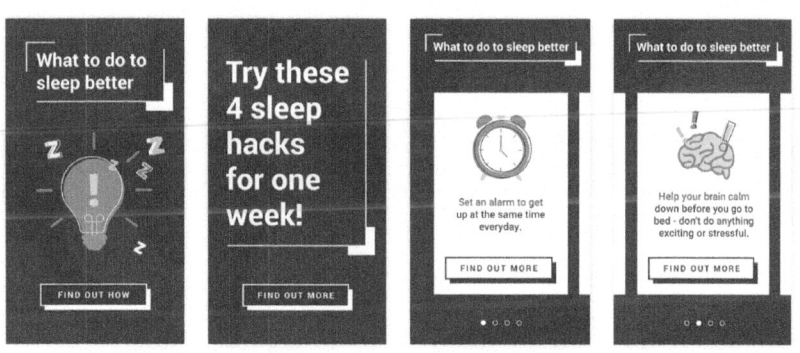

Most popular Sleep Solved medium fidelity mock-up as chosen by teens

  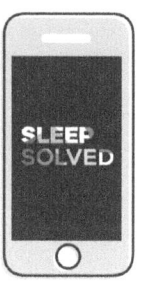 

Sleep Solved medium fidelity app icon mock-ups

Third Iteration: Coded App for Testing (high-fidelity)
App interactions and engagement objectives

Interaction Type	Objective
Text	keep it informative, minimal, but do not oversimplify it
Menu	need for a visible menu with progress bar (or task completion checkboxes)
Points/Rewards	addition of a points system to make the experience more rewarding
Related sleep apps	need for more relatability to Phone Downtime and Teen SHUTi (sister apps) for tracking, metrics and notifications

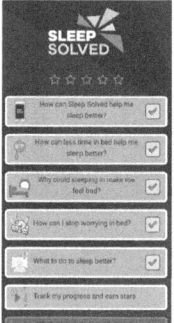 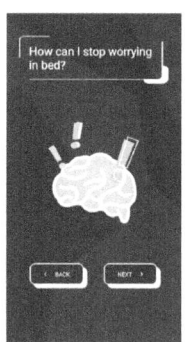 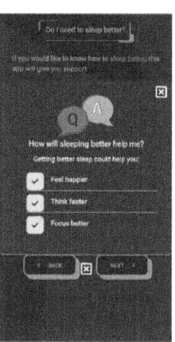 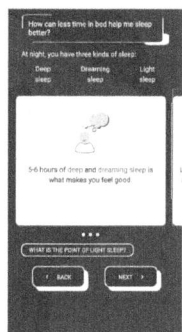

Sleep Solved coded beta app (high fidelity)

Appendix 3

Video walkthrough: The Virtual Co-design of Sleep Solved: Case Study on an Educational Sleep App for Teens

https://www.youtube.com/watch?v=DTLhyuhwQTQ.

References

1. Carmona, N.E., Usyatynsky, A., Kutana, S., et al.: A transdiagnostic self-management web-based app for sleep disturbance in adolescents and young adults: feasibility and acceptability study. JMIR Form Res. **5**, e25392 (2021)
2. Werner-Seidler, A., Wong, Q., Johnston, L., et al.: Pilot evaluation of the sleep Ninja: a smartphone application for adolescent insomnia symptoms. BMJ Open **9**, e026502 (2019)
3. Ali, N., Rigney, G., Weiss, S.K., et al.: Optimizing an eHealth insomnia intervention for children with neurodevelopmental disorders: a Delphi study. Sleep Health **4**, 224–234 (2018)
4. Neher, T., Green, J., Puzia, M., Huberty, J.: Describing the use of a mindfulness-based app for sleep and mental well-being, across age, in children. Child Youth Care Forum **51**, 749–768 (2022)
5. Ahuja, M.: Perceived credibility in mHealth apps : a case study on a sleep scheduling app for insomnia. University of Twente (2018)
6. Alami, H., Gagnon, M.-P., Fortin, J.-P.: Digital health and the challenge of health systems transformation. Mhealth **3**, 31 (2017)
7. Rowland, S.P., Fitzgerald, J.E., Holme, T., et al.: What is the clinical value of mHealth for patients? NPJ Digit. Med. **3**, 4 (2020)
8. E-Health Market Analysis. In: Grandview Research (2023). http://www.grandviewresearch.com/industry-analysis/e-health-market. Accessed 12 Oct 2023
9. Global digital health market report 2020: market is expected to witness a 37.1% spike in growth in 2021 and will continue to grow and reach USD 508.8 billion by 2027. In: Globe Newswire (2020). https://www.globenewswire.com/news-release/2020/11/25/2133473/0/en/Global-Digital-Health-Market-Report-2020-Market-is-Expected-to-Witness-a-37-1-Spike-in-Growth-in-2021-and-will-Continue-to-Grow-and-Reach-US-508-8-Billion-by-2027.html. Accessed 25 Sep 2023
10. Ospina-Pinillos, L., Davenport, T., Mendoza Diaz, A., et al.: Using participatory design methodologies to Co-design and culturally adapt the spanish version of the mental health eClinic: qualitative study. J. Med. Internet Res. **21**, e14127 (2019)
11. Hetrick, S.E., Robinson, J., Burge, E., et al.: Youth codesign of a mobile phone app to facilitate self-monitoring and management of mood symptoms in young people with major depression, suicidal ideation, and self-harm. JMIR Ment. Health **5**, e9 (2018)
12. Roberts, C., Freeman, J., Samdal, O., et al.: The health behaviour in school-aged children (HBSC) study: methodological developments and current tensions. Int. J. Public Health **54**(Suppl 2), 140–150 (2009)
13. Mugford, J.: Development and usability testing of an eHealth sleep intervention program for Youth. Mount Saint Vincent University (2019)
14. Cherenshchykova, A., Miller, A.D.: Sociotechnical design opportunities for pervasive family sleep technologies. In: Proceedings of the 14th EAI International Conference on Pervasive Computing Technologies for Healthcare, pp. 11–20. Association for Computing Machinery, New York, NY, USA (2021)
15. Tougas, M.: A user-centered approach in the development of an eHealth sleep intervention for adolescents with and without recurrent pain (2021)
16. Egilsson, E., Bjarnason, R., Njardvik, U.: Usage and weekly attrition in a smartphone-based health behavior intervention for adolescents: pilot randomized controlled trial. JMIR Form Res. **5**, e21432 (2021)
17. Peabody, J.O., Miller, D.C., Linsell, S., et al.: 192 Wisdom of the crowds: use of crowdsourcing to assess surgical skill of robot-assisted radical prostatectomy in a statewide surgical collaborative. Eur. Urol. Suppl. **2**, e192–e192a (2015)

18. Thomason, J.: Big tech, big data and the new world of digital health. Glob. Health J. **5**, 165–168 (2021)
19. Benis, A., Tamburis, O., Chronaki, C., Moen, A.: One digital health: a unified framework for future health ecosystems. J. Med. Internet Res. **23**, e22189 (2021)
20. Petrakaki, D., Hilberg, E., Waring, J.: The cultivation of digital health citizenship. Soc Sci Med **270**, 113675 (2021)
21. Powell, J., Deetjen, U.: Characterizing the digital health citizen: mixed-methods study deriving a new typology. J. Med. Internet Res. **21**, e11279 (2019)
22. Temiz, S.: Open innovation via crowdsourcing: a digital only hackathon case study from Sweden. J. Open Innov. Technol. Mark. Complex. **7**, 39 (2021)
23. Oyebode, O., Alhasani, M., Mulchandani, D., et al.: SleepFit: a persuasive mobile app for improving sleep habits in young adults. In: 2021 IEEE 9th International Conference on Serious Games and Applications for Health(SeGAH). ieeexplore.ieee.org, pp. 1–8 (2021)
24. Huberty, J., Green, J., Glissmann, C., et al.: Efficacy of the mindfulness meditation mobile app 'calm' to reduce stress among college students: randomized controlled trial. JMIR Mhealth Uhealth **7**, e14273 (2019)
25. Pulantara, I.W., Parmanto, B., Germain, A.: Development of a just-in-time adaptive mhealth intervention for Insomnia: usability study. JMIR Hum. Factors **5**, e21 (2018)
26. Tan-MacNeill, K.M., Smith, I.M., Weiss, S.K., et al.: An eHealth insomnia intervention for children with neurodevelopmental disorders: results of a usability study. Res. Dev. Disabil. **98**, 103573 (2020)
27. Takeuchi, H., Suwa, K., Kishi, A., et al.: The Effects of objective push-type sleep feedback on habitual sleep behavior and momentary symptoms in daily life: mhealth intervention trial using a health care internet of things system. JMIR Mhealth Uhealth **10**, e39150 (2022)
28. Leichman, E.S., Gould, R.A., Williamson, A.A., et al.: Effectiveness of an mHealth intervention for infant sleep disturbances. Behav. Ther. **51**, 548–558 (2020)
29. Aji, M., Gordon, C., Stratton, E., et al.: Framework for the design engineering and clinical implementation and evaluation of mHealth apps for sleep disturbance: systematic review. J. Med. Internet Res. **23**, e24607 (2021)
30. Yardley, L., Ainsworth, B., Arden-Close, E., Muller, I.: The person-based approach to enhancing the acceptability and feasibility of interventions. Pilot Feasibility Stud. **1**, 37 (2015)
31. Brabham, D.C., Ribisl, K.M., Kirchner, T.R., Bernhardt, J.M.: Crowdsourcing applications for public health. Am. J. Prev. Med. **46**, 179–187 (2014)
32. Dawson, R., Bynghall, S.: Getting results from crowds (2012)
33. Créquit, P., Mansouri, G., Benchoufi, M., et al.: Mapping of crowdsourcing in health: systematic review. J. Med. Internet Res. **20**, e187 (2018)
34. Pedgley, O.: Capturing and analysing own design activity. Des. Stud. **28**, 463–483 (2007)
35. Yang, Q., Cranshaw, J., Amershi, S., et al.: Sketching NLP: a case study of exploring the right things to design with language intelligence. In: Proceedings of the 2019 CHI Conference on Human Factors in Computing Systems, pp. 1–12. Association for Computing Machinery, New York, NY, USA (2019)
36. E-ACT Multi-Academy Trust. In: E-ACT (2017). https://www.e-act.org.uk/. Accessed 31 Mar 2024
37. Association of Colleges. In: Association of Colleges (2021). https://www.aoc.co.uk/. Accessed 31 Mar 2024
38. The Sleep Charity. In: The Sleep Charity (2020). https://thesleepcharity.org.uk/. Accessed 31 Mar 2024
39. The McPin Foundation. In: The McPin Foundation (2023). https://mcpin.org/. Accessed 31 Mar 2024

40. Young People Improving Research. The Bristol Young People's Advisory Group (YPAG). In: Generation R, Young People Improving Research. https://generationr.org.uk/bristol/. Accessed 20 Mar 2024
41. Supporting patient and public involvement in research. In: National Institute for Health and Care Research. https://www.nihr.ac.uk/explore-nihr/campaigns/supporting-patient-and-public-involvement-in-research.htm. Accessed 20 Mar 2024
42. Clarke, V., Braun, V.: Thematic analysis. In: Encyclopedia of Critical Psychology, pp. 1947–1952. Springer, New York, NY (2014)
43. Taylor, A., Brigden, A., Loades, M., Crawley, E.: Exploring the experience of young people with chronic fatigue syndrome (CFS)/myalgic encephalomyelitis (ME) and depression using qualitative methodology. In: SAGE Research Methods Cases: Part 2 (2018)
44. Barony Sanchez, R.H., Bergeron-Drolet, L.-A., Sasseville, M., Gagnon, M.-P.: Engaging patients and citizens in digital health technology development through the virtual space. Front Med. Technol. **4**, 958571 (2022)
45. Duffy, A., Christie, G., Riadi, I., Boroumandzad, N., Moreno, S.: Examining challenges to the incorporation of end users in the design of digital health interventions: systematic review. J. Med. Internet Res. 50178 (2024). https://doi.org/10.2196/50178. https://preprints.jmir.org/preprint/50178
46. Rumsfeld, J.S., Brooks, S.C., Aufderheide, T.P., et al.: Use of mobile devices, social media, and crowdsourcing as digital strategies to improve emergency cardiovascular care: a scientific statement from the American heart association. Circulation **134**, e87–e108 (2016)
47. AirOps. In: AirOps. https://www.airops.com/nlp-guide/how-to-classify-instagram-social-media-posts-with-generative-ai. Accessed 23 May 2024
48. Guo, C., Ashrafian, H., Ghafur, S., et al.: Challenges for the evaluation of digital health solutions—a call for innovative evidence generation approaches. npj Digit. Med. **3**, 1–14 (2020)

mHealth and Telemonitoring

H2Office: A Smartwatch and Water-Gauge System for Facilitating Hydration of Knowledge Workers

Shashank Ahire$^{(\boxtimes)}$ [ID], Abdalrazak Almahayni [ID], and Michael Rohs [ID]

Human-Computer Interaction, Leibniz University Hannover, Hanover, Germany
{shashank.ahire,michael.rohs}@hci.uni-hannover.de,
almahayni@stud.uni-hannover.de

Abstract. Consistent hydration is paramount for health and well-being. For knowledge workers, it also has an impact on overall productivity. Unfortunately, many knowledge workers experience insufficient hydration during busy working hours. We conducted interviews (N = 10) to investigate the causes of inconsistent hydration during work and explore the expectations of knowledge workers regarding intervention systems to improve their hydration habits. Based on the results of the interview study we designed the H2Office system, a comprehensive approach comprising a water gauge and a smartwatch app. A comparative field study over 10 days (N = 7) of the H2Office system shows its effectiveness in motivating knowledge workers to increase their water intake substantially (by 61%). The combination of auditory and vibration intervention effectively reminded them without causing any work distractions. In the evaluation of H2Office we identify detailed water consumption patterns of users concerning the time of day, sip interval, and sip quantity. Lastly, we found that knowledge workers desired a holistic approach (tracking consumption of other beverages) for delivering hydration interventions.

Keywords: Hydration · Interventions · Auditory icon · Office · Health · Well-being · Knowledge worker

1 Introduction

Water is essential for our day-to-day functioning. It accounts for 60% of an adult body weight [8]. It helps in building material for cells and carriers for tissues [10]. Hydration helps in regulating body temperature, aids brain function, helps to restore fluids, breathing, sweating, and the removal of waste [9]. Irregular hydration leads to a decrease in alertness and concentration, and a significant increase in headaches and tiredness [11,12]. Hence, it is important to have consistent and adequate intake of water during work.

As knowledge workers, individuals invest a significant portion of their daily lives in the workplace, dedicating 8–10 hours each day. They are found across

H. Kondylakis and A. Triantafyllidis (Eds.): PervasiveHealth 2024, LNICST 612, pp. 31–47, 2025.
https://doi.org/10.1007/978-3-031-85575-7_2

multiple professions, where they are expected to innovate and solve complex problems in their respective fields [27]. Considering the entirety of our lifespan, work emerges as the second most time-consuming activity after sleep [13]. On average, a working individual located in Europe or the USA allocates 1350–1750 hours per year to working [14]. Given the demands of their busy schedules and workloads, knowledge workers often overlook the importance of maintaining adequate hydration.

Water intake reminders after a regular interval were one of the desired features of work assistance [16]. To overcome dehydration knowledge workers have been relying on various techniques to hydrate themselves regularly. Examples include mobile applications like "Water Minder" [20] and "Water Reminder" [21] as well as smart water bottles like "HidrateSpark" [25]. However, none of the current water intake apps and devices have been specifically designed considering the challenges and requirements of the knowledge workers while at work.

The initial phase of this research involved conducting interviews with 10 knowledge workers, with a specific focus on determining challenges related to regular water intake at the workplace. The objective was to identify the expectations of knowledge workers with regard to a water reminder system. Subsequently, we developed the "H2Office" system, which comprises a water-gauge device and a smartwatch watchface and app. The water-gauge device was designed for precise measurement of water consumption over time, while the smartwatch app aimed to deliver interventions, update the water intake state within the app, set goals, and motivate knowledge workers to achieve their daily hydration targets.

Following the development phase, we executed a 10-day comparative field study involving 7 knowledge workers. The results demonstrate a significant increase in water consumption among knowledge workers when using H2Office in comparison to their baseline (Table 1). The auditory icon of a water-pouring sound was well-suited to a formal office setting, effectively capturing their attention without distracting them or their colleagues. Additionally, feedback from knowledge workers highlighted H2Office effectiveness in increasing daily water intake. Furthermore, the participants gave suggestions for improving the system's design and considering holistic approach for H2Office interventions.

Our contributions can be summarized as follows: (1) We identified the factors associated with the inconsistent hydration of knowledge workers and elicited their expectations with regard to a water reminder system. (2) We designed and developed the H2Office system for office settings to actively promote and support consistent hydration. (3) We conducted an evaluation of H2Office through a field study, determining the system's potential and identifying hydration patterns of knowledge workers.

2   Related Work

Different intervention techniques have been used with the objective of ensuring hydration during work. To increase hydration, intervention techniques can broadly be divided into two approaches: The gamification approach uses points and penalties in the interface to motivate users to drink more water. Another approach involves group-based motivation strategies, which are based on collective encouragement.

2.1 Intervention and Gamification Approaches for Hydration

Graphical and ambient intervention techniques have been frequently implemented to remind users to drink water. In the 'Mug-Tree' experiment [7], Ko et al. designed a playful mug linking water consumption to nurturing a virtual tree. Similarly, 'WaterCoaster' [5] introduced a virtual fish character in a fish tank, relying on regular water intake for the virtual creature's survival. Another approach, 'GROW' [6], presented an ambient water bottle unveiling a cherry tree silhouette. The act of drinking water determined the visibility of branches and leaves, tracking progress towards the hydration goal. 'MossWater' [17] employed an empathetic approach, with the system performing the action of watering moss to remind users to drink.

'WorkFit' [3] utilized voice interventions techniques for reminding knowledge workers to drink water. Voice interactions were successful in reminding and motivating knowledge workers in drinking water. Moreover, in 'Dual-intervention' [2] strategy Ahire et al. asked knowledge workers to rank their modality preference for nutrition intervention. They ranked vibration, ring, graphical and auditory icon and their preferred mode for primary intervention and followed by voice reminder as secondary mode of intervention.

'Hydroprompt' [19] utilized three approaches within its system: historical information, enabling users to compare their water intake levels; implicit feedback, providing subtle cues to users; and explicit prompting, attempting to remind participants when hydration falls below acceptable levels. Gouko et al. [18] developed a coaster that prompted desk workers to hydrate by emitting periodic sounds. Their investigation revealed that a 15-min interval was optimal for maximizing work efficiency. Hamatani et al. [26] investigated the use of smartwatch sensors to gauge water intake by analyzing drinking duration. They employed a macro-activity classifier to differentiate drinking from other activities and a micro-activity classifier to identify sequential micro-actions like holding the bottle, drinking, and putting the bottle down.

2.2 Collective Water Consumption

In an effort to promote collective water consumption among office workers, the 'Playful Bottle' study [4] compared a single-user 'Tree' with multi-user 'Forest' strategies for encouraging water intake. Social reminders were found to be more effective than single-user prompts. Additionally, 'Wwall' [15] employed an ambient display to offer individual yet collective feedback in office settings, promoting cooperation and shared goals over individual objectives. Visuals on the wall held significance when all participants achieved their personal objectives. Although prior literature has evaluated multiple approaches, it is essential to investigate whether proactive autitory interventions can encourage knowledge workers to drink water and, if so, how effective those are.

2.3   Commercial Applications and Devices for Hydration

Knowledge workers are also opting for different water reminder and water intake tracking applications like "Water Minder" [20] and "Water Reminder – Daily Tracker" [21]. However this applications delivers a reminder and requires users to estimate their consumption and update it regularly. Similar these apps, some smartwatches also offer water intake reminding and tracking[1]. However these typically rely on the user for updating the hydration state. Likewise, the HidrateSpark water bottle [25] features an integrated gauge for monitoring water intake. It sends reminders to the user's smartphone and enables water consumption tracking through a dedicated app. All applications and devices are dependent on mobile phones for delivering interventions. This reliance means users must consistently check their phones for updates on their hydration intake, potentially leading to increased screen time and distraction while at work.

3   Interview Study

To gather insight into the hydration behavior of knowledge workers and the associated challenges, we conducted semi-structured interviews. In particular, the aim was to understand the causes of inconsistent hydration during work hours and to gather knowledge workers expectations concerning a hydration reminder system.

3.1   Participants

We conducted interviews with 10 knowledge workers. All the participants were male. The age range of the participants was between 24 and 30. On average the participants worked 7.2 h per day. They self-reported that during their workday, they drank between 2 to 3.3 cups of water per day. We recruited the participants using snowball sampling and by advertising the study on university forums. Three participants also had experience using water reminder apps such as WaterMinder [20] and Aqualert [24].

3.2   Method

We initiated our interviews by investigating the problems that knowledge workers face in achieving consistent hydration. Following this, we inquired them about their expectation of a system that would support them in achieving consistent hydration.

Audio recordings of post-study interviews underwent transcription and coding. Codes were devised to encapsulate the essence of the data and convey its

---

[1] https://www.youtube.com/watch?v=U8MTy0VV4gc.

concepts and ideas. Inductive thematic analysis was employed to uncover emerging themes. Patterns, similarities, and connections among codes were scrutinized to delineate distinct themes, each of which was described and labeled. To uphold rigor, the first and second author independently cross-checked the identified themes [22].

3.3   Findings: Causes of Inconsistent Hydration

From the interviews, we identified four important causes of inconsistent hydration.

Forgetfulness Amidst Demanding Work Routines. Knowledge workers function within tight schedules and engage in challenging and demanding tasks. Participant P4, P6, and P9 highlighted that their heavy workload and deep engagement in tasks often led to forgetfulness regarding water consumption. In some instances, back-to-back meetings consumed their time, causing them to overlook their health needs. The demanding and fully scheduled nature of their work routines resulted in many users forgetting to prioritize and consume an adequate amount of water.

Reduced Hydration: Consequence of Habitual Consumption of Other Beverages. Participants P6, P1, and P7 noted that their habitual consumption of coffee made them less prone to feeling thirsty, resulting in limited water intake each day. The regular consumption of other beverages, such as tea, coffee, and energy drinks, often eliminated their explicit thirst for water. This consistent intake of alternative beverages contributed to a reduced overall consumption of water in their daily routine.

Challenges with Existing Water Reminder Apps. Participants P2, P8, and P3, who had prior experience with water reminder apps, expressed their views on the effectiveness of such apps. While acknowledging the utility of reminder and tracking apps, they pointed out a significant drawback – the reliance on users for inputting data. The dependence on users to manually log water intake updates was perceived as tedious and added cognitive load, as it required consistent input each time. Additionally, participants felt that manual logging introduced inaccuracies, making it challenging to estimate their actual water intake. These inaccuracies, in turn, led to demotivation over the long term.

Dilemma of Reminder and Distractions. Many water reminder applications depend heavily on mobile notifications for hydration reminders. However while working if the mobile device is set aside due to distractions, then there is a risk of forgetting to drink water. However, if the mobile phone is kept nearby, the knowledge worker may face additional distractions from other notifications such as social media notifications. This situation presents users with a dilemma, as they must choose between being distracted by the phone and receiving water intake notifications, thereby creating a challenging decision-making scenario.

3.4   Requirements: Expectations of the System

In this section, we discuss two essential expectations of the participants concerning the hydration intervention system.

Effortless and Automatic. In contrast to existing applications, participants suggested a system featuring an automated water measurement mechanism. They proposed that the system would monitor their water intake timing, send notifications at regular intervals, record water consumption, and compile a total of daily water intake. Additionally, participants expressed their desire to establish a daily water intake goal, utilizing the water reminder system to assist them in achieving this objective. *"I do not want to give too much effort every time I use the device or the app. I only want to get notification and motivation."* -P1. Moreover, the participants expressed the desire for the system to send reminders every 45–60 min.

Non-disruptive and Unobtrusive Interventions. Some participants preferred a non-intrusive water reminder in the form of a pop-up rather than an app that requires active opening and tracking. They wished for the water app to be consistently visible on the front of the screen of their smartphone, serving as a subconscious prompt for water intake without distracting them consistently. The app should also automatically display progress in a subtle manner to without breaking their workflow, removing the need to open the app each time to check intake and progress. One participant specifically mentioned his preference to show the information on the front screen, stating, *"I am too busy to open the app and see my progress every time and I might end up forgetting about the app."* -P2 Furthermore, unlike commercial intervention systems that use distractive reminders, participants desired a system that was subtle and non-intrusive.

4   Development and Testing of H2Office

In this section, we explain the development of H2Office, its components, and software for development. Further, we also discuss the process of testing the H2Office water-gauge.

4.1   Water Gauge

The water gauge utilizes a load cell sensor HX711, which functions as an analog-to-digital converter (ADC), primarily employed for object scaling[2]. The primary

---

[2] https://www.digikey.com/htmldatasheets/production/1836471/0/0/1/hx711.html.

function of the water gauge is to calculate water consumption after each sip. This involves determining the weight of the bottle or glass both before and after consumption. The water gauge calculates the water quantity by analyzing the difference in bottle weight before and after consumption, converting grams to milliliters ($1\,g = 1$ ml). The HX711 comprises four relevant pins: GND, VCC, DT, and SCK. GND and VCC are responsible for powering the circuit, while communication with the Raspberry Pi is realized via DT and SCK.

4.2   Raspberry Pi

A Raspberry Pi serves as the integral component for calculating water intake and for recording date, time, and user identifier. It connects to the Internet via WiFi and uploads the data to a Firebase database.

4.3   Firebase Database

Firebase, a back-end service by Google[3], operates as a real-time database, in which data is stored and retrieved in JSON format. The Firebase database is utilized to store the water intake (in milliliters), date, time, and user identifier. The measurements sent to the database are subsequently forwarded to the H2Office smartwatch app, to update the water intake information. The Firebase database maintains a persistent record of each user's water intake behavior.

4.4   Smartwatch

The smartwatch was chosen as the users interaction device for its close proximity to the user, thereby being effective in capturing attention and delivering voice interventions. The likelihood of users not noticing voice interventions due to focused work is minimized when delivered through a smartwatch. Additionally, smartwatches facilitate multimodal interactions, encompassing graphical, voice, and tactile outputs, enabling users to engage through diverse modes. As found in the interviews (Sect. 3.3) unlike mobile phones, smartwatches do not pose a significant source of distraction for knowledge workers. We used the Samsung Galaxy 4[4] smartwatch for app deployment (Fig. 2).

H2Office App. The smartwatch app was created to administer interventions and synchronize user's water intake consumption from the cloud. Users are required to log in to their profile, configure the water intake interval, and set their working hours and working days within the app. Additionally, the app provides a display of weekly statistics (Fig. 3) of daily water consumption.

---

[3] https://firebase.google.com/.
[4] https://www.samsung.com/global/galaxy/galaxy-watch4/specs/.

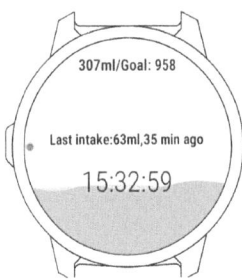 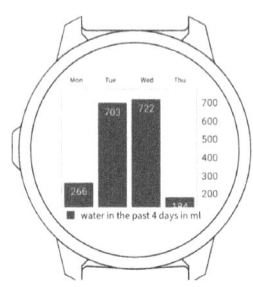 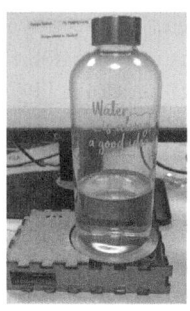

Fig. 1. H2Office watch-face: showcasing achieved goal, overall intake target, last water intake timer, and last water consumption

Fig. 2. H2Office app stats page, showing the consumption of last 4 days

Fig. 3. H2Office gauge system at the in-situ settings

H2Office Watchface. Prior literature has shown that smartwatch users prefer's to update about their activity in glance without consuming more time and is perceivable at the periphery of users attention [1]. Watchface enables users to quickly glance the activity status. Moreover, watchface helps motivating smartwatch users and encourage them in achieving their goals [23]. Therefore, we used a watchface so that the water reminder is always upfront and explicit. This enables users to monitor this information in a short glimpse and not get distracted from the on-going task. The watchface must meet aesthetic requirements and can only display one app at a time due to limited space. Because it must be easy to read at a glance and space is limited, it cannot accommodate a large amount of information. Additionally, it must still allow users to easily read the current time.

As shown in Fig. 1, we designed the watchface as an animated water tank. The water level increases after each sip. The watchface also displays the total amount of water that was consumed during the day as well as the goal the user set for the day. It displays the water consumption during the last intake and time (in minutes) since last consumption.

H2Office Interventions. While designing the interventions for H2Office, we focused on keeping the attention required by the knowledge workers at a minimum in order to prevent distracting them too much. We decided to deliver the intervention using an auditory icon and a vibration. For the auditory icon we selected the sound of pouring water, which can be easily associated with drinking water. Further, the sound of pouring water is subtle and non-intrusive to knowledge workers and their colleagues. The sound of auditory icon[5]. A vibration intervention combine with audio can serve as an additional reminder if the

---

[5] https://drive.google.com/file/d/1tt0TSe0_7HIKTa0Q2YnWfr_cyiO8LYvi/view?usp=sharing.

audio fails to capture the user's attention or if the smartwatch is set on low volume.

4.5   Testing H2Office

In the testing phase, we assessed the precision of water intake measurements by cross-referencing them with a kitchen weighing scale. To ensure the calibration of the gauge, a known weight was placed on it to establish a reference unit. Subsequently, this value was incorporated into the code. Our calibration process involved using 1 kg food packets, weighing them on a standard scale, and calibrating the gauge accordingly. Through multiple gauge tests, we observed a standard error of ± 3 grams for every 1 kg. This deviation is deemed acceptable, equating to an error of 0.3%. As a verification step, we utilized a measuring jar to validate the accuracy of the calculated value in milliliters.

5   Field Study

5.1   Participants

The participant group consisted of 6 males and 1 female, all falling within the age range of 24 to 30. This group included both full-time and part-time knowledge workers. All the six male participants had also participated in our interview study. Participants were requested to complete the consent form. To maintain the integrity of the study, we ensured that participants were not utilizing any other intervention system for water intake, and their drinking behavior habits remained uninfluenced.

5.2   Method

The study was conducted for a duration of 10 working days, equivalent to two work weeks. The initial 5 days constituted the baseline condition, followed by the second 5 days dedicated to the evaluation of the H2Office prototype. Throughout the baseline condition, participants were instructed to independently record their daily water intake using measuring jugs and submit the data at the end of each day. In the evaluation phase, participants were requested to use our prototype, which consisted of the H2Office water gauge system and a smartwatch app. It was emphasized that the smartwatch should be consistently worn throughout the study period, as the H2Office app would only deliver interventions when the smartwatch was securely fastened to the wrist.

The study was conducted in the month of May 2023 and all the participants were located in Hannover, Germany. After the field evaluation we conducted interviews with the participants. Post-study interview recordings were transcribed, coded, and analyzed using thematic analysis. Patterns and connections among codes were examined to define distinct themes, cross-checked independently by the second author [22].

Table 1. Mean values of each participant's data, including baseline water consumption, water intake with the H2Office intervention, percentage increase, total number of sips, intake per sip, and sip frequency using H2Office.

Participant	Baseline (ml)	H2Office (ml)	Increase (%)	Total Sips	Intake per Sip (ml)	Sip Interval (minutes)
P1	1080	1196.4	10.8	48	112	42
P2	515	1068.0	107.3	41	126	59
P3	290	494.4	70.4	49	122	44
P4	1350	1708.6	26.6	69	128	50
P5	500	1032.8	106.6	35	71	50
P6	1500	1975.4	31.7	196	51	12
P7	560	980.2	75.0	35	140	63
Mean	828	1208.0	61.2	68	107	46

6 Results

6.1 Quantitative Findings

Overall, the system recorded 473 sips of water by the seven participants. The total number of sips per participant ranged from 35 to 196, with a mean of 68 sips per participant. Similarly, water consumption per sip for participants ranged from 51 to 140 ml, with a mean of 107 ml per sip. During interviews participants desired the sip interval to be 45–60 min (Sect. 3.4). Nevertheless, except for P6 all participants had sip intervals between 42 and 63 min. During the baseline condition, participants consumed an average of 827 ml, whereas with the H2Office intervention, the average water consumption increased to 1207 ml, indicating a 61% increase.

In the evaluation we found an average increase in water intake of 61.2%. The smallest increase was by 10.8% for participant P1. The maximum increase was by 107.4% for participant P2. It was unexpected to discover that participants P4 and P6, despite having a substantial baseline intake of 1350 and 1500ml, exhibited notable increases of 26.6% and 31.7%, respectively, in the H2Office condition. A paired t-test showed a significant difference in water consumption between the H2Office condition and the baseline condition ($p < 0.05$).

The comparative bar graph of baseline and H2Office for each participant is presented in Fig. 4, revealing a substantial increase in water consumption for each participant. The distribution of water intake for all participants is shown in the histogram in Fig. 5. Notably, the frequency of intakes within the 40–80 ml range surpasses that of all other intake values. Additionally, Fig. 6 illustrates the overall water intake for each hour. Notably, there is an observed increase in the frequency and water intake amount from 12 pm to 4 pm, indicating higher and more frequent water consumption in the afternoon compared to the morning.

As the results show, H2Office substantially increases the water consumption of the participants during the work hours. Thus H2Office is an effective intervention for achieving higher water intake among the participants. This outcome underscores the positive impact of H2Office on encouraging individuals to consume more water, which can have important implications for overall health and well-being.

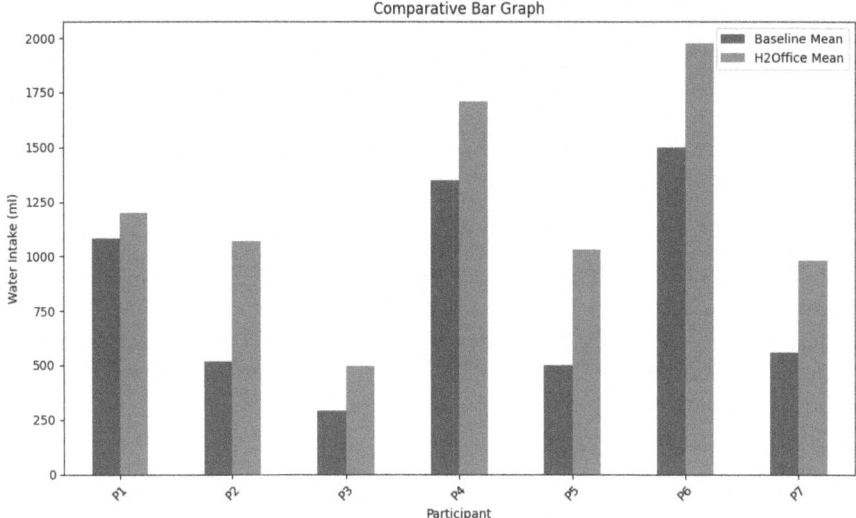

Fig. 4. Means water intake under the baseline condition (blue) and the H2Office condition (orange) for each participant. The intervention leads to a clear increase in average water intake. (Color figure online)

6.2   Qualitative Findings

Auditory Icons and Vibrations Proved to Be Effective. Several participants stated that auditory intervention combined with vibration was well-suited for the formal office setting. It was able to effectively catch their attention but at the same time did not distract them significantly from work. As the intervention was an auditory icon of pouring water, they could easily distinguish the H2Office notification from the other notifications. Furthermore, the auditory intervention was not extensively loud and did not capture the attention of neighboring colleagues. Because of the smartwatch's proximity to the user, they could distinctly feel the vibration during the intervention. As a result, the combination of both modalities effectively reminded them to stay hydrated.

Count-Up Timer Serves as a Hydration Reminder. Several participants expressed that the count-up timer (Fig. 1, line 2), which shows the time since the last water intake was effective in motivating them to consume water. Participant 1 specifically stated, *"The count-up timer was more helpful than the notification"* emphasizing that observing the time elapsed since the last water intake proved beneficial. Often, participants did not wait for the interventions, but drank water after having a glimpse at the last intake time. In the interview, P6 stated *"I didn't receive so many notifications to drink water, as I looked at the count-up timer and frequently drank water."*

Building Trust: Importance of Accuracy in Water Intake. Participants observed that precision of H2Office during water consumption was particularly intriguing. H2Office demonstrated proficiency in calculating water intake, providing updates in milliliters that were not rounded off to conventional values like 50 ml or 100 ml. Instead, the displayed measurements were precise, such as 58 ml or 67 ml, aligning closely with the actual amount of water consumed with each sip. This non-rounded approach contributed to participant's trusting the device's calculations, leading them to take their water intake more seriously. As one participant, P6, expressed, *"I was skeptical at first: Does the device really measure the amount of water? I drank from the glass and estimated the water intake, then compared it with the given result on the watchface. It is really doing its job."* This firsthand verification highlighted the accuracy of the device and reinforced the participants' confidence in its functionality.

Holistic Approach: Extending Beyond Water. Some participants suggested adopting a holistic approach that involves tracking the intake of beverages (such as coffee, tea, soft drinks, and juices) and subsequently recommending water intake. The interest in tracking these beverages stemmed from their habitual consumption of these drinks, unlike water, which often required external triggers and motivation. Participants, however, were concerned about the health implications of their habitual consumption of beverages containing caffeine and sugar. Since these beverages also contribute to overall fluid intake, participants proposed incorporating a comprehensive approach to hydration recommendations. Additionally, participants pointed out specific times during the workday, such as the start and post-lunch period, when coffee and tea intake was crucial for functioning and integral to their daily routine. They suggested

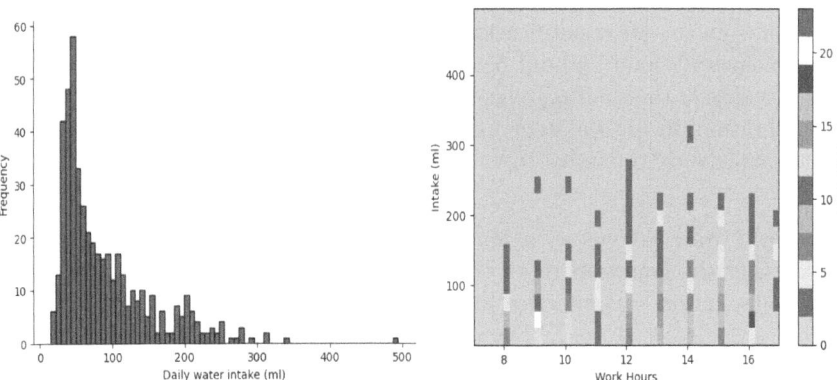

Fig. 5. Distribution of intake amounts (in ml).

Fig. 6. Overall water intake for each hour and frequency of intake per hour.

H2Office to consider these factors before recommending water intake to align with their established beverage consumption patterns.

Recommending Water Intake Goal Based on a Health Issue. Few participants recommended taking into account individual health considerations related to dehydration. They emphasized the importance of recognizing the critical role of consistent water consumption, acknowledging that while it might be a routine for some, for others, it is crucial for maintaining their health. One participant, P2, expressed a desire for the H2Office to not only monitor but also to recommend a goal based on health issues related to hydration. *"I want it [H2Office] to determine the needed amount of water based on health issue."* This suggestion illustrates the participants' interest in personalized health monitoring and the potential role of technology in addressing individual hydration needs.

Desire for Gamification Based on Points and Penalties. Most Participants expressed a desire for a more gamified experience to enhance their interest and engagement. Participants suggested incorporating gamification elements such as earning coins or points daily upon achieving the set water intake goals.

This approach was seen as a potential means to encourage consistency in daily water consumption and increase overall participant engagement. Additionally, the idea of rewarding them for the goal completion and penalizing if them for not consistently hydrating them was considered valuable fostering a more serious approach. Participant P7 highlighted this sentiment, stating, *"I think the amount of water that I have consumed was enough, but I need to mention that I would like to have more games if it is possible."* Participant 5 echoed this sentiment, expressing, *"The idea is great, but I need more games. Water tank alone is good, but I need something more, like coins to buy something in the game."*

Optimized Design and Aesthetic of the Device. Some participants recommended optimizing the design of H2Office, noting its current size was somewhat bulky for placing on a desk. They proposed a redesign, emphasizing the need to consider the clutter typically found on desks. Specifically, the participants suggested shaping the prototype to resemble a coaster in terms of size and thickness.

In addition, participants advised taking into account the average empty space available on desks during the design process. One participant, P3, commented, *"The idea and the device itself are well designed, but I don't have enough space on my desk, although I can find some space for it."* Another participant, P5, highlighted the significance of the device's shape and design, stating, *"The device shape and design are very important to me, as the office is a formal setting."* These statements underscored the participants emphasis on practicality, aesthetics, and the integration of the device into their professional work environment.

7   Discussion

As knowledge workers have a busy schedule, it was important to find a balance between attention seeking, interventions, and distractions. Users expected our H2Office system to be non-intrusive and not distracting. In H2Office, we implemented a technique involving auditory interventions, GUI notifications, and vibration. Using this combination, users felt that the intervention was not distracting. Users highlighted that the "last intake timer" feature increased their awareness of their drinking habits and made them more attentive to their hydration behavior.

We found that hydration interventions proved beneficial to the users and were able to significantly increase the water intake in comparison to their baseline. We uncovered drinking patterns of the users by considering their time intervals between sips and amount of water consumption. We found that water intake was higher in the period between noon and 4 pm than in the period between 8 am and noon. There can be multiple reasons for this. Knowledge workers generally consume coffee or tea in the morning, which may lead to the less water intake in the early morning. Another reason could be weather conditions, since the study was conducted in the month of May, in which the temperature rises after noon, which may lead to higher consumption. During the afternoon, knowledge workers may demonstrate an increased awareness of water consumption compared to the morning, resulting in a rise in the frequency of intake and overall consumption.

In the WorkFit study [3], proactive voice interventions in office environments faced challenges such as lack of agency, privacy concerns, and intrusiveness to colleagues. However, in our study, auditory interventions proved advantageous by delivering subtle audio cues audible only to the users, ensuring they were non-intrusive to their colleagues. Moreover, the use of auditory icons did not raise privacy or agency concerns among knowledge workers in a formal office setting. In 'Dual-Intervention' [2] study, vibration was ranked as most preferred modality for nutritional intervention, similarly we found vibration modality provide beneficial for delivering hydration intervention in work setting.

In previous studies, penalties were implemented using various methods such as a tree wilting [7], moss drying up [17], and in the "Water Coaster" system [5], the water level in the fish tank decreased when there was insufficient water intake, potentially endangering the fish. Although we built an interactive system for water intake, H2Office does not have a provision for assigning penalties for missing the water intake. Like the collective water consumption and drinking techniques [4,15], participants expressed a desire for gamification and for inculcating a competitive approach for achieving their daily goals. This could encourage users to compete and achieve their goals with more dedication.

While HidrateSpark [25] employs a similar approach, its limitations include dependency on the HidrateSpark water bottle exclusively for tracking and reminders of water consumption. Moreover, it carries a hefty price tag, ranging from \$54–\$79 per bottle, and requires meticulous care in both cleaning and usage. In contrast, H2Office users have the flexibility to use day-to-day items like glasses, water bottles, or cups according to their needs. Additionally, Hidrate-

Spark water bottles and intervention are not specifically designed and developed for office settings and knowledge workers.

Accuracy was judged as an important feature of H2Office. Accuracy of the amount of water consumed helped in building trust and maintain the participants' interest towards H2Office. Further, users were also impressed that H2Office not only delivered interventions, but that it also delivered and calculated their consumption automatically. An average working day of a knowledge workers comprises various drinks, such as water, coffee, juice, and tea. Beverages like coffee and tea were judged as essential for their work day productivity. Furthermore, for some knowledge workers who were habitual to drinking coffee, this was also a growing concern for them. These knowledge workers desired to minimize their coffee intake during their work day. They requested to also measure their coffee consumption and to help them to minimize it and increase their water intake.

7.1   Limitations and Future Work

We would like to discuss the limitations of our paper. Our sample size is highly dominated by male participants. However, we do not think that this invalidates the results of the study. As the study was conducted in the month of May in Hannover, Germany, the drinking patterns are affected by the location, duration, and weather during the study. In the future, we would like to develop a model that provides recommendations to knowledge workers based on weather, gender, age and health conditions. Further, we aim to implement a holistic approach to monitor the intake of other beverages and help knowledge workers to limit them. Also, we would like to optimize and improve the design of H2Office with respect to the size and available place on the knowledge worker's desk. Lastly, since the users appreciated the ability to quickly glance at the watch to see the time interval size the last sip, we would like to improve the visualization of the time interval to enable glanceability [1].

8   Conclusion

We commenced our research by examining the factors contributing to inconsistent hydration among knowledge workers. Our findings highlight that demanding work schedules, habitual consumption of other beverages and challenges with distractions and reminders in existing apps were key contributors to dehydration. In exploring our participant's expectations, we identified a preference for a device that is effortless, performs automated calculations and interventions, and sustains their interest in the long term. In response to these insights, we developed the H2Office system, comprising a water gauge and a smartwatch watchface and app. We used auditory icon as an intervention for hydration reminder. Results of the field study indicate that H2Office effectively reminds knowledge workers to consistently rehydrate during work. Notably, H2Office substantially enhanced hydration levels compared to the baseline (by 61%). Importantly, we identified the drinking patterns of knowledge workers and in particular quantified the water intake intervals, consumption in milliliters and hourly consumption.

References

1. Gouveia, R., Pereira, F., Karapanos, E., Munson, S.A., Hassenzahl, M.: Exploring the design space of glanceable feedback for physical activity trackers. In: Proceedings of the 2016 ACM International Joint Conference on Pervasive and Ubiquitous Computing, pp. 144–155. Association for Computing Machinery (2016). https://doi.org/10.1145/2971648.2971754

2. Ahire, S., Othman, S., Rohs, M.: Dual-mode interventions: giving agency to knowledge workers in proactive health interventions. In: Proceedings of the 6th ACM Conference on Conversational User Interfaces, p. 37. Association for Computing Machinery, New York (2024). https://doi.org/10.1145/3640794.3665578

3. Ahire, S., Simon, B., Rohs, M.: WorkFit: designing proactive voice assistance for the health and well-being of knowledge workers. In: Proceedings of the 6th ACM Conference on Conversational User Interfaces, p. 5. Association for Computing Machinery, New York (2024). https://doi.org/10.1145/3640794.3665561

4. Chiu, M.-C., et al.: Playful bottle: a mobile social persuasion system to motivate healthy water intake. In: Proceedings of the 11th International Conference on Ubiquitous Computing (UbiComp 2009), pp. 185–194. Association for Computing Machinery, New York (2009). https://doi.org/10.1145/1620545.1620574

5. Lessel, P., Altmeyer, M., Kerber, F., Barz, M., Leidinger, C., Krüger, A.: Water-Coaster: a device to encourage people in a playful fashion to reach their daily water intake level. In: Proceedings of the 2016 CHI Conference Extended Abstracts on Human Factors in Computing Systems, CHI EA 2016, pp. 1813-1820. Association for Computing Machinery, New York (2016). https://doi.org/10.1145/2851581.2892498

6. Kaner, G., Genç, H.U., Dinçer, S.B., Erdoğan, D., Coşkun, A.: GROW: a smart bottle that uses its surface as an ambient display to motivate daily water intake. In: Extended Abstracts of the 2018 CHI Conference on Human Factors in Computing Systems, pp. 1–6. Association for Computing Machinery, New York (2018). https://doi.org/10.1145/3170427.3188521

7. Ko, J.C., Hung, Y.P., Chu, H.H.: Mug-Tree: a Playful Mug to encourage healthy habit of drinking fluid regularly (2007)

8. The Nutrition Source (2019). https://www.hsph.harvard.edu/nutritionsource/water/

9. Doherty, T.: The importance of good hydration. Nutr. Rev. **63**(Suppl. 1), 6–9 (2003)

10. Jéquier, E., Constant, F.: Water as an essential nutrient: the physiological basis of hydration. Eur. J. Clin. Nutr. **64**(2), 115–123 (2009). https://doi.org/10.1038/ejcn.2009.111

11. Shirreffs, S.M., Merson, S.J., Fraser, S.M., Archer, D.T.: The effects of fluid restriction on hydration status and subjective feelings in man. Br. J. Nutr. **91**(6), 951–958 (2004). https://doi.org/10.1079/BJN20041149

12. Cian, C., Koulmann, N., Barraud, P.A., Raphel, C., Jimenez, C., Melin, B.: Influence of variations in body hydration on cognitive function. J. Psychophysiol. **14**(1), 29–36 (2000). https://doi.org/10.1027//0269-8803.14.1.29

13. Ortiz-Ospina, E., Giattino, C., Roser, M.: Time Use. Our World in Data (2020). https://ourworldindata.org/time-use

14. Giattino, C., Ortiz-Ospina, E., Roser, M.: Working Hours. Our World in Data. https://ourworldindata.org/working-hours

15. Yıldız, M., Coşkun, A.: Wwall: a public water dispenser system to motivate regular water intake in the office environment. In: DIS 2019 Companion, pp. 347–352. Association for Computing Machinery(2019). https://doi.org/10.1145/3301019.3323890

16. Ahire, S., Rohs, M., Benjamin, S.: Ubiquitous work assistant: synchronizing a stationary and a wearable conversational agent to assist knowledge work. In: 2022 Symposium on Human-Computer Interaction for Work, p. 3. Association for Computing Machinery (2022). https://doi.org/10.1145/3533406.3533420

17. Zhou, Y., Chen, Y., Zhou, L., Luo, S.: MossWater: a living media interface for encouraging office workers' daily water intake. In: Extended Abstracts of the 2021 CHI Conference on Human Factors in Computing Systems, p. 355. Association for Computing Machinery (2021). https://doi.org/10.1145/3411763.3451648

18. Gouko, M., Arakawa, Y.: A coaster robot that encourages office workers to drink water. In: Proceedings of the 5th International Conference on Human Agent Interaction, pp. 447–449. Association for Computing Machinery (2017). https://doi.org/10.1145/3125739.3132584

19. Neves, D., Costa, D., Oliveira, M., Jardim, R., Gouveia, R., Karapanos, E.: Motivating Healthy Water Intake through Prompting, Historical Information, and Implicit Feedback. CoRR, abs/1603.01367 (2016). http://arxiv.org/abs/1603.01367

20. WaterMinder. Track your daily water intake with Waterminder (2023). https://waterminder.com/

21. Water Reminder. Water reminder - daily tracker (2023). https://apps.apple.com/us/app/water-reminder-daily-tracker/id1221965482

22. Hochheiser, H., Feng, J.H., Lazar, J.: Research Methods in Human Computer Interaction (Second Edition). Morgan Kaufmann Publishers (2017)

23. Gouveia, R., Epstein, D.A.: This watchface fits with my tattoos: investigating customisation needs and preferences in personal tracking. In: Proceedings of the 2023 CHI Conference on Human Factors in Computing Systems, p. 327. Association for Computing Machinery (2023). https://doi.org/10.1145/3544548.3580955

24. Aqualert. Aqualert App (2024). https://www.aqualertapp.com#about

25. Hidrate Inc. Smart Water Bottle - HidrateSpark Bluetooth Water Bottle + Tracker App (2023). https://hidratespark.com/

26. Hamatani, T., Elhamshary, M., Uchiyama, A., Higashino, T.: Poster: smartwatch knows how much you drink. In: Proceedings of the 15th Annual International Conference on Mobile Systems, Applications, and Services, p. 162. Association for Computing Machinery (2017). https://doi.org/10.1145/3081333.3089306

27. Drucker, P.F.: Knowledge-worker productivity: the biggest challenge. Calif. Manag. Rev. **41**(2), 79–94 (1999). https://doi.org/10.2307/41165987

A Gamified Smartphone Application to Improve the Adherence to the Mediterranean Diet in Cardiac Patients: A Usability and Feasibility Study

Wald Habets[1]([⊠]) [iD], Linqi Xu[2] [iD], Paul Dendale[3], and Karin Coninx[1] [iD]

[1] Human-Computer Interaction and eHealth, Faculty of Sciences, Hasselt University, Hasselt, Belgium
wald.habets@uhasselt.be
[2] Faculty of Medicine and Life Sciences, Hasselt University, Hasselt, Belgium
[3] Heart Centre Hasselt, Jessa Hospital, Hasselt, Belgium

Abstract. Background. The Mediterranean diet is highly recommended for most patients in cardiac rehabilitation and secondary prevention, but compliance is often poor. This study aimed to evaluate the usability and feasibility of NutriQuest, a gamified smartphone application aimed at supporting patients' adherence to the Mediterranean diet. **Methods.** The study used mixed-methods: consisting of a usability study and a six-week, single group intervention with patients (n = 21) following a programme for cardiac rehabilitation. Patients were requested to utilize the smartphone application and complete questionnaires to evaluate its usability and acceptance, as well as its impact on modified MedDietScore, knowledge, and self-efficacy. **Results.** 15 out of 21 patients completed the full six-week trajectory. Patients were accepting the application and general impressions were positive. They mostly made use of the logbook-component and reacted positively towards the dietitian's feedback. The study did not find any significant improvement in the patients' modified MedDietScore, knowledge and self-efficacy after the intervention. **Conclusion**. The study reveals patients' acceptance of the NutriQuest application and usability improvements. The accuracy of measuring MedDietScore using a daily and digital approach versus weekly questionnaires remains inconclusive. The study provides insights in user preferences for and engagement with different components of the NutriQuest application, which could inform design of dietary management applications.

Keywords: Gamification · Smartphone · Mediterranean diet · Nutrition · Cardiovascular diseases · Intervention

© ICST Institute for Computer Sciences, Social Informatics and Telecommunications Engineering 2025
Published by Springer Nature Switzerland AG 2025. All Rights Reserved
H. Kondylakis and A. Triantafyllidis (Eds.): PervasiveHealth 2024, LNICST 612, pp. 48–69, 2025.
https://doi.org/10.1007/978-3-031-85575-7_3

1   Introduction

According to the World Health Organisation (WHO), cardiovascular diseases (CVD) remain worldwide the leading causes of death in 2021 [3]. Secondary prevention has been shown to reduce mortality, cardiovascular events and re-hospitalization [25]. Consequently, it is considered a class 1A recommendation for patients suffering from CVD by the European Society of Cardiology (ESC) [25]. Secondary prevention mainly involves medication optimization and modification of lifestyle-related risk factors through physical activity, smoking cessation and dietary changes. Diet is one of the most important factors modifiable by lifestyle changes and influences CVD risks via lipids, blood pressure, body weight and diabetes mellitus [11].

A targeted diet is therefore recommended for most cardiac patients. The *Dietary Approaches to Stop Hypertension* (DASH) aims to lower blood pressure in people suffering from hypertension [27]. The Healthy Nordic diet adheres to current dietary guidelines (Nordic Nutrition Recommendations [4]) and includes foods that are locally produced or traditionally used in Nordic countries, such as oily fish like salmon and herring, berries (e.g. blueberries) and fruits (e.g. apples) [24]. The *Mediterranean Diet* consists primarily of fish, unsaturated fats, whole grains, fruits, and vegetables [33]. It is important to promote the Mediterranean diet among patients with CVD, as there is well-established evidence of the cardiovascular benefits, and it may be more efficient at reducing long-term CVD outcomes compared to the DASH diet [8,17].

However, changing dietary patterns, and behaviour change in general, is especially difficult when one is stuck in unhealthy habits. Other aspects, such as lack of motivation or limited knowledge about healthy diets, can create additional barriers in the behaviour change process.

Mobile health apps may play a positive role in promoting lifestyle change, increasing motivation, and providing education to CVD patients [7,20]. They have the capacity to break barriers by presenting trustworthy information on dietary choices, supporting communication with the dietitian and facilitating persuasive techniques to increase motivation and promote behaviour change [7,20]. Gamification has been integrated into health apps as a way to boost motivation and engagement. Increasing evidence is currently emerging in this area [16,30,34].

To improve cardiac patients' adherence to the Mediterranean diet, researchers developed the mobile application "NutriQuest", which includes persuasive principles, gamification, behaviour tracking, goal setting and an information repository. The aim of this study is to evaluate the usability and feasibility of the "NutriQuest" application and its different components. The study sets out to investigate which components of the application are preferred by patients and how they use these components. It also evaluates intrinsic motivation during application use and habit formation. Additionally, the study aims to make a preliminary assessment of the effect of the intervention with the gamified application on the Modified MedDietScore (MMDS) (a modified version of the Med-DietScore, which includes salt and sugar intake and considers an alcohol consumption of 0 as positive [14]), knowledge and self-efficacy in cardiovascular patients.

2   Materials and Methods

2.1   Study Design

The application was first evaluated through a usability study, followed by a single group intervention study. There was no overlap in participants for these two parts. Eligible cardiac patients were requested to use "NutriQuest" for six weeks, alongside their usual cardiac rehabilitation program. A mixed-method design was used to explore both quantitative and qualitative results of the intervention. The study has been approved by the ethical committee of Jessa Hospital (2022/058).

2.2   Recruitment

Cardiac patients were recruited on a voluntary basis during their introduction to the cardiac rehabilitation program at the Jessa Hospital in Hasselt, Belgium. Interested patients were assessed for eligibility by an experienced dietitian and, after approval, referred to the research team. The investigator informed the patient of the study details and asked the patient to sign the informed consent form.

Patients were eligible if (1) they were adults (age $\geq$ 18); (2) they had a history of cardiovascular disease with or without intervention; (3) they had a history of current or past cardiac rehabilitation in the recruitment hospital; (4) their current treatment required them to follow the Mediterranean diet plan. For the full list of inclusion and exclusion criteria, see Appendix A, Table 8.

2.3   The NutriQuest App

The primary purpose of NutriQuest is to help patients increase their adherence to the Mediterranean diet through persuasive principles and gamification, behaviour tracking, goal setting and an information repository. The app featured three major components:

– A logbook, which was monitored by dietitians, who would leave comments on the entries. Based on the entries in the logbook, the Modified MetDietScore (MMDS) was calculated, and a weekly progress report was generated, showing for which food categories the patient performed well or not. To enter a meal, patients could take a picture, enter a description and indicate portion quantities for the MMDS food categories.
– Goal-setting, which automatically updates the goals based on the logbook entries. Patients could choose a goal from a predefined list, or create their own custom goals.
– The ability to search for brand-products in the OpenFoodFacts database and retrieve nutritional and guideline-based information (based on the *The European Cook Book* [1]).

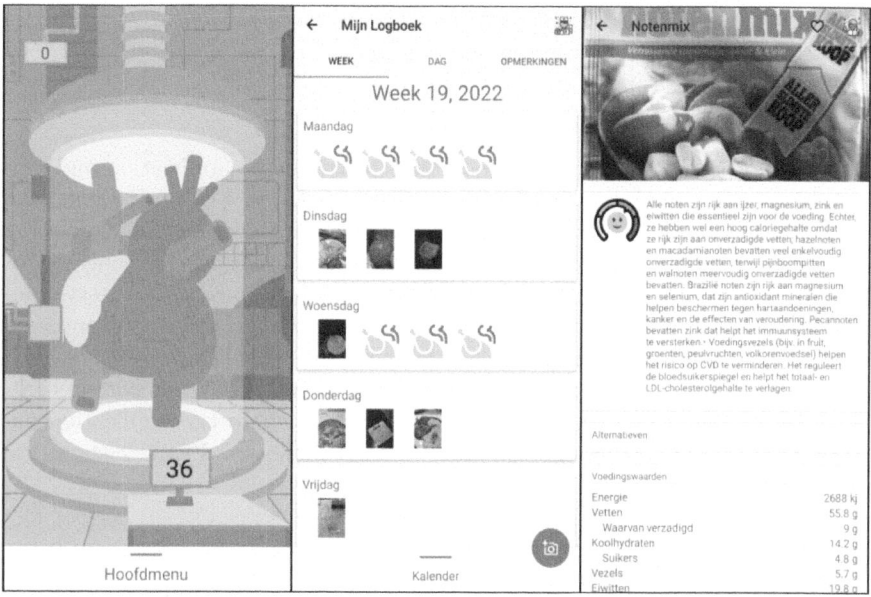

Fig. 1. Screenshots of the NutriQuest application. From left to right: the home screen, a week-overview from the logbook, and an overview page of a product with advice.

The home-screen featured a visualisation of a heart. It would show healthier or unhealthier based on the current MMDS of the patient, thus emphasizing the healthiness of the patient's current eating habits. The goal setting was gamified: selected goals were assigned to an "adventurer", which would be sent on a "quest" once the goal was activated. Each time the patient progressed towards a goal, a system notification with a progress bar was shown. When the user completed a goal, the app showed a notification indicating that the adventurer found treasures. Additionally, there was a small chance that adventurers would uncover wisdom, which was a tip on how to live healthier that could be consulted on a separate screen.

Patients would start with only one adventurer. By collecting enough treasures, patients buy more adventurers, therefore stimulating patients to start small and become more ambitious in their goals when they are performing well.

Finally, patients were able to watch educational videos on cardiovascular disease and how to live healthier.

2.4   Usability Study

Before the intervention, the "NutriQuest" application was evaluated in a usability study involving 8 participants, that would not take part in the intervention study later on. Participants were invited for a one-hour session, in which they received an explanation of the "NutriQuest" application and were asked to complete various tasks. The outcomes of this usability study were used to further improve the application before the intervention.

2.5   Intervention

Participants received an explanation of the "NutriQuest" application and were asked to use the app for six weeks (Screenshots shown in Fig. 1). Patients were encouraged but not forced to make use of the full feature set of the application. Application usage was tracked by the application for retrospective analysis, but no further follow-up of application usage was performed during the intervention period, except for dietitians monitoring and responding to the logbook entries of the patients. These dietitians are associated with the rehabilitation centre where the patients receive care and are well-trained in providing care for patients with CVD. Before the study, the dietitians were introduced to the application and taught how to leave comments on the patients' logbooks. Figure 2 shows the various stages for a single patient.

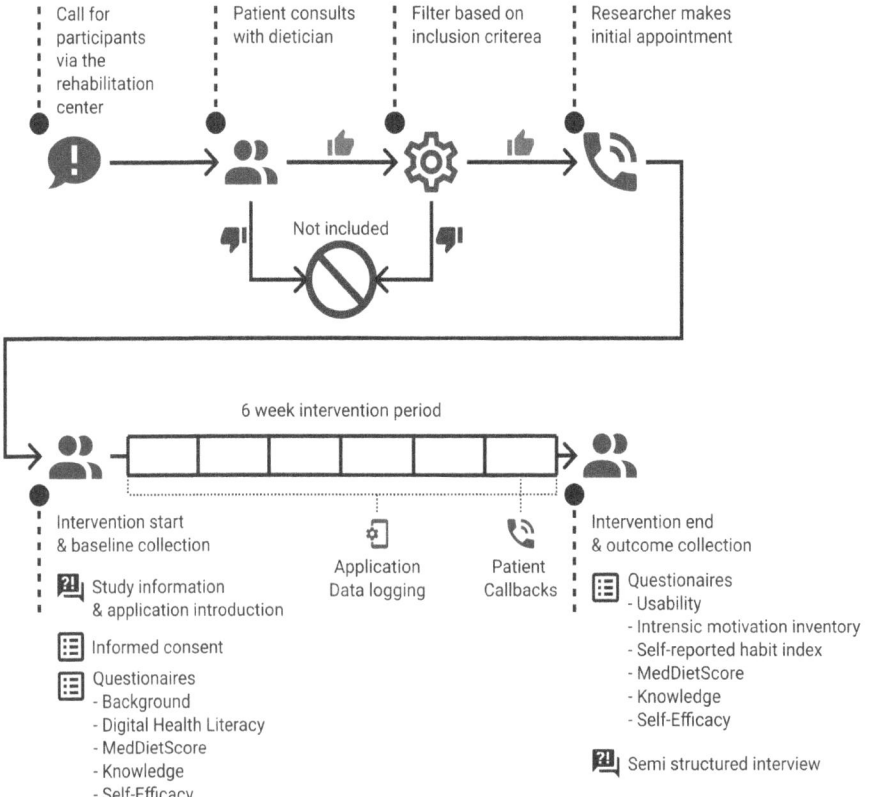

Fig. 2. Study-timeline showing the various stages for a single patient.

2.6 Measurements

Quantitative Data. Socio-demographic information (age, gender, education, and employment) and information on the *Digital Health Readiness* level [28] were collected at the start of the study.

All patients were asked to finish questionnaires on the Modified MedDietScore (MMDS) [14], Nutrition Knowledge questionnaire [14] and Nutrition Self-Efficacy scale [29], before and after the six-week intervention. At the end of the intervention, patients completed a 22-item version of the Intrinsic Motivation Inventory (IMI) [9], the Self-Report Habit Index (SRHI) [31], and an ad-hoc usability questionnaire.

The MMDS we used in this study is an adaption of the MedDietScore [21] in which parameters about salt and sugar intake are added to the score, and an intake of zero alcohol is considered positive (in contrast to the MedDietScore, which allows limited alcohol consumption). The score was developed by the H2020 CoroPrevention [2] research team, but was not yet validated in earlier studies [14]. The Nutrition knowledge questionnaire was created by the cardiac rehabilitation research team from Jessa Hospital and Hasselt University, together with in-house cardiac rehabilitation dietitians. The questionnaire assesses knowledge about heart-healthy food [14]. The usability questionnaire asks patients to evaluate various screens of the application based on perceived usefulness, ease of use and ease of understanding. It also assesses visual attractiveness and contains various questions specific to the features on each screen. An ad-hoc questionnaire was preferred over a standardised usability questionnaire (such as the System Usability Scale), as it allowed us to get in-depth feedback for each screen and identify possible reasons for (under)utilisation, as well as provide insights in how to improve future iterations of the application.

During the intervention, usability data was collected through data logging within the application and a usability questionnaire at the end of the study. The logging counted the number of visits to the application and the specific pages, as well as data about the logbook entries and goals that were set. An ad-hoc usability questionnaire queried the visual attractiveness, ease of use, ease of understanding and usefulness, as well as some other aspects specific to each component of the application (such as assigning goals, clarity of the advice for a product, etc.).

Qualitative Data. Patients were also invited to a short semi-structured interview (that lasted approximately 20 min) at the end of the usability study and at the end of the intervention. With the patients' consent, we recorded the interview. The questions mostly concerned the patients' usage of, and experience with the application, asking for example: "What features did you think were exceptionally useful?", "What aspects or features do you think need to be improved?", "What do you consider a must-have feature for diet applications in general?", etc. The interview evaluated acceptance through questions such as "If given the option, would you keep on using the application?", "Would you recommend the application to friends or family?" and "If you had to pay for the application, would you do so and how much would you be willing to pay?".

2.7 Data Analysis

For the quantitative data, continuous variables were described by mean and standard deviation. Categorical variables were described as frequencies and percentages. Shapiro-Wilk test was used to test for normality. For before-and-after comparison, the paired t-test was performed if the data was normally distributed. Correlation was analysed using the Pearson correlation coefficient. For qualitative data, all audio recordings were transcribed into text format and were then analysed for recurring themes.

2.8 Handling of Missing Data

No data was missing, except for one patient included in the final analysis that did not use the application. The answers to the questionnaires and semi-structured interview of this patient were included in the analysis. In the calculations of total and average application and page visits, this patient was excluded, as well the calculations of total and average logbook entries and goals set. When calculating correlations between application visits, page visits logbook entries or goals set with other outcomes, the patient was included and the values for the former mentioned parameters were considered 0.

3 Results

Between June 2022 and September 2022 a total of 110 patients were screened (Fig. 3): 24 of which did not show any interest in participating and 65 who did not meet the inclusion criteria. Out of the 21 patients who started the intervention, 15 were included in the final analysis. One patient could not be reached, and another patient forgot to use the application, and no longer wanted to complete the final questionnaires. Four patients dropped out citing personal issues; they did not attribute their dropout to the application. Since no outcomes were available for the dropped-out patients, they were not included in the final analysis. Of those patients included in the final analysis, 20% (n = 3) were female. The mean age was 63.27 and 53.3% held a higher education degree (a detailed description of patient characteristics can be found in Appendix B, Table 9).

3.1 Usability and Usage

Logging and Usability Questionnaire. With 1386 page views, the logbook was the most popular component. A total of 1447 entries were added to the logbook. The highest number of entries by a single patient was 195 entries on 43 separate days. The lowest number was 17 entries on 12 separate days (excluding the one patient who forgot to use the application). The goal-setting component

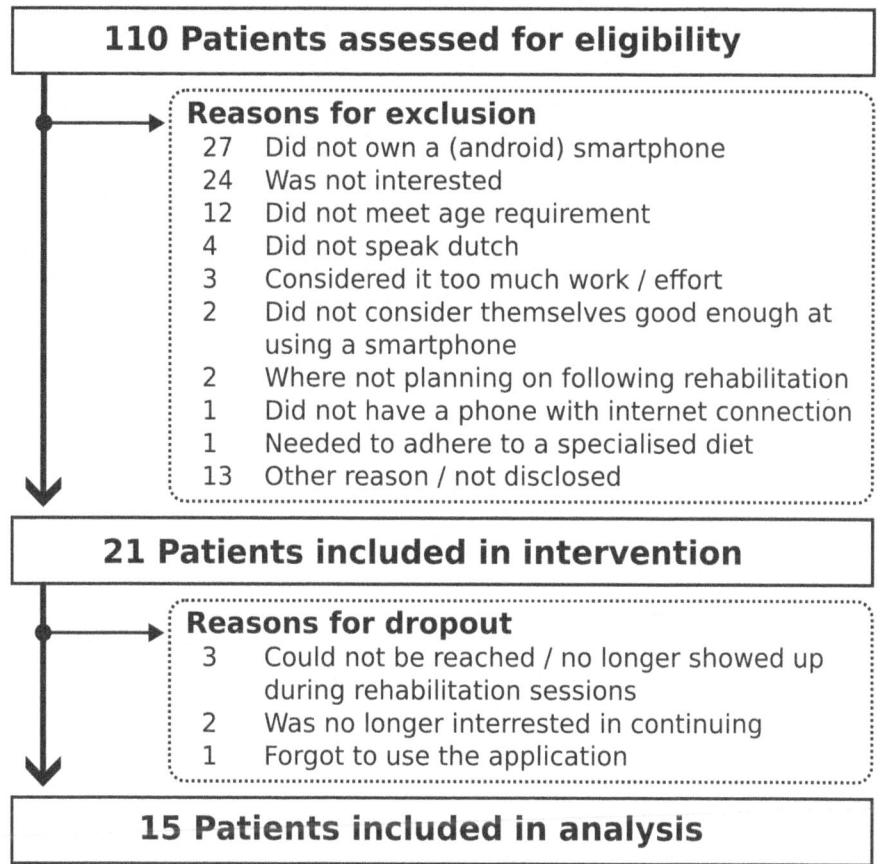

Fig. 3. Inclusion diagram. 110 patients were assessed for eligibility, 15 were eventually included in the analysis.

received 404 page-views. However, over the 15 patients, only 63 goals were set, with one patient being responsible for 21 of those goals. 66.7% (10/15) of the patients set 2 or fewer goals over the intervention period. Considering goals had to be set on a weekly basis, actual usage of the goal feature is relatively low. Table 1 describes visits to each component, Table 2 describes interaction with the logbook and goal-setting components.

Table 3 shows the average response to the usability questions. Across all dimensions, patients scored the application lower in the intervention study compared to the usability study. The questionnaire results and interviews indicate that patients found the logbook most useful and easiest to understand, which is in line with the amount of interaction the component received.

Analysing the usability data for correlations with the number of page-views (using Spearman's rho) for each component yielded a weak correlation between the page-views and their perceived ease-of-understanding ($rho = 0.211$,

Table 1. Visits to the application and its components.

	Total	Average	Min	Max	N^b
Application Visits	1124	80.29	16	226	14
Logbook Page	1386[a]	99.00	26	223	14
Logbook Entry Page	749	53.50	2	229	14
Goal-setting Page	404	28.86	3	180	14
Search Page	94	6.71	1	20	14
Product Page	81	5.79	0	20	14
Video Page	57	4.07	0	17	14

[a]Patients can visit a component multiple times within a single visit.
[b]One patient did not use the application but returned for the questionnaires and interview.

Table 2. Patients' interaction with the logbook and goal-setting components.

	Total	Average	Min	Max	N^a
Total entries in logbook	1447	96,47	17	195	14
Number of days reports were made	434	28,93	12	45	14
Total number of goals set by the user	63	4,5	0	21	14

[a]One patient did not use the application but returned for the questionnaires and interview.

$p = 0.046$). No correlation was found between page-views and *ease of use* or *usefulness*.

When queried about the comments left by the dietitians, 10 out of 15 patients agreed or completely agreed with the sentiment that those comments were useful to them, while the rest were neutral. Seven out of 15 patients found the comments motivating, with only one patient disagreeing and the other patients responding neutrally. Finally, eight patients indicated that the comments helped them learn about healthy nutrition, with all other patients except one being neutral.

Intrinsic Motivation Inventory. The study analysed four subscales of the Intrinsic Motivation Inventory [9]: interest-enjoyment (when using the application), perceived competence (in using the application), effort-importance (of using the application) and tension-pressure (perceived during application use). The scores are presented in Table 4.

Strong correlations between the IMI and the number of application visits were found for the dimensions interest-enjoyment ($r = 0.760$, $p = 0.003$), perceived competence ($r = 0.780$, $p < 0.001$) and effort-importance ($r = 0.698$, $p = 0.004$).

3.2   Acceptance

Semi-structured Interviews. Patients were asked three questions in the semi-structured interview related to their acceptance of the application: "Would you

Table 3. Average score for the usability dimensions of the components (percentage) for the usability study (US) and intervention study (IS).

	Ease of use		Ease of understanding		Usefulness	
	US[a]	IS[b]	US[a]	IS[b]	US[a]	IS[b]
Logbook Page	2.88	2,27	3.13	2,67	3.00	2.67
Logbook Entry Page	3.25	2,60	3.25	2.60	2.88	2,47
Goal-setting Page	3.25	2,40	3.00	2,20	3.00	2,47
Search Page	3,38	2,33	3.25	2,27	3.13	2,07
Product Page	3.38	2,40	3.25	2,33	3.25	2,07
Video Page[c]	-	2,27	-	2,33	-	2,40
Progress	3,13	2,07	3,13	2,07	3,25	2,47

[a]$n = 8$.
[b]$n = 15$.
[c]The video page was not evaluated during the usability study.

Table 4. Dimensions of the IMI and their scores. $N = 15$.

Dimension	Score
Interest-enjoyment[a]	20.4/35 (58.3%)
Perceived competence[a]	19.8/35 (56.6%)
Effort-importance[a]	17.0/28 (60.7%)
Tension-pressure[b]	11.8/28 (42.1%)

[a]Higher is better.
[b]Lower is better.

be interested in continuing using this system in the future?", "In case this was a commercial application for which you needed to pay, would you pay for it?" and "Would you recommend this application to friends or family?". Figure 4 shows the distributions of answers to the three questions.

Self-reported Habit Index. Acceptance was also measured as the perceived habits of using the application using the validated Self-Report Habit Questionnaire (SRHI) [31]. SRHI is composed of questions that assess three domains of habits: history of repetition (frequency of application use), lack of awareness (e.g. "by force of habit") and lack of control (to which degree patients control when they use the application). The latter two together can be considered "automaticity". The average scores of the three sub-scales, as well as the total combined score of the SRHI are described in Table 5.

Furthermore, strong correlations were found for all dimensions of the SRHI with the amount of application visits: History of repetition ($r = 0.832$, $p < 0.001$), Lack of awareness ($r = 0.803$, $p < 0.001$), Lack of control ($r = 0.772$, $p < 0.001$) and the Total score ($r = 0.859$, $p < 0.001$).

Would you be interested to continue using this system in the future?

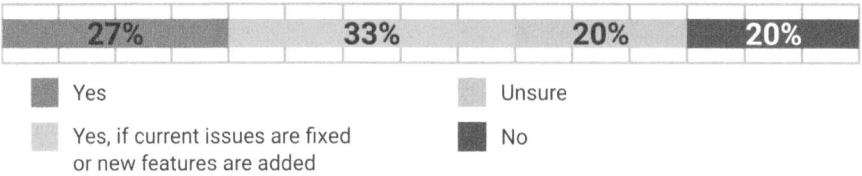

| 27% | 33% | 20% | 20% |

■ Yes   □ Unsure

□ Yes, if current issues are fixed   ■ No
   or new features are added

In case this was a commercial application for which you needed to pay, would you pay for it?

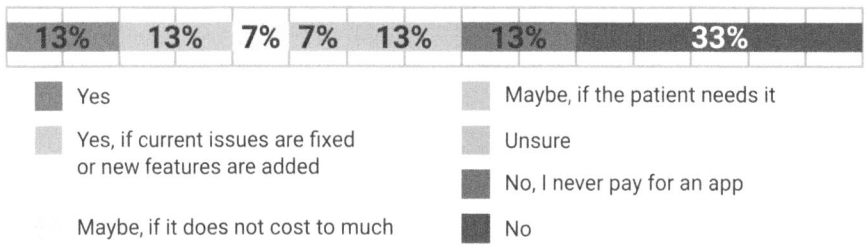

| 13% | 13% | 7% | 7% | 13% | 13% | 33% |

■ Yes   □ Maybe, if the patient needs it

□ Yes, if current issues are fixed   □ Unsure
   or new features are added
                                                   ■ No, I never pay for an app
   Maybe, if it does not cost to much
                                                   ■ No

Would you recommend this application to friends or family?

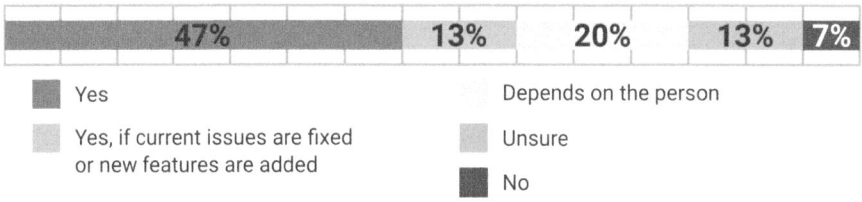

| 47% | 13% | 20% | 13% | 7% |

■ Yes   □ Depends on the person

□ Yes, if current issues are fixed   □ Unsure
   or new features are added
                                                   ■ No

Fig. 4. Patients (n = 15) responses to the three questions related to acceptance, categorised by sentiment.

3.3 Effects on Modified MedDietScore, Self-efficacy and Knowledge

After the six-week intervention study, no significant differences were found between the Modified MedDietScore (MMDS), knowledge and self-efficacy before and after the intervention. Table 6 shows the values at baseline and six weeks.

The study did not reveal any correlation between the differences in MMDS, knowledge or self-efficacy and the total amount of application visits (Table 7).

No correlations were found between the *application visits*, IMI, SRHI and the differences in MMDS, self-efficacy or knowledge; except for a negative correlation between tension-pressure (IMI) and the MMDS ($r = -0.614$, $p = 0.015$).

Table 5. Average scores of the Self-reported Habit Index and its subscales.

Dimension	Average scores
History of repetition	3.87/7 (55.24%)
Lack of awareness	3.80/7 (54.29%)
Lack of control	3.20/7 (45.71%)
Total	3.67/7 (52.46%)

Table 6. Average scores for the Modified MedDietScore (MMDS), self-efficacy and knowledge at baseline and outcome assessment. No significant difference was found.

	Baseline	Six-weeks	P-value
MMDS (questionnaire)	45.7 ± 4.25	46.9 ± 4.22	0.131
MMDS (application)	41.4 ± 6.77	41.1 ± 3.92	0.555
Self-efficacy	14.8 ± 2.01	14.7 ± 2.02	0.865
Knowledge	6.80 ± 1.97	7.33 ± 1.71	0.135

3.4 The Differences in Modified MedDietScore Measured by Questionnaire and Application

The Modified MedDietScore (MMDS) questionnaires were finished by patients at the start of the intervention and at 6 weeks, which requires patients to recall their dishes from the previous week. However, the "NutriQuest" application also calculated the MMDS on a weekly basis according to the patients' daily logbook entries of that week. We compared these two different measuring methods, by comparing the first full week reported in the application to the baselines and the last full week to the questionnaire results at the end of the intervention. It was found that there is a significant difference between the MMDS measured by the questionnaire and that by the application ($t = 2.36$, $P < 0.05$). The "first" and "last" full weeks are defined as the first and last weeks in which the patient used the app from Monday to Sunday (for example, if the patients started their intervention on a Thursday, we would take the results of the next week) and for which the amount of reported meals was within the standard-deviation of their average amount of reported meals per week. It is important to note that if patients did not report all meals in the logbook, or did not

Table 7. Correlation-matrix showing the correlations between application visits and differences between patient reported Modified MedDietScore (MMDS), knowledge and self-efficacy.

	MMDS difference	Knowledge difference	Self-efficacy difference
Visits	r = 0,342	r = 0,289	r = 0,080
	p = 0,2012	p = 0,295	p = 0,777

report truthfully, the MMDS calculated by the application will also deviate from its true value. Additionally, using this method, we did not make a one-to-one comparison of weeks. Nonetheless, the difference in the MMDS reported digitally via the application and questionnaire is an interesting finding of this study. We will further elaborate on this in the Discussion.

4   Discussion

This study is one of the few to evaluate a smartphone application with the purpose of increasing adherence to the Mediterranean diet among patients with cardiovascular disease (CVD) specifically. A 2019 systematic review by Villinger et al. indicated that mobile app interventions are increasingly developed for nutrition behaviours and are proven effective in improving nutrition behaviours and nutrition-related health outcomes [32]. However, the studies included in the review concern mostly obese patients, evidence of its efficacy in cardiovascular disease is still emerging.

Our study primarily investigated the usability of the NutriQuest application. On average, patients scored the components of this application neutral to positive for the "Ease of use", "Ease of understanding" and "Usefulness". Although the scores are lower than those given during the usability study, they still show that patients see merit in the use of the application. Furthermore, the general view of patients towards the application was positive. Four patients were interested in continuing to use the application, and seven patients would recommend it to friends or family. Many patients would join this sentiment if some of their current issues with the application would be fixed.

The correlation of the SRHI and its various subdomains with the amount of application visits means that for patients that frequently used the application, it likely became a habit. This finding is important, as it indicates a positive level of acceptance. Additionally, the presence of habit formation might lead to better adherence over longer periods. In general, the results suggest that this type of application is somewhat welcomed in patients' daily life. However, in terms of efficacy, the study did not find any significant difference in the Modified Med-DietScore (MMDS), knowledge and self-efficacy of patients during the limited six-week intervention period.

4.1   Feature Preference

In a 2016 study, Franco et al. [12] evaluated the 13 most popular nutrition apps and found that most included some form of food diary (often focusing on recording caloric intake). Analysis of the NutriQuest application logs revealed that patients mostly made use of the logbook feature. Only a few patients actively used the product search and goal-setting functions in our application. This might play a role in the efficacy of the application. Nonetheless, one patient mentioned that "Logging my meals helps me think about what I eat". This kind of self-reflection is valuable in itself. Self-monitoring and self-evaluation appear in behaviour change models such as the *Self-Regulation Theory* [15]. The use of only the logbook could therefore still prove beneficial for some patients.

4.2   Strengths and Shortcomings of the Application

A study by Bonaccio et al. found that nutrition knowledge is positively associated with a higher adherence to the Mediterranean diet [6]. Rosenstock's *Health Belief Model* also describes perceived susceptibility, severity, benefits, and barriers as the primary beliefs that determine the likelihood of action. [26]. However, our application might not have reached its full educational potential, due to low interaction with the product search (and information accompanying the products) and the informative videos.

The current information provided alongside the results of the product search was taken from the European Cookbook [1] and offered a broad and nuanced description of the product category and its general effects on health. However, patients indicated that they wanted more detailed and specific information, which clearly indicates why the product was (not) recommended for them.

In our study, personal feedback was delivered to the patients in the form of the dietitians' comments. Patients considered this as a major benefit. One patient told the interviewer that the idea that someone was monitoring their eating habits encouraged him, and that if the comments were generated automatically by the system, they would be less persuasive. Another participant believed it is a must-have in the context of diet applications to have someone motivating you by confirming you are doing well.

Personalised advice was also a centre-point for two different RCTs by Recio-Rodriguez et al. and Gonzalez-Ramirez et al., evaluating the EVIDENT II and Salbi Educa applications respectively. In both studies, the patients could use the respective application to log their food intake and the application would generate personalised recommendations on how to improve their diet. Both studies found a significant improvement in adherence to the Mediterranean diet after three months for the patients of the intervention group [13,23]. (However, neither study found a between-group difference.)

Considering the patients' statements lauding the human feedback, and the results of our study contrasted to those of the EVIDENT II and Salbi Educa studies, it is unclear to which degree patients actually considered the feedback provided by the dietitians in the NutriQuest app, whether the differences in results are due to the length of the study or due to other feature-differences between the three applications.

A separate study by Kaihara et al. evaluated the use of a chat app in a 12-week RCT [14]. Patients would send pictures of all their meals to dietitians during weeks one, four, and eight; which in turn would provide feedback. The study found a significant increase in the Nutrition- and knowledge scores. The premise of this study is similar to our logbook, in which the patients could upload pictures and dietitians could leave feedback in the form of comments. However, there are two key differences: (1) in our app, uploading pictures was optional and (2) patients could not respond to the dietitians' comments. We hypothesise that the ability to create a dialogue in which dietitians can rectify misconceptions might play a key role in the learning effect.

The lack of use of the goal-setting feature in NutriQuest was mainly attributed to two reasons: (1) patients thought they did not need it, and (2) patients found the feature confusing and hard to understand because of the gamification elements and the terminology that was used. While the latter is easier to fix, the former indicates that the application should better promote the feature and benefits, as goal setting remains an important technique for behaviour change, playing into theories such as *The Theory of Planned Behaviour* [5] and the *Trans-theoretical Model of Behaviour Change* [22]. Nonetheless, our application was innovative in its inclusion of goal-setting in a healthy nutrition context. A study by McAleese et al. evaluated the presence of behaviour change techniques in mobile apps for the Mediterranean diet. Out of the 55 analysed apps, none of them included any features related to goals; most were limited to providing instructions as well as information on behaviour, health risks and consequences [19].

4.3   Improvements

In general, patients concluded that the NutriQuest app offered many features, which was overwhelming for several participants. Patients indicated that some application components would have been useful to them, but admitted that they forgot about their existence during the study. The correlation of "perceived-competence" with "application visits" and "ease of understanding" with "page-views" suggests that for many participants, the app was still too complex. On the other hand, the correlation of "effort-importance" with "application visits" suggests that the app should make more effort in highlighting its benefits.

Nonetheless, the efficacy of the application is likely hampered by the lack of use of its various components, specifically the goal setting and weekly progress report. We hypothesise that the application should more actively guide patients towards these components (for example, by automatically redirecting them when context requires so) and promote their use. Additionally, we hypothesise that education related components should provide higher levels of detail and personalisation might have to be interwoven more strongly into the other components (for example, education could be provided in the weekly progress report).

4.4   Viability of the Modified MedDietScore for Reporting

Two issues arise when using the Modified MedDietScore (MMDS) (and by extension the MedDietScore) as a reporting tool for the logbook in the NutriQuest app. First, there is a significant difference between the MMDS reported by the questionnaires and the application. The questionnaires reported significantly higher MMDS. The application tracks the patient's diet daily in the logbook interface, whereas the questionnaire requires the patient to recall their diet for the week. Studies found that the amount of memorised information and episodic detail richness declined with retention interval [10], therefore daily reporting of measurements may be more accurate, but it depends on the patient's ability and willingness to consistently and accurately record the data. Further studies are needed to fully explore which of the measuring methods is more accurate and effective. Secondly, patients reported their meals to the application by indicating how many portions of each category of the MMDS the meal contained. The same descriptions and clarifications for the categories as the questionnaire were available in the app. However, almost all patients indicated that, even with the extra information, this limited list of categories was often confusing to use for accurate reporting of the meal. They were unsure to what category an ingredient would belong, found it hard to estimate how many portions they had consumed, and were wondering if they had to log it at all. They mentioned they would prefer an exhaustive list of categories that would take longer to browse, over a shorter but quicker one.

Both issues bring up the question about the suitability of the MMDS (and by extension the MedDietScore) to log meals via the app. Confusion about the categories, as well as having to reflect on the past week, could easily lead to unreliable reports.

4.5   Limitations

The small sample size of the study may limit its statistical power, meaning that the results may not be able to detect small but meaningful differences. Further research with larger sample sizes may be needed to confirm the findings of the current study. Two participants also mentioned that they did not complete their logbook themselves, but that their partners completed it for them, since they would decide about the meal and prepare it. It is unclear whether this situation also applied to other participants. It must also be noted that the proportion of male to female participants (12 to 3) might affect results. Since participation was voluntary, a selection bias might be present: included patients might have had higher motivation, or better adherence to a healthier diet. A minor technical limitation is the fact that this study was only conducted with Android phones, which might cause selective bias.

With a study length of only six weeks, the study was relatively limited in duration. However, the goal was to assess the initial effect on behaviour change. Lally et al. indicated that it takes on average 9 weeks (more precisely an average of 66 days, ranging from 18 to 254 days) for automacy in habit formation to plateau [18].

This suggests that behaviour change and habit formation is a gradual process. Therefore, we assume that if the application had influenced behaviour, signs of increased effort regarding diet habit formation could have been detected as early as after 5 or 6 weeks. Furthermore, the timing of six weeks aligned with a follow-up consultation with the dietitian in usual care. The current study was relevant to assess feasibility and usability, but more permanent behaviour change can only be detected in a longer follow-up study.

5   Conclusions

This study evaluated NutriQuest: a gamified smartphone application for promoting adherence to the Mediterranean diet in cardiovascular patients. The study revealed that patients generally accepted and liked the application, and suggested some usability improvements. After six weeks, no significant effect was found for the Modified MedDietScore (MMDS), knowledge and self-efficacy to the baseline measurement. Participants primarily utilized the logbook feature and neglected the goal-setting and educational components, citing application complexity and lack of awareness as reasons for neglecting these components. An interesting finding is that the study is inconclusive on whether the MMDS is the most suitable method for logging meals in a digital application in the context of behaviour change. Significant differences occurred in scores calculated based on daily logbook entries in the app, and those calculated based on reflections on the past week collected via questionnaires. We believe the findings of this study provide pointers to guide the design of future applications, such as patients' preferences towards the logbook, appreciation of monitoring by dietitians, or the need to actively promote application features.

Acknowledgements. The authors want to acknowledge the contributions of the following people in different stages of the research. Dietitians **Anne Gijbels** and **Inge Gielen** guided the patients during the intervention. **Maarten Falter** contributed to the ethical committee submission. **Sebastiaan Weytjens** was involved in part of the software development.

Author contributions. Contributions according to the Contributor Roles Taxonomy. **W.H.**: Conceptualisation, Methodology, Software, Formal analysis, Investigation, Resources, Data Curation, Writing - Original Draft, Visualisation, Project administration. **L.X.**: Methodology, Formal analysis, Investigation, Resources, Writing - Original Draft. **P.D.**: Writing - Review & Editing, Supervision, Funding acquisition. **K.C**: Writing - Review & Editing, Supervision, Funding acquisition.

Funding. The author(s) disclosed receipt of the following financial support for the research, authorship, and/or publication of this article: The research presented in this paper was supported by grants from the CoroPrevention project, which has received funding from the European Union's Horizon 2020 research and innovation programme under grant agreement No 848056.

Ethical Approval. The study was conducted in accordance with the Declaration of Helsinki, and approved by the Institutional Review Board (or Ethics Committee) of Jessa Hospital (approval number 2022/058 on 2022-05-08).

A   Appendix

Table 8. Inclusion & exclusion criteria

Inclusion criteria
The patient is an adult (age $\geq$ 18)
The patient has a history of cardiovascular disease with or without intervention.
The patient has a history of current or past cardiac rehabilitation in the recruitment hospital.
The patient their current treatment requires them to follow the Mediterranean diet plan.
The patient is willing and physically able to follow an application-based healthy nutrition program and other study procedures in a six-week follow-up period.
There is evidence of a personally signed and dated informed consent, indicating that the subject (or a legally recognized representative) is informed of all pertinent aspects of the study.
The patient has access to the internet through their smartphone.
The patient is in possession of and/or able to use an Android-based smartphone (version 6 or higher).
The patient speaks and understands the Dutch language.
Exclusion criteria
The patient was a pregnant female.
The patient suffers from diabetes or severe kidney disease.
The patient participated in other cardiac rehabilitation program trials, focusing on diet outcome.
The patient participated recently, or at the time, in other technology-supported programs, even when not directly targeting nutrition.
The patient suffered from any condition which in the opinion of the investigator would make it unsafe or unsuitable for the patient to participate in this study.
The patient had a life expectancy of less than six months based on the investigator's judgement.

B   Appendix

Table 9. Patient characteristics

Characteristic **General characteristics**	Recruited sample (n = 21)	Analysed sample (n = 15)
Age, years	62.86 ± 9.96	63.26 ± 8.71
Gender (female)	4/21 (19.00%)	3 (20.00%)
Body weight	81.05 ± 15.18	79.35 ± 15.13
Body mass index, kg/m2	26.57 ± 3.70	26.04 ± 3.92
Heart Rate (bpm)	71.20 ± 12.46	75.07 ± 11.78
Systolic blood pressure (mmHg)	127.43 ± 19.10	128.13 ± 21.01
Diastolic blood pressure (mmHg)	78.29 ± 11.76	77.67 ± 12.34
Triglycerides (mmg/dL)	123.76 ± 53.29	131.69 ± 56.58
HDL Cholesterol (mmg/dL)	47.59 ± 13.25	46.92 ± 14.53
LDL cholesterol (mmg/dL)	88.83 ± 49.40	100.46 ± 49.32
Diagnosis		
Coronary heart disease	11/21 (52.38%)	8 (53.33%)
Atrial Fibrillation	5/21 (23.80%)	4 (26.67%)
Congenital or acquired cardiac malformation or valve injury	2/21 (9.52%)	2 (13.33%)
Heart failure	3/21 (14.29%)	1 (6.67%)
Other factors		
Diabetes	6/21 (28.57%)	3 (20.00%)
Hyperlipidemia	15/21 (71.43%)	12 (80.00%)
Arterial hypertension	11/21 (52.38%)	7 (46.77%)
Prior coronary revascularisation (percutaneous coronary (PCI), coronary artery bypass grafting (CABG), none)	9/20 (45.00%)	6 (40.00%)
Family history of cardiovascular disease	14/21(66.67%)	11(73.33%)
History of Smoking		
Current	4/20 (20.00%)	4 (28.57%)
Former	8/20 (40.00%)	7 (50.00%)
None	8/20 (40.00%)	3 (21.43%)
Digital Health Readiness		
Digital access	15.62 ± 2.73	15.80 ± 2.81
Usage of digital technology	19.95 ± 4.82	20.67 ± 4.39
Digital Literacy	12.90 ± 2.00	12.80 ± 2.11
Digital Health Literacy	9.33 ± 2.94	9.20 ± 2.60
Learnability	20.33 ± 3.48	20.80 ± 3.21

References

1. European society of cardiology launches heart-friendly cookery book (2010). https://www.escardio.org/The-ESC/Press-Office/Press-releases/European-Society-of-Cardiology-launches-heart-friendly-cookery-book
2. Coroprevention – preventing coronary heart disease with research (2020). https://www.coroprevention.eu/
3. Who on cardiovascular diseases (2021). https://www.who.int/news-room/fact-sheets/detail/cardiovascular-diseases-(cvds)
4. Nordic nutrition recommendations 2022 (2022). https://www.helsedirektoratet.no/english/nordic-nutrition-recommendations-2022
5. Ajzen, I.: From intentions to actions: a theory of planned behavior. In: Kuhl, J., Beckmann, J. (eds.) Action Control. SSSSP, pp. 11–39. Springer, Heidelberg (1985). https://doi.org/10.1007/978-3-642-69746-3_2
6. Bonaccio, M., et al.: Nutrition knowledge is associated with higher adherence to mediterranean diet and lower prevalence of obesity. results from the moli-sani study. Appetite **68**, 139–146 (2013). https://doi.org/10.1016/j.appet.2013.04.026. https://www.sciencedirect.com/science/article/pii/S0195666313001657
7. Coorey, G.M., Neubeck, L., Mulley, J., Redfern, J.: Effectiveness, acceptability and usefulness of mobile applications for cardiovascular disease self-management: Systematic review with meta-synthesis of quantitative and qualitative data. Eur. J. Prev. Cardiol. **25**(5), 505–521 (2020). https://doi.org/10.1177/2047487317750913
8. Critselis, E., et al.: Comparison of the mediterranean diet and the dietary approach stop hypertension in reducing the risk of 10-year fatal and non-fatal cvd events in healthy adults: the attica study (2002–2012). Public Health Nutr. **24**(9), 2746–2757 (2021). https://doi.org/10.1017/S136898002000230X
9. Deci, E.L., Ryan, R.M.: Intrinsic Motivation and Self-Determination in Human Behavior. Springer, New York (1985). https://doi.org/10.1007/978-1-4899-2271-7
10. Diamond, N.B., Armson, M.J., Levine, B.: The truth is out there: accuracy in recall of verifiable real-world events. Psychol. Sci. **31**(12), 1544–1556 (2020)
11. Eilat-Adar, S., Sinai, T., Yosefy, C., Henkin, Y.: Nutritional recommendations for cardiovascular disease prevention. Nutrients **5**(9), 3646–3683 (2013). https://doi.org/10.3390/nu5093646. https://www.mdpi.com/2072-6643/5/9/3646
12. Franco, R.Z., Fallaize, R., Lovegrove, J.A., Hwang, F.: Popular nutrition-related mobile apps: a feature assessment. JMIR mHealth uHealth **4**(3) (2016). https://doi.org/10.2196/mhealth.5846
13. Gonzalez-Ramirez, M., et al.: Short-term pilot study to evaluate the impact of Salbi Educa nutrition app in macronutrients intake and adherence to the mediterranean diet: randomized controlled trial. Nutrients **14**(10) (2022)
14. Kaihara, T., et al.: The impact of dietary education and counselling with a smartphone application on secondary prevention of coronary artery disease: a randomised controlled study (the telediet study). Digit. Health **9**, 20552076231164101 (2023). https://doi.org/10.1177/20552076231164101
15. Kanfer, F.H., Gaelick-Buys, L.: Self-management methods, pp. 305–360. Pergamon general psychology series, vol. 52., Pergamon Press, Elmsford (1991)
16. Kim, J., Castelli, D.M.: Effects of gamification on behavioral change in education: a meta-analysis. Int. J. Environ. Res. Public Health **18**(7), 3550 (2021)
17. Klonizakis, M., Bugg, A., Hunt, B., Theodoridis, X., Bogdanos, D.P., Grammatikopoulou, M.G.: Assessing the physiological effects of traditional regional diets

targeting the prevention of cardiovascular disease: a systematic review of randomized controlled trials implementing mediterranean, new nordic, japanese, atlantic, persian and mexican dietary interventions. Nutrients **13**(9) (2021). https://doi.org/10.3390/nu13093034. https://www.mdpi.com/2072-6643/13/9/3034

18. Lally, P., van Jaarsveld, C.H.M., Potts, H.W.W., Wardle, J.: How are habits formed: modelling habit formation in the real world. Eur. J. Soc. Psychol. **40**(6), 998–1009 (2010). https://doi.org/10.1002/ejsp.674. https://onlinelibrary.wiley.com/doi/abs/10.1002/ejsp.674

19. McAleese, D., Linardakis, M., Papadaki, A.: Quality and presence of behaviour change techniques in mobile apps for the mediterranean diet: a content analysis of android google play and apple app store apps. Nutrients **14**(6) (2022)

20. Neubeck, L., Lowres, N., Benjamin, E.J., Freedman, S.B., Coorey, G., Redfern, J.: The mobile revolution-using smartphone apps to prevent cardiovascular disease. Nat. Rev. Cardiol. **12**(6), 350–360 (2015)

21. Panagiotakos, D.B., Milias, G.A., Pitsavos, C., Stefanadis, C.: Meddietscore: a computer program that evaluates the adherence to the mediterranean dietary pattern and its relation to cardiovascular disease risk. Comput. Methods Programs Biomed. **83**(1), 73–77 (2006). https://doi.org/10.1016/j.cmpb.2006.05.003. https://www.sciencedirect.com/science/article/pii/S0169260706001052

22. Prochaska, J.O., DiClemente, C.C.: Transtheoretical therapy: toward a more integrative model of change. Psychother. Theory Res. Pract. **19**, 276–288 (1982). https://doi.org/10.1037/h0088437

23. Recio-Rodriguez, J.I., et al.: Short-term effectiveness of a mobile phone app for increasing physical activity and adherence to the mediterranean diet in primary care: a randomized controlled trial (EVIDENT II Study). J. Med. Internet Res. **18**(12), e331 (2016)

24. Risérus, U.: Healthy nordic diet and cardiovascular disease. J. Intern. Med. **278**(5), 542–544 (2015)

25. Roffi, M., et al.: 2015 ESC guidelines for the management of acute coronary syndromes in patients presenting without persistent ST-segment elevation: task force for the management of acute coronary syndromes in patients presenting without persistent ST-segment elevation of the european society of cardiology (ESC). Eur. Heart J. **37**(3), 267–315 (2016). https://doi.org/10.1093/eurheartj/ehv320

26. Rosenstock, I.M.: Historical origins of the health belief model. Health Educ. Monogr. **2**(4), 328–335 (1974). https://doi.org/10.1177/109019817400200403

27. Sacks, F.M., et al.: Effects on blood pressure of reduced dietary sodium and the dietary approaches to stop hypertension (dash) diet. N. Engl. J. Med. **344**(1), 3–10 (2001). https://doi.org/10.1056/NEJM200101043440101. pMID: 11136953

28. Scherrenberg, M., et al.: Development and internal validation of the digital health readiness questionnaire: prospective single-center survey study. J. Med. Internet Res. **25**, e41615 (2023)

29. Schwarzer, R., Renner, B.: Health-specific self-efficacy scales (2009)

30. Suleiman-Martos, N., et al.: Gamification for the improvement of diet, nutritional habits, and body composition in children and adolescents: a systematic review and meta-analysis. Nutrients **13**, 2478 (2021). https://doi.org/10.3390/nu13072478

31. Verplanken, B., Orbell, S.: Reflections on past behavior: a self-eport index of habit strength. J. Appl. Soc. Psychol. **33**, 1313–1330 (2003). https://doi.org/10.1111/j.1559-1816.2003.tb01951.x

32. Villinger, K., Wahl, D.R., Boeing, H., Schupp, H.T., Renner, B.: The effectiveness of app-based mobile interventions on nutrition behaviours and nutrition-related

health outcomes: A systematic review and meta-analysis. Obes. Rev. **20**(10), 1465–1484 (2019)

33. Widmer, R.J., Flammer, A.J., Lerman, L.O., Lerman, A.: The mediterranean diet, its components, and cardiovascular disease. Am. J. Med. **128**(3), 229–238 (2015). https://doi.org/10.1016/j.amjmed.2014.10.014

34. Yang, H., Li, D.: Health management gamification: Understanding the effects of goal difficulty, achievement incentives, and social networks on performance. Technol. Forecast. Soc. Change **169**, 120839 (2021). https://doi.org/10.1016/j.techfore.2021.120839. https://www.sciencedirect.com/science/article/pii/S0040162521002717

mCARE: Integrating Mobile Phones, Caregivers, and Health Practitioners to Provide Regular Monitoring and Care for the Children with ASD in Bangladesh

Md M. Haque[1(✉)], Md Ishrak Islam[2], Masud Rabbani[2], Dipranjan Das[2],
Amy Schwichtenberg[3], Naveen Bansal[2], Tanjir Rashid Soron[4], Shaheen Akhter[5],
Shahana Parveen[6], Azima Begum[4], Mohammad Shaha A. Patwary[1], Austin Schmidt[1],
Syed Ishtiaque Ahmed[7], and Sheikh Iqbal Ahamed[2]

[1] Butler University, Indianapolis, IN 56208, USA
mhaque@butler.edu
[2] Marquette University, Milwaukee, WI 53233, USA
[3] Purdue University, West Lafayette, IN 47907, USA
[4] Telepsychiatry Research and Innovation Network Ltd, Dhaka, Bangladesh
[5] Institute of Paediatric Neurodisorder and Autism, Dhaka, Bangladesh
[6] National Institute of Mental Health, Dhaka, Bangladesh
[7] University of Toronto, Toronto, ON M5S1A1, Canada

Abstract. Designing technologies for the people with mental health challenges in the Global South has largely remained a neglected area in HCI and related fields. However, the overwhelming adoption of mobile phones in Bangladesh has created an unprecedented opportunity to overcome the various social-cultural-financial constraints that deprive Children with Autism Spectrum Disorder (CWA) of regular monitoring, care, and support. To leverage this opportunity, we designed, developed, and evaluated mCARE, a mobile application that integrates Experience Sampling Method (ESM) with the local healthcare practice by putting the caregivers in the loop. This paper reports: (a) mCARE helped the mental health professionals, but was dependent on the collaboration between them and the caregivers; (b) mCARE provided a novel platform to assess the impact of COVID-19 on CWA, and; (c) the impact of mCARE was shaped by the familial values. We also discuss the broader implications of these findings for the HCI scholarship.

Keywords: Autism Spectrum Disorder · symptom monitoring · COVID-19

1 Introduction

Autism Spectrum Disorder (ASD) is a highly prevalent neurodevelopmental disorder affecting about one percent of the population in the U.S. and abroad [1, 2], including Bangladesh [3–5]. The worldwide predominance of (ASD) has expanded 20 to 30-fold during the last 50 years [6]. Most of the previous research on autism has been

© ICST Institute for Computer Sciences, Social Informatics and Telecommunications Engineering 2025
Published by Springer Nature Switzerland AG 2025. All Rights Reserved
H. Kondylakis and A. Triantafyllidis (Eds.): PervasiveHealth 2024, LNICST 612, pp. 70–88, 2025.
https://doi.org/10.1007/978-3-031-85575-7_4

limited to western or wealthy Asian countries [2, 7–10]. Research in the domain of ASD in the Low- and Middle-Income Countries (LMICs) is mostly done in the area of screening [11–13]. Although a few mHealth tools exist that, in a limited capacity, serve for monitoring mental health diseases in LMICs [14, 16], those cannot accommodate the rich variety, individual nuances, and the uncertain patterns of ASD. Also, most mHealth applications are built assuming that the health data will be collected by physicians or health care workers [17–20]. Moreover, values embedded in a cultural setting impact the perception, diagnosis, and treatment of ASD [21–23]. Thus, a carefully designed mHealth application that considers the socio-cultural values, norms and perception of ASD, and can be easily used by caregivers (based on literacy level and mobile use experience) themselves to address the aforementioned constraints, is an important need.

Regardless of gaining remarkable progress in ASD screening and raising awareness in recent years, the healthcare support system is limited for families raising children with ASD (CWA) in Bangladesh [24]. Like many other low and middle- income countries (LMICs), social-cultural-financial constraints and a scarcity of mental health professionals (MHPs) have deprived CWA from regular monitoring, care, and support in Bangladesh. Approximately 200 psychiatrists and 50 psychologists are currently available for 160 million people in Bangladesh [25]. The situation is even worse in rural areas. Also, existing practices depend on traditional 'on spot' evaluations of the behavior of CWA or caregiver recollections during their occasional and infrequent visits affect the evidence-based decision making of MHPs resulting in inaccurate and unreliable care.

The objective of our work is to dynamically improve the care system with an accessible and easy-to-use mobile-based application called mCARE for evidence-based decision making. mCARE designed to address three major constraints in the care system – financial hardship for parents to arrange frequent visits and to accurately report to MHPs, lack of availability of MHPs, and lack of availability of longitudinal data of behavioral changes. mCARE, developed following the socio-cultural and existing care protocol, has been used by 8 mental health professionals (MHPs) and 300 caregivers of CWA for over a year. Caregivers of CWA use mCARE (mCARE-APP/mCARE-SMS version) to routinely submit selected behavioral and developmental progress parameters. MHPs utilize the web-based data visualization tool mCARE-DMP (Data Management Platform), to view the submitted data and support evidence-based decision making.

The contribution of this paper to HCI literature is threefold. First, this paper describes the design, development, and evaluation of mCARE, which is the first mobile-based tool to routinely report behavior and developmental parameters of CWA in LMICs by caregivers. The evaluation of this application demonstrates how the collaborations between the care professionals and caregivers are crucial for such technologies to work properly. Second, this paper reports a novel way to capture the impact of COVID-19 on CWA by using mCARE. We report how COVID-19 had a wide range of impact on various CWA based on their familial circumstances, socioeconomic condition, and geographic location. Finally, this paper describes how the impact of such digital behavior monitoring platform is shaped by familial values of the children and caregivers. We demonstrate how the use of this application was impacted by the patriarchal social structure and other social norms. Thus, this paper makes an important contribution in the HCI scholarship on designing mental health technologies with the people in LMICs (especially in the Global South).

2   Related Work

In recent years, the popularity of using smartphones to monitor CWA has been increased [17, 20–28]. Besides smart-phone technology, several other technologies are also used to monitor and support children with ASD [9, 25]. Our thorough review revealed the use of different technologies as follows: (i) wearable devices like a smartwatch [29, 30], wrist/chest/ankle bands [31–33], GPS [34], head-mounted displays [35], and cameras [36, 37] (51 papers); (ii) Tablet [38, 39], iPad [40, 41] or mobile applications [27, 28, 42] (58 papers); (iii) Virtual Reality (VR) [35] (11 papers), and; (iv) Robots [43] (14 papers). Multiple web-based mobile health (mHealth) apps are proposed to continuously monitor the symptoms and progress of children with ASD including My JAKE (Janssen Autism Knowledge Engine) [28, 44].

Early identification of ASD symptoms is crucial for the ASD treatment process [11, 12] and hence research in the domain of ASD in LMICs is mostly done in the area of screening [11–13]. Examples of this category include Prottoy [14], Autism Barta [11], Autism Severity Assessment App [45] (Bangladesh), Autism&Beyond [46] (South Africa), 12 m [47] (India, Pakistan, Zambia), ACCESS [48] (Uganda, Sri Lanka), AHC-DMAT [49] (Cambodia), and MDAT [50] (Malawi). A 2018 cross-sectional study [51] in Bangladesh emphasized the importance of early detection and decentralization of healthcare service delivery in the domain of ASD care.

mCARE addresses the shortcomings of the aforementioned projects in multiple ways: i) it has been developed considering the socio-cultural-financial aspects of the population; ii) it includes module to be used by both caregivers and MHPs; iii) to include the mass population, both app and SMS version of mCARE are developed and deployed in 4 institutes (public and private), and; iv) it monitors both behavioral and milestone parameters using locally accepted scales. Successful completion of this project served as a proof of concept that persons living in an LMIC can effectively use a carefully designed mHealth application and that such applications can improve overall outcomes and quality of care of ASD.

3   Methodology

Any tool to support ASD in LMICs needs involvement of both caregivers and MHPs from the very beginning of the development. In this paper, considering Bangladesh as a case study, we completed multiple field studies to understand the hidden dynamics of the stake holders which will be crucial in designing the technological intervention.

3.1   Challenge Identification

First, we interviewed 20 parents of children with ASD (12 female, 8 male) in Bangladesh and learned about their challenges in understanding their child's progress and in reporting those to the MHPs. Snowball sampling [52] was used to recruit these participants and continued until a saturation point [53] is reached. Since it was difficult to reach the participants in person, who are distributed all over the country, we used phone or Viber calls for the interview that lasted for 22 min on average. The mean age of the parents was 37.1 and the mean age of children with ASD was 10.7 [54].

Second, we conducted 4 focus groups discussion (FGD) sessions in Dhaka and Chittagong, Bangladesh from May 2017 to July 2017 to identify the challenges faced in the current treatment process and find the potential of an mHealth tool to address these challenges. 28 MHPs, 2 government officials, and 10 parents of CWA participated in these sessions. The MHPs were selected on a random basis from the convenience-sampled institutions [55]. One of the clinical coordinators of the research team moderated the FGDs which are audio recorded and later transcribed and analyzed.

These FGDs frequently highlighted the current situation of scarcity of skilled MHPs. We qualitatively analyzed the interview and FGD notes using thematic analysis [56] and grounded theory [57]. The interviews and FGD sessions revealed the following challenges faced by the caregivers on a regular basis: 1) lack of time during visits to express the condition of their children; 2) lack of regular communication with practitioners, and; 3) lack of knowledge in general (what to focus on, what to achieve next etc.). In contrast, that of the practitioners were: 1) lack of data points to get the whole picture; 2) irregular visits with commonly exaggerated information; 3) failure to answer questions with clarity; 4) limited time window during visits, and; 5) lack of communication (no feedback) between visits. From heretofore, we will use PC# and CC# to refer to practitioners' or caregivers' challenge number. Along with the aforementioned challenges, three themes came up again and again as the major constraints in the care system for children with ASD in resource scarce contexts - a) financial hardship for parents to arrange frequent visits (a visit to major cities typically requires patients to spend BDT 800–1600 (approximately USD 10–20) [54]) and to accurately report to MHPs; b) lack of availability of MHPs, and; c) lack of availability of longitudinal data of behavioral changes. We included participants from the family welfare department of the Government of Bangladesh to take their input in terms of Government's willingness to make it a scalable and sustainable project in future. One interesting observation from this two step challenge identification process was the unanimous acceptability among the caregivers of an mHealth tool that might help them to improve the quality of care. As one caregiver said: "*I always carry phone with me. Actually, all the adult members of my family have mobile phones. If spending some minutes from my son help me to get better treatment, get better attention, and doctors are ok with it..why not?*".

3.2 Identification of Parameters

This project adopted a systematic and comprehensive procedure for identifying a set of demographics, behavioral and developmental progress parameters (also known as milestone parameters) that - i) are feasible to incorporate in existing treatment practice and ii) might help the practitioners in decision making if monitored longitudinally.

Identification of Behavioral Parameter: With the help of a group of ASD care practitioners (n = 7) and parents (caregivers) (n = 9), we identified a set of questions to put into the preliminary data (e.g., demographic and contact information, height, weight, sibling information, ASD severity, and number of years of being diagnosed) and a set of behavior parameters based on two internationally recognized autism monitoring routines (Indian Scale for Assessment of Autism (ISAA) [58] and DSM-5 [57]). Both DSM-5 and Indian Scale of Autism Assessment (ISAA), used for developing the list of behavior parameters to be monitored, are validated in Bangladesh. ISAA has already been adapted by Bangladesh government for autism screening. The data collected using mCARE followed the same unit and scale as suggested in ISAA to avoid confusion.

Fine Tuning Behavioral Parameters: Later we used a Qualtrics survey to receive feedback from the MHPs and caregivers on the necessity of selected parameters and frequency of submission (daily/weekly/monthly). Based on the 39 recorded responses (detailed in Table 1), we updated the language of the questions asked, frequency of input, and other features (e.g., addition of a free form field for caregivers to provide context against any parameter) as summarized below:

Table 1. Qualtrics participants summary.

Gender			Role			Years of experience			
M	F	Unidentified	Professional	Parents	Unidentified	0–1	1–3	3–6	> 6
15	10	14	17	7	15	4	6	1	6

Identification of Developmental Progress/Milestone Parameters: Based on Vineland-II adaptive behavior scale [59], the MHPs and parents also identified a set of developmental progress/milestone parameters categorized by age in the domain of communication (e.g., says first and last name when asked), daily living skills (e.g., brushes teeth), socialization (e.g., shares toys), and motor skills (e.g., color simple shapes).

The Vineland scale has been validated and used frequently in India for similar settings [60]. The MHPs and parents discarded/altered multiple developmental progress parameters mentioned in Vineland-II as those either do not culturally fit or are not considered as priority. For example, most of the caregivers discarded the 'memorize the address' parameter saying "*…we never let our kid go outside the house alone. Even the gate is under lock and key all the time. So, I don't think it is that important.*" Also, sometimes the MHPs and caregivers have conflicting opinion in terms of importance of certain parameters. As one of the MHPs said: "*We consider self-hygiene (like cleaning themselves after pooping), self-eating, or getting dressed very important whereas many parents think that these will be learnt by the kids later because it is very common for parents in Bangladesh to do these things for their kids (even for normal ones) for long period of time. Parents are more concerned about education (learning colors, alphabet etc.).*"

Number of parameters adapted from Vineland-II adaptive behavior scale and selected for each age group is summarized in Table 2.

Table 2. Number of developmental progress/milestone parameters by categories.

Domain	Age (3–6)	Age (6–9)
Communication	13	11
Daily living skill	9	10
Socialization	6	5
Motor skill	10	6

3.3 Study Site and Population

The mCARE study took place in 4 major institutes of Bangladesh in two geographical locations - Dhaka and Chittagong. We collaborated with two of the largest government ASD research and treatment institutes, National Institute of Mental Health (NIMH) and Institute of Pediatric Neuro-disorder & Autism (IPNA), to recruit 100 caregivers of CWA from each. The participants are divided into two groups - mCARE-APP (50) and mCARE-SMS (50) who will be later using the app and SMS version of mCARE. Each group is further divided in test (25) and control (25) groups. Typically, in Bangladesh, families with low and high socioeconomic resources receive treatment from public and private organizations respectively. To include participants from all socioeconomic classes, we included two private organizations - Nishpap (means sinless) and AWF (Autism Welfare Foundation). 50 participants are chosen from each of these schools divided into test (25) and control (25) groups only for the mCARE-APP study. Our FGD sessions revealed that all the parents/caregivers of these children have smartphones and so mCARE-SMS is not applicable in this scenario. A total of 16 MHPs used the web-based mCARE data management platform (mCARE-DMP) to monitor and utilize the data submitted by the caregivers in their treatment process (Table 3).

Table 3. Participants overview (P: Mental Health Professional, C: Caregiver).

	NIMH	IPNA	Nishpap	AWF
mCARE-SMS	50 (C)	50 (C)		
mCARE-APP	50 (C)	50 (C)	50 (C)	50 (C)
mCARE-DMP	5 (P)	5 (P)	3 (P)	3 (P)
Status	Public	Public	Private	Private
Location	Dhaka	Dhaka	Chittagong	Dhaka

3.4 Eligibility, Recruitment, and Enrollment

This project included 300 children, aged 3 to 9. We incorporated diversity in terms of age, sex, ASD severity, and family socioeconomic resources. We did not use children with serious illnesses, or who are otherwise unable to participate. The recruitment was performed over a period of 7 months from Mar'19 to Sep'19. The participants are classified into mCARE-APP or mCARE-SMS group based on their access to type of mobile phones and comfortability using mobile apps. Later they are randomly classified into either test or control group. The consent and data collection methods were approved by Bangladesh Medical Review Council (BMRC). All the test group subjects were given 50 BDT ($0.60 USD) per month as data cost.

3.5 Preliminary Data Collection

We performed the following tasks with one MHP/clinical coordinator (clinical coordinators are MHPs who are assigned as supervisor for each site) and one researcher:

i) **Demographic data:** Each caregiver filled out a demographic questionnaire with 28 questions categorized in two domains: socio-demographic information of the child (10 questions) and birth and developmental history (18 questions).

ii) **Baseline value of behavioral and milestone parameters**: At this step MHPs selected 6−23 behavioral parameters that are appropriate for the child in question and would be most helpful if longitudinally monitored. This required 6–8 min by the MHPs. Majority of the caregivers are assigned 6 ~ 13 parameters (67%) with varied frequency of submissions (daily/weekly/biweekly/monthly) as requested by the MHPs. Later, based on the discussion with each caregiver, MHPs selected one or two developmental progress/milestone parameters from each of the four categories (communication, daily living skills, socialization, and motor skills). The frequency of submission for milestone parameters is selected as monthly and justified by MHP 9 saying:

"These developmental progress parameters do not change in days or weeks. So, monthly should be fine. Also, we don't exactly need too many data points on these since we do not use them for treatment purpose unlike behavioral parameters."

Finally, demographic and baseline values of behavioral and milestone parameters are collected from all 300 participants. For behavioral parameters the scale was from 0 to 10 (0 means never and 10 means almost always as mentioned in the ISAA scale) and for developmental progress parameters the scale was from 0 to 2 (with 0, 1, and 2 stands for never, sometimes, and always respectively as mentioned in Vineland-II scale). While the MHP was recording this information in paper, one researcher recorded the values in the mCARE database. Along with this, we also collected baseline information regarding satisfaction level (towards MHPs and quality of care), basic knowledge of ASD, and travel time and cost for each visit from all participants. This portion was done by the researcher only since we felt that the caregivers would not feel comfortable providing the satisfaction level for MHPs/quality of care in the presence of an MHP. The same set of data is also collected from all 300 participants at the end of the study.

3.6 Data Collection and Coordination Methodology

All the test group caregivers (mCARE-APP or mCARE-SMS) submitted data from Nov. 2019 to Nov. 2020. All the researchers and MHPs met every week for 30 min to discuss the day-to-day operations of the study. A larger (2 h) group discussion was scheduled quarterly to discuss the experience of long-term use of mCARE-DMP and its impact on the quality of care of CWA. We also had an end of study interview with 30 caregivers to collect their experience of using mCARE-APP or mCARE-SMS.

4 mCARE Development

4.1 Design and Development of mCARE

mCARE adopted the three-step methodology of Value Sensitive Design (VSD) for the design process. For the 'Conceptual' (identify the stakeholders and their cultural values based on theoretical concepts/previous studies/stories from local people) and 'Empirical' (collect empirical data to underpin the understanding of local values and practices of the stakeholders) step, we relied on exhaustive field visits, FGD discussions, face to face and phone interviews, online surveys, and long experience of the mCARE team members in providing care to children with ASD, and designing, developing mHealth applications for targeted communities in Bangladesh [7, 9, 12, 16, 21, 23, 26–28, 51]. For 'Technical' (build technologies according to the stakeholders' values, deploy the technology with them, and gradually improve the system based on feedback from the users) step, we developed mCARE-APP and mCARE-SMS following a user-centered and evolutionary approach (Agile development method) [61] constantly integrating feedback from users [4]. mCARE has adapted Fogg's Behavior Model (FBM) by providing bi-weekly reports and hopes of better care as 'motivations', its simple as possible design ensures 'ability' to use, and regular prompt for reminders acts as 'trigger'.

mCARE-APP: We developed mCARE-APP for parental monitoring of behavior and milestone parameters of CWA. Caregivers used mCARE-APP to submit selected parameter values, send urgent SMS to the MHPs, and view bi-weekly summary report.

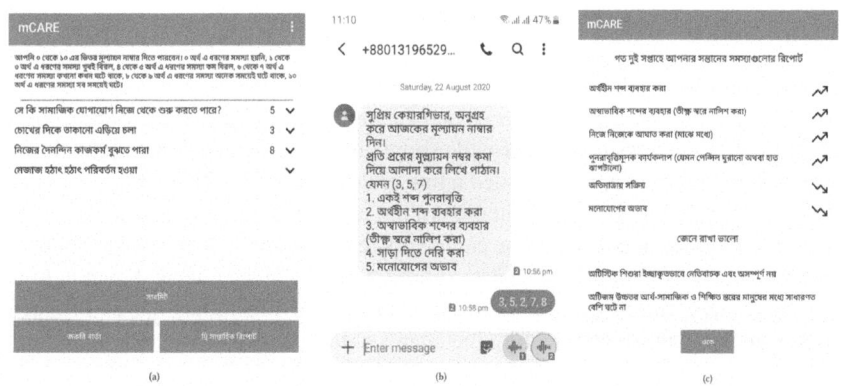

Fig. 1. Screenshot of (a) mCARE-APP (b) mCARE-SMS (c) Bi-weekly report.

mCARE-SMS: An SMS is sent to the caregivers with the name of the parameters for which values need to be submitted for that day and the caregivers are needed to reply with the sequential values separated by comma. Figure 1 shows the sample screenshots of mCARE-APP and mCARE-SMS.

mCARE-DMP: mCARE-DMP is developed as a visualization and analyzing tool for the MHPs based on the data submitted by the caregivers. The details of the development and User Centered Design challenges has been left out of the scope of this paper.

5 Discussion and Lessons Learned

5.1 "What's My Benefit" and Data Submission Adherence

After the initial enthusiasm of getting involved in a new project was over, we saw a sharp decline in terms of data submission adherence. Though the benefits of participating were articulated during the consent signing, many of the caregivers echoed the following sentiment of a caregiver (Nishpap 14): *"I have been submitting the data for 3 months now. But I don't see any noticeable improvement in my child's behavior. I somehow thought there would be a miracle and my son would get better once I start. Also, it is too many (parameters)."*

Based on this, MHPs asked 20 caregivers (10 mCARE-APP and 10 mCARE-SMS test users) two specific questions: i) what number of parameters they would feel comfortable submitting and ii) what we can do to help them benefited. Then we discussed the findings during our weekly meeting (with all researchers and MHPs) and made the following changes in our protocol: i) maximum number of parameters to be monitored would be restricted to $5-7$ parameters; ii) Monthly call from clinical coordinators, and; iii) Monthly free face to face meeting with senior mental health professionals (director of IPNA and NIMH) who served as site principal investigators. We also trained the clinical coordinators to repeat the benefits during their conversation. For example, the clinical coordinator of NISHPAP explained to one of the caregivers as follows:

"We know it is hard to see any notable improvement in behavioral parameters in short period. But as you see when I call you, I know the exact status of your kid since you have submitted data regularly. Others do not get calls from us. Please take the opportunity to meet with Professor X (the senior MHP overlooking NISHPAP participants) end of the month. Also, you can send me SMS (text) and get help of any situation instantaneously."

Finally, MHPs suggested us to provide some kind of instant feedback right after the caregivers submit data. So, we provided a link once data is submitted which, if clicked, would show the longitudinal representation of the submitted data for the last 7 days. This would provide instant feedback to the caregivers regarding how their child is doing. All these steps helped us to improve the data submission adherence rate as shown in Fig. 2. Prior to these steps, the average data submission rate over 4 institutes was 39.05% (Nov 2019–Apr 2020). After implementing the changes, the corresponding rate increased to 54.43% over the period of six months (May 2020–Oct 2020).

5.2 Milestone Parameter – The 'Sense of Achievement'

One of the challenges mentioned by the caregivers is that they do not have an idea of what to achieve next (CC3). As a solution, we added milestone parameters as part of the longitudinal monitoring. These would be used as individualized milestones to be achieved

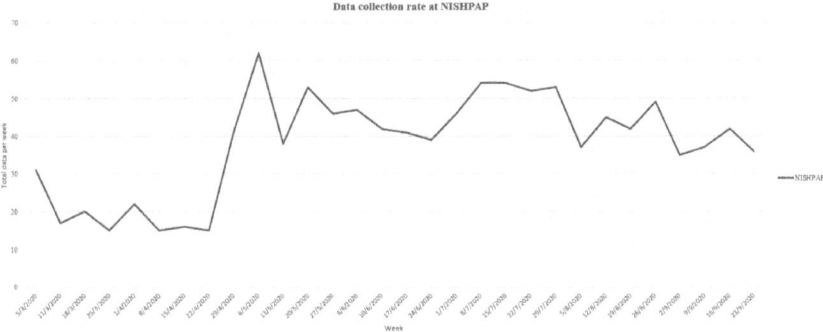

Fig. 2. Data collection rate at Nishpap over the study period.

by the caregivers and once the milestone parameter is reached to 2 (which represents always), MHPs would replace these with new target, thus continuously engaging the caregivers with small targets. Each caregiver was given 8 developmental progress/milestone parameters (2 from each of the 4 categories mentioned in Vineland II scale) to work on. During the monthly call, clinical coordinators specifically asked about the progress on milestone parameters and guided the caregivers regarding how to achieve the next level for the selected parameters. Caregiver NIMH 03 said:

"I have tried really everything to improve (the symptoms) but I don't see much (for behavioral parameters). But for these (milestone parameters), I try to teach them and take advise from the madam (clinical coordinator of NIMH). I taught my son the name of 5 colors. I felt that I really accomplished something, some positive change that I can see. I think this is helping me not to lose hope and carry on."

Overall, out of total 1200 (150 test group participants X 4 domains X 2 parameters per domain) developmental progress/milestone parameters selected for mCARE test group members, improvement was seen in 732 of them (61%) and the rest (39%) remain unchanged (neutral). This analysis is based on comparing the data collected at the end of the study with the baseline value. If the baseline value of the selected parameter changed from 0 to 1 or from 1 to 2, we have considered that as an improvement (with 0, 1, and 2 stands for never, sometimes, and always respectively as mentioned in Vineland-II). For mCARE control group, the percentage of parameters that improved (over all 4 domains) is 21.05%. The changes in milestone parameters are shown in Table 4.

As seen from Table 4, the average percentage level of participants with improved milestone parameters for mCARE test group (78.82%) is significantly higher compared to that of the mCARE control group (21.05%). Unlike the mCARE-APP test group, mCARE-APP control group did not submit regular data or receive calls from the clinical coordinators with suggestions regarding how to work on the selected milestone parameters. This indicates the impact of mCARE in improving the milestone parameters.

Table 4 gives an interesting insight about the focus of the caregivers. The percentage of mCARE test participants (all four sites) with improved milestone parameter is 34.33 (Communication), 73.53 (Daily Living Skills), 47.2 (Socialization), and 55.6 (Motor Skills). The corresponding values for the mCARE control group are 8.87 (Communication), 22.13 (Daily Living Skills), 10.47 (Socialization), and 14.67 (Motor Skills). This

Table 4. Percentage of participants with improved milestone parameters.

	Communication		Daily Living Skills		Socialization		Motor Skills	
	Test	Control	Test	Control	Test	Control	Test	Control
NIMH	19.9	1.4	20.4	8.1	19.0	3.6	21.3	6.3
IPNA	10.9	2.2	34.8	12	15.2	1.1	20.7	3.3
AWF	13.8	9.7	17.2	9.7	15.9	11	13.8	9
Nishpap	6.9	0.0	37.9	3.4	20.7	0.0	27.6	3.4

indicates that caregivers from both test and control groups put priority in 'Daily Living Skills' followed by 'Motor Skills'. Caregiver (AWF 17) said the following:

"I have tried for his other skills (like eye contact) but I am mostly focusing on the basic things so that he can do these things by himself. I want to make sure he can have his food by himself, dress by himself, can hold a pencil etc. These are the must need for him. I am worried what would happen to him when I am not here if he doesn't know these skills."

5.3 Evidence Based Decision Making

Lack of data over time has been identified as the single most important factor hindering the evidence-based management of ASD care (PC1). This is now available through mCARE-DMP, and so MHPs can make more informed, data driven decisions. During the quarterly group sessions with participating MHPs, we identified cases where longitudinal data (or other features of mCARE-DMP) helped them in making evidence-based decisions. These quarterly sessions are centered around 4 questions: i) Do you think it is helping you in managing your patients? ii) Can you give a case example for each feature you used? iii) Can you give any example where mCARE-DMP helped you in making evidence-based decision making? iv) Can you please elaborate and compare your experience pre and post deployment of mCARE in terms of patient management?

Along with the availability of longitudinal data, MHPs identified four specific visit scenarios, that they regularly experience, where mCARE-DMP was helpful. Some use case scenarios are given below that came up during these discussions:

Case 1: Focusing Only On Certain Parameters: According to the MHPs, many parents are only interested to talk about certain parameters or issues that they think important. This happens due to socio-cultural impact and personal belief. As MHP 2 said:

"Many of the parents come to me and spend the whole-time on couple of specific issues like does he respond when called by name or does he smile socially or does he avoid eye contact. These are important parameters, but their kids have other important issues to talk about too. But they are simply not interested."

When we asked certain caregivers about this, we got the following context.

"I live in an extended family and people want to make sure kids respect the seniors. As you know, in our culture not to smile or respond when a senior calls is considered as very rude, I want to make sure my child learn these first. Also, it is not the case that I do not want to discuss the others (parameters). They (MHPs) simply do not have that time. If I have 5 min, I first like to talk about these priority points." - Nishpap 11.

But now, MHPs can simply select the other important parameters and monitor them using mCARE.

Case 2: Suppressing Certain Parameters: Many times, MHPs fail to notice some important features during caregiver visits. This is because sometimes parents do not want to show things that they find embarrassing and even coach their children not to do those things during visits. MHP 3 detailed one specific experience as follows:

"..I was about to finish the visit and then all on a sudden this kid banged his forehead so hard in my table that I was afraid his skull has been fractured. But I saw his parents were not that much concerned. This gave me an idea that this is not the first time. They never reported this issue before and hence I did not select this parameter to be monitored. Then I asked them to be open with me. Initially, the father said that it is not a big deal but later he said he did not want others to know about this issue specially when the door is open and others in line just outside my door can see. Once they are submitting the values from their home, they are typically honest (since no one else is seeing that except me)."

Case 3: Over Emphasizing Symptoms/Outliers: Caregivers travel to IPNA and NIMH from all around the country typically 3 or 4 times a year (according to our field study). There is this common belief among caregivers that they would get better attention and treatment if they exaggerate the values. Also, they inadvertently highlight certain parameters due to recall bias. MHP 7 summarized this common experience as:

"Any parameter that the caregivers like to prioritize, would get a higher value. And you know, whatever they say that is the gold standard. Sometimes I am not sure what to do (to stick with my feeling or accept what the caregiver is saying). But now I can verify the actual average of any parameter looking at the historical data (mCARE-DMP)."

MHP 6 shared her experience with outlier values saying:

"This caregiver (mother) spent half of the visit time talking about aggressive behavior. But when I checked the longitudinal history, I was confused since I did not see high values there. When I shared this, she explained that the kid was really aggressive on the way here. And they took 3 transports (bus, rickshaw and scooter) and the bus was full of people. She also mentioned that some people in the bus were even taunting her son. Because, this has happened just prior to the visit, she was upset and wanted to focus on this. Without the longitudinal history feature of mCARE-DMP, I would never be able to verify this."

Case 4: The Complete Picture: During our field visit, the lack of data resulting from infrequent visits came up again and again. MHPs mentioned the term 'complete picture' which they often miss but crucial for treating CWA. MHP 1 said the following:

"Sometimes I used to feel shaky to prescribe since I was not confident to prescribe with so few and seemingly exaggerated or vague (PC2, PC3) information (received during the face-to-face visits). But now I can see the whole timeline of how it went once

they left my office last time. Also, if I feel, I can simply add a new parameter or discard a parameter not needed anymore. I feel more powered and more confident."

5.4   Proactive Agent of Change

MHPs reported that they have found the caregivers, who submit data regularly, are relatively more aware of their child's situation and many times act proactively. This includes asking for change based on specific contextual scenario, taking actions based on their judgement (helped by longitudinal data), recording changes of abnormal behavior etc. According to MHP 11:

"I see that these parents are much more knowledgeable and proactive now. They are asking me questions with examples. Like, my child ate rich food and the next day he had these issues. Should I be aware of this? Even one mother came with a notebook showing me that when she notices some abnormal value (while entering that value in mCARE), she tries to record what happened that day to show me. I have not seen this before."

Caregiver of AWF 21 said how mCARE is boosting the positive behavior as:

"I regularly check the longitudinal graph of my children and take necessary steps accordingly. This also helps us keep our motivation high in taking care of our child. If you check (mCARE data), you will see that I followed the advises of the doctor and after months my kid started making eye contacts. I made sure I keep continue doing the things that helped him in achieving this (as shown in Fig. 3)."

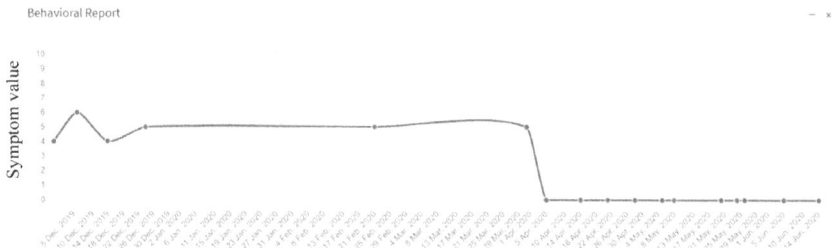

Fig. 3.   The behavioral data report for AWF 21 on 'Avoid eye contact'.

5.5   Improvement in Satisfaction

Overall, we found that the average satisfaction level towards quality of care and MHPs has been improved for both mCARE-APP and mCARE-SMS test group participants (compared to baseline data) as detailed in Fig. 4.

The average satisfaction level on quality of care and MHPs has been improved by 0.8 for mCARE-SMS users whereas that of mCARE-APP users stand at 1.69 and 1.84 respectively. The answer lies in the mindset of these two groups of users who come from very different socio-economic class. mCARE-SMS users, belonging to the lower socio-economic class, were happy even to see a MHP in public hospital whereas

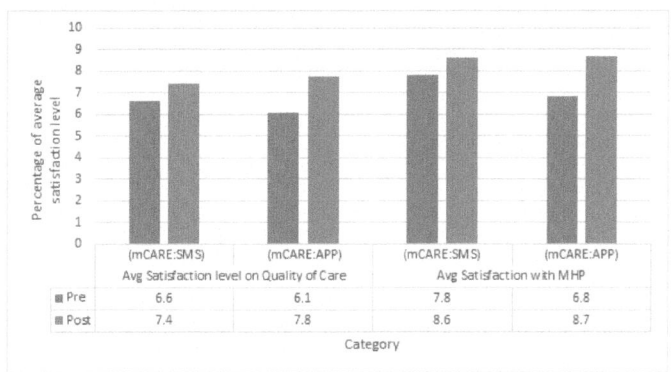

Fig. 4. Change in satisfaction level pre and post deployment of mCARE.

mCARE-APP users always expected more compared to what they receive in public hospitals. As a result, there was a big gap in the satisfaction level between these two groups prior to the deployment of mCARE (6.6 vs 6.08 and 7.8 vs 6.85). mCARE-SMS users simply submitted selected behavioral parameter values with no other features. Hence, their satisfaction level improved by a simple margin (0.8) post deployment. But mCARE-APP provided many features (longitudinal view of submitted data, biweekly report, milestone parameters etc.) that helped the mCARE-APP users resulting in a big jump for satisfaction level (average satisfaction improved by 1.69 and 1.84 respectively).

6   Impact of COVID-19

The first outbreak of COVID-19 was detected in March 2020 in Bangladesh [62]. The Government of Bangladesh declared an emergency and lock down (except emergency situations) was enforced starting end of March. The hospitals closed almost all non-emergency services including mental health services (or running with very limited support). But during this lockdown period, mCARE played a very effective role.

6.1   Impact on ASD Status: Better or Worse?

One of the questions discussed during the interview with caregivers was the impact of COVID-19 on the CWA. Interestingly we found that COVID-19 impacted the health outcomes of CWA in both positive and negative ways as detailed below:

Negative Impact: Case 1: *"Due to not going outside for the corona virus, my child was at home all the time. He really missed going to the school or park. For this reason, my child shouted and cried loudly. His tendency of screaming really went up. We are being locked down in our congested (small) apartment, and our neighbor's house is very close to our flat. They complained to us when my child got hyper, and sometimes they quarreled with us. For, many nights, I could not sleep"* - (Father of IPNA 167) (Fig. 5).

Negative Impact: Case 2: Multiple caregivers reported of stress due to financial situations because of COVID-19. At least 5 head of households lost their jobs due to the

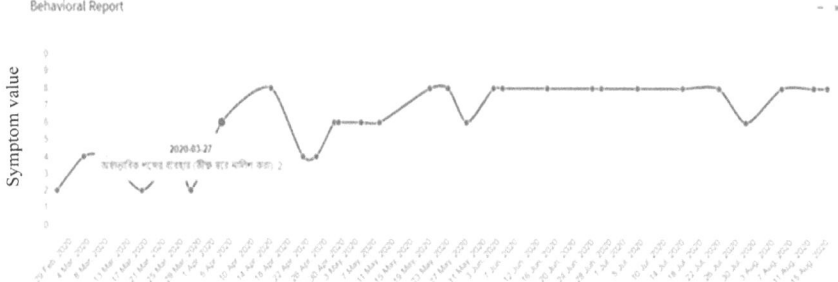

Fig. 5. The behavioral data report for IPNA 167 on 'Use of unnatural sounds' showing worsening of the symptom value during covid time.

pandemic. Majority of the participating families are affected in some way. For many families, survival became the priority and that hampered the care of the CWA. Mother of NIMH 97 (whose husband lost job) said the following:

"… my husband lost his job. It became impossible to talk with him. He is continuously thinking how to support the family. We don't have enough savings. He shouts at home and always in irritated mode. I also don't have the money to buy medicine. All these have impacted my son. He became more aggressive in his behavior (as shown in Fig. 6)."

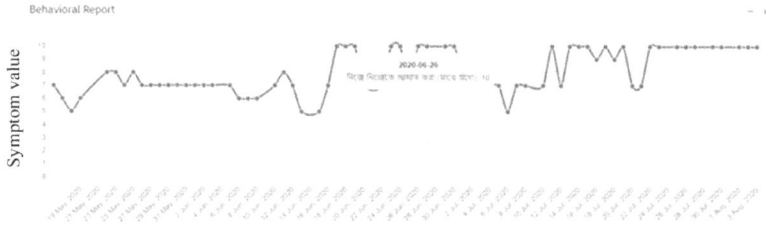

Fig. 6. The behavioral data report for NIMH 97 on 'Self-injurious behavior'.

Positive Impact: Case 1: *"This COVID was actually a good thing in disguise for me. I worked remotely from home. I was able to spend quality time with my kid. Before, I would leave for the office early morning and came back late in the evening. Also, I would be too tired. But now I am talking and playing with him regularly. Sometimes, we go to the roof in the afternoon. I think all these helped him to do better."* - (Father of AWF 24).

Positive impact: Case 2: *"We came to the village (hometown) because it is much cheaper here (you don't need to pay rent). My husband has started a small shop here. We have a large family here. My kid is playing with her cousins and getting the chance to spend time with her grandparents. There is also big field here for him to play. I would say my kid is doing better overall during this period."* - (Caregiver of IPNA 49).

7 Conclusion

This paper describes the design, development, and evaluation of mCARE - a novel sociotechnical system for systematically monitor the behavioral and developmental progress of the CWA. We demonstrate how the success of mCARE was dependent upon the collaboration between the MHPs and the caregivers. We also discussed how mCARE performed as a reliable tool for measuring the impact of COVID-19 on the CWA. The reported data demonstrated how the CWA's situation during the COVID-19 was dependent on their family members. Further, we also showed how the data collected through mCARE from the home settings helped to gather accurate, reliable data overcoming bias and promote proactiveness among the caregivers. This paper also discusses the deep-rooted socio-cultural-economic norms/beliefs, their impact on ASD care and how mCARE was adjusted/accommodated to adhere those situations. Thus, this paper helps the future designers and practitioners in HCI understand the complex landscape of designing mental health technologies in the LMICs in the Global South.

Acknowledgment. This work is partially supported by an NIH grant (1R21MH116726-01).

References

1. Facts About ASDs. CDC - Facts about Autism Spectrum Disorders – NCBDDD (2014). http://www.cdc.gov/ncbddd/autism/data.html
2. Lai, M., Lombardo, M.V., Baron-Cohen, S.: Autism. Lancet **383**, 896–910 (2014). https://doi.org/10.1016/S0140-6736(13)61539-1
3. Golden, R., Wardlaw, T.: Monitoring Child Disability in Developing Countries: Results from the Multiple Indicator Cluster Surveys. UNICEF, University of Wisconsin-Madison, New York (2008)
4. Mullick, M.S.I., Goodman, R.: The prevalence of psychiatric disorders among 5–10 year olds in rural, urban and slum areas in Bangladesh. Soc. Psychiatry Psychiatr. Epidemiol. **40**(8), 663–671 (2005)
5. Rabbani, M.G., et al.: Prevalence of mental disorders, mental retardation, epilepsy and substance abuse in children. Bang J. Psychiatry **23**(1), 1–54 (2009)
6. Soron, T.R.: Technology to take care of autism. Autism Open Access **7**, 205 (2017)
7. Fombonne, E.: The changing epidemiology of autism. J. Appl. Res. Intellect. Disabil. **18**(4), 281–294 (2005)
8. Fombonne, E.: Epidemiology of autistic disorder and other pervasive developmental disorders. J. Clin. Psychiatry **66**, 3 (2005)
9. Klein, T.J., Al-Ghasani, T., Al-Ghasani, M., Akbar, A., Tang, E., Al-Farsi, Y.: A mobile application to screen for autism in Arabic-speaking communities in Oman. Lancet Glob. Health **3**, S15 (2015)
10. Online: Autism Tracker Pro: Track and Analyze ASD. https://itunes.apple.com/us/app/autism-tracker-pro-track-and-analyze-asd/id478225574?mt=8. Accessed 24 Aug 2020
11. Bardhan, S., et al.: Autism Barta—a smart device based automated autism screening tool for Bangladesh. In: 5th International Conference on Informatics, Electronics and Vision (ICIEV) 2016, pp. 602–607. IEEE (2016)
12. Dumont-Mathieu, T., Fein, D.: Screening for autism in young children: the modified checklist for autism in toddlers (M-CHAT) and other measures. Ment. Retard. Dev. Disabil. Res. Rev. **11**(3), 253–262 (2005)

13. Khan, N.Z., et al.: Validation of rapid neurodevelopmental assessment for 2-to 5-year-old children in Bangladesh. Pediatrics **131**(2), e486–e494 (2013)
14. Satu, S., et al.: Prottoy: a smart phone based mobile application to detect autism of children in Bangladesh. In: 4th International Conference on Electrical Information and Communication Technology (EICT), pp. 1–6 (2019)
15. Chipps, J., Brysiewicz, P., Mars, M.: Effectiveness and feasibility of telepsychiatry in resource constrained environments? a systematic review of the evidence. Afr. J. Psychiatry **15**(4) (2012)
16. Saraceno, B., et al.: Barriers to improvement of mental health services in low-income and middle-income countries. Lancet **370**(9593), 1164–1174 (2007)
17. Dell, N.L., Venkatachalam, S., Stevens, D., Yager, P., Borriello, G.: Towards a point-of-care diagnostic system: automated analysis of immunoassay test data on a cell phone. In: Proceedings of the 5th ACM Workshop on Networked Systems for Developing Regions, pp. 3–8 (2011)
18. DeRenzi, B., Dell, N., Wacksman, J., Lee, S., Lesh, N.: Supporting community health workers in India through voice- and web-based feedback. In: Proceedings of the 2017 CHI Conference on Human Factors in Computing Systems, pp. 2770–2781 (2017)
19. Luk, R., Ho, M., Aoki, P.M.: Asynchronous remote medical consultation for Ghana. In: Proceedings of the SIGCHI Conference on Human Factors in Computing Systems, pp. 743–752 (2008)
20. Ramachandran, D., Canny, J., Das, P.D., Cutrell, E.: Mobileizing health workers in rural India. In: Proceedings of the SIGCHI Conference on Human Factors in Computing Systems, pp. 1889–1898 (2010)
21. Ennis-Cole, D., Durodoye, B.A., Harris, H.L.: The impact of culture on autism diagnosis and treatment: considerations for counselors and other professionals. Fam. J. **21**(3), 279–287 (2013)
22. Guralnick, M.J.: The developmental systems approach to early intervention. Brookes Pub. (2005)
23. World Health Organization et al.: World Report on Disability 2011. World Health Organization (2011)
24. Soron, T.R.: Autism, stigma and achievements of Bangladesh. J. Psychiatry **18**(5) (2015)
25. Soron, T.R.: Telepsychiatry for depression management in Bangladesh. Int. J. Ment. Health **45**(4), 1–2 (2016)
26. Haque, M.M., et al.: A machine learning approach to inform developmental milestone achievement for children with autism. JMIR Med. Inform. (2021)
27. Haque, M., et al.: Towards developing a mobile-based care for children with autism spectrum disorder (mCARE) in low and middle-income countries (LMICs) like Bangladesh. In: IEEE 44th Annual Computers, Software, and Applications Conference (COMPSAC), pp. 746–753 (2020)
28. Haque, M.M., et al.: Grant report on mCARE: mobile-based care for children with autism spectrum disorder (ASD) for low-and middle-income countries (LMICs). J. Psychiatry Brain Sci. **6** (2021)
29. Gomez, J., Torrado, J.C., Montoro, G.: Using smartwatches for behavioral issues in ASD. In: Proceedings of the XVII International Conference on Human Computer Interaction, pp. 1–2 (2016)
30. O'Brien, A.M., Schlosser, R.W., Yu, C., Allen, A.A., Shane, H.C.: Repurposing a smartwatch to support individuals with autism spectrum disorder: Sensory and operational considerations. J. Spec. Educ. Technol. 0162643420904001 (2020)
31. Cabibihan, J.-J., Javed, H., Aldosari, M., Frazier, T.W., Elbashir, H.: Sensing technologies for autism spectrum disorder screening and intervention. Sensors **17**(1), 46 (2017)
32. Chen, H., Xue, M., Mei, Z., Oetomo, S.B., Chen, W.: A review of wearable sensor systems for monitoring body movements of neonates. Sensors **16**(12), 2134 (2016)

33. Chong, P.L.H., Abel, E., Pao, R., McCormick, C.E.B., Schwichtenberg, A.J.: Sleep dysregulation and daytime electrodermal patterns in children with autism: a descriptive study. J. Genetic Psychol. 1–14 (2021)

34. Sumi, A.I., Zohora, M.F., Mahjabeen, M., Faria, T.J., Mahmud, M., Kaiser, M.S:. fASSERT: a fuzzy assistive system for children with autism using Internet of Things. In: Wang, S., et al. Brain Informatics. BI 2018. Lecture Notes in Computer Science(), vol. 11309, pp. 403–412. Springer, Cham (2018). https://doi.org/10.1007/978-3-030-05587-5_38

35. Newbutt, N., Bradley, R., Conley, I.: Using virtual reality head-mounted displays in schools with autistic children: views, experiences, and future directions. Cyberpsychol. Behav. Soc. Netw. 23(1), 23–33 (2020)

36. Leo, M., et al.: Computational assessment of facial expression production in ASD children. Sensors 18(11), 3993 (2018)

37. Tsuji, A., Sekine, S., Matsuda, S., Yamamoto, J., Suzuki, K.: Towards modeling of interpersonal proximity using head-mounted camera for children with ASD. In: Miesenberger, K., Manduchi, R., Covarrubias Rodriguez, M., Peňáz, P. (eds.) Computers Helping People with Special Needs. ICCHP 2020. Lecture Notes in Computer Science(), vol. 12377, pp. 104–111. Springer, Cham (2020). https://doi.org/10.1007/978-3-030-58805-2_13

38. Hong, E.R., et al.: A meta-analysis of single-case research on the use of tablet-mediated interventions for persons with ASD. Res. Dev. Disabil. 70, 198–214 (2017)

39. O'malley, P., Lewis, M.E.B., Donehower, C.: Using tablet computers as instructional tools to increase task completion by students with autism. Online Submission (2013)

40. King, A.M., Thomeczek, M., Voreis, G., Scott, V.: IPad¬Æ use in children and young adults with autism spectrum disorder: an observational study. Child Lang. Teach. Therapy 30(2), 159–173 (2014)

41. King, M.L., Takeguchi, K., Barry, S.E., Rehfeldt, R.A., Boyer, V.E., Mathews, T.L.: Evaluation of the iPad in the acquisition of requesting skills for children with autism spectrum disorder. Res. Autism Spectrum Disorders 8(9), 1107–1120 (2014)

42. Aburukba, R., Aloul, F., Mahmoud, A., Kamili, K., Ajmal, S.: AutiAid: a learning mobile application for autistic children. In: IEEE 19th International Conference on e-Health Networking, Applications and Services (Healthcom) 2017, pp. 1–6. IEEE (2017)

43. Huijnen, C.A.G.J., Lexis, M.A.S., Jansens, R., de Witte, L.P.: Roles, strengths and challenges of using robots in interventions for children with autism spectrum disorder (ASD). J. Autism Dev. Disord. 49(1), 11–21 (2019)

44. Bangerter, A., et al.: Caregiver daily reporting of symptoms in autism spectrum disorder: observational study using web and mobile apps. JMIR Mental Health 6(3), e11365 (2019)

45. Soron, T.R., Rabbani G., Despande N., Chokraborti, S.: Development of Bangla autism assessment mobile application. In: International Association of Child and Adolescent Psychiatry and Allied Professions (IACAPAP) 23rd Congress Prague, Czech Republic, pp. 23–27 (2018)

46. Kumm, A.J.: Feasibility of a smartphone application to identify young children at risk for Autism Spectrum Disorder in a low-income community setting in South Africa. Master's thesis, University of Cape Town (2018)

47. Biasini, F.J., et al.: Development of a 12 month screener based on items from the Bayley II scales of Infant development for use in low middle income countries. Early Human Dev. 91(4), 253–258 (2015)

48. Wirz, S., Edwards, K., Flower, J., Yousafzai, A.: Field testing of the ACCESS materials: a portfolio of materials to assist health workers to identify children with disabilities and offer simple advice to mothers. Int. J. Rehabil. Res. 28(4), 293–302 (2005)

49. Ngoun, C., Stoey, L.S., van't Ende, K., Kumar, V.: Creating a Cambodia-specific developmental milestone screening tool-a pilot study. Early Hum. Dev. 88(6), 379–385 (2012)

50. Gladstone, M., et al.: The Malawi Developmental assessment tool (MDAT): the creation, validation, and reliability of a tool to assess child development in rural African settings. Plos Med. 7(5), e1000273 (2010)

51. Akhter, S., Hussain, A., Shefa, J., Kundu, GK., Rahman, F., Biswas, A.: Prevalence of Autism Spectrum Disorder (ASD) among the children aged 18–36 months in a rural community of Bangladesh: a cross sectional study. F1000 Res. 4(7), 424 (2018). https://doi.org/10.12688/f1000research.13563.1. PMID: 30026928; PMCID: PMC6039957

52. Goodman, L.A.: Snowball sampling. Ann. Math. Stat. 148–170 (1961)

53. O'reilly, M., Parker, N.: Unsatisfactory saturation': a critical exploration of the notion of saturated sample sizes in qualitative research. Qual. Res. 13(2), 190–197 (2013)

54. Ehsan, U., et al.: Confronting autism in urban Bangladesh: unpacking infrastructural and cultural challenges. EAI Endorsed Trans. Pervasive Health Technol. 4(14) (2018)

55. Sedgwick, P.: Convenience sampling. BMJ 347, f6304 (2013)

56. Aronson, J.: A pragmatic view of thematic analysis. Qual. Report 2(1), 1–3 (1995)

57. Edition, F., et al.: Diagnostic and statistical manual of mental disorders. Am. Psychiatric Assoc. 21, 21 (2013)

58. Chakraborty, S., Thomas, P., Bhatia, T., Nimgaonkar, V.L., Deshpande, S.N.: Assessment of severity of autism using the Indian scale for assessment of autism. Indian J. Psychol. Med. 37(2), 169 (2015)

59. Fombonne, E.: Epidemiology of pervasive developmental disorders. Pediatr. Res. 65(6), 591–598 (2009)

60. Manohari, S.M., Raman, V., Ashok, M.V.: Use of Vineland adaptive behavior scales-II in children with autism-an Indian experience. J. Indian Assoc. Child Adolesc. Ment. Health 9(1), 5–12 (2013)

61. Agile Software Development (2017). https://en.wikipedia.org/wiki/Agile_software_development. Accessed 30 Apr 2024

62. Ahmed, S., Tazmeem, F.: First case diagnosed with both COVID-19 and dengue virus infections in Bangladesh: possible dengue prevention strategies amid COVID-19 outbreak. Public Health 191, 39 (2021)

Gamifying a Chronic Pain Management mHealth Intervention: Do's and Don'ts

Maxwell Szymanski$^{(\boxtimes)}$ 📵, Leen Van Houdt📵, Robin De Croon📵,
Katrien Verbert📵, and Vero vanden Abeele📵

Department of Computer Science, KU Leuven, Leuven, Belgium
{maxwell.szymanski,leen.houdt,robin.croon,
katrien.verbert,vero.abeele}@kuleuven.be

Abstract. Mobile health (mHealth) interventions hold promise for chronic pain management, but suffer from high user attrition. Using motivational features to support users in adhering to their intervention has been a widely studied field, but their effectiveness in mHealth often varies due to a lack of standardised frameworks. This is particularly concerning for chronic musculoskeletal pain management, where poorly implemented elements could instil anxiety or promote negative coping mechanisms. Recognising this gap, we design an extensive list of 24 motivational features based on a recent framework, tailored for chronic pain musculoskeletal mHealth apps and conducted focus groups with health coaches and employees (potential users) to evaluate them. Results favour positive reinforcement strategies (i.e. praise, goal-setting) while highlighting concerns about pressure-inducing elements (time limits, leaderboards). Participants also emphasise the need for careful information presentation to avoid potential catastrophising and the importance of privacy when considering social features. Our findings offer initial guidelines for the ethical and user-centred implementation of motivational features in chronic musculoskeletal pain mHealth interventions.

Keywords: Gamification · motivational features · motivational design · mHealth · chronic pain management

1 Introduction

With the prevalence of smartphones, mHealth has increasingly been used to offer health interventions in timely and accessible manners, with positive outcomes. These interventions span from nudging users towards healthier lifestyles based on behaviour tracking [17], to aiding users in monitoring their glucose levels [23]. Recently, the domain of chronic disease and pain management has

---

K. Verbert and V. vanden Abeele—Authors contributed equally.

© ICST Institute for Computer Sciences, Social Informatics and Telecommunications Engineering 2025
Published by Springer Nature Switzerland AG 2025. All Rights Reserved
H. Kondylakis and A. Triantafyllidis (Eds.): PervasiveHealth 2024, LNICST 612, pp. 89–103, 2025.
https://doi.org/10.1007/978-3-031-85575-7_5

received increased attention, supporting patients in monitoring, understanding and managing their chronic condition [9,14,27] via mobile applications and related sensors.

However, mHealth interventions suffer from high attrition rates [25], with interventions experiencing a dropout rate up to 40% for randomised controlled trials (RCTs), and up to 50% in real-world settings. Several *motivational features* have been researched, encompassing behaviour change techniques and persuasive principles, to address these high attrition rates and increase intervention adherence [13]. Gamification is one example subdomain that involves the use of game-like elements in non-game environments, such as points, badges, leaderboards and personalised avatars [6,8]. Another example is social support, where features like community forums or the ability to share progress with others can offer a sense of belonging and accountability [22]. These elements can be powerful motivators, especially when users feel connected and supported by those facing similar health challenges.

As these motivational features within mHealth often aim to support positive behavioural change, about half of the interventions guide their development through motivational theories and frameworks. For example, half of the mHealth studies promoting physical activity rely on theories or frameworks to implement motivational techniques, with Self-Determination Theory - focusing on intrinsic motivation and the conditions under which it flourishes - being the most common framework (32%), followed by Behavioural Economics - understanding and modifying behaviour through external consequences - being second (20%).

While studies employing motivational features have shown positive outcomes, such as supporting increased physical activity, several surveys also show mixed [35] to positive no results [32] across interventions. This can be attributed due to guidelines stemming from heterogeneous studies and intervention types [20,35] or a lack of rigorous and standardised frameworks denoting which techniques are appropriate for certain interventions [5,24]. Recent work of Geuens et al. tried to bridge the gap between the motivational features being employed, as well as the underlying psychological theories driving them, with a set of 'dyadic lenses' [13]. Subsequently, they applied these lenses by reviewing mobile apps for managing chronic arthritis, and found that features providing system credibility were amongst the most implemented, whereas social features turned out to be the least implemented [16]. However, they did not find a link between the features being implemented or not, and the actual rating of the intervention, leading to inconclusive results regarding the efficacy of the implemented techniques.

As for the adjacent field of mHealth interventions addressing chronic musculoskeletal pain, there has been budding work investigating an app design with few gamification elements from a health expert perspective, with promising results [18], but still lacking any concrete design guidelines. As chronic musculoskeletal pain is a very prevalent problem amongst Belgian employees, with 60% experiencing pain on a frequent basis, and one third of them even being on prolonged sick-leave due to these pain complaints [7], the need to develop interventions with high adherence rates is high. Therefore, using the work of Geuens et al. as a cornerstone, we set out to design motivational features for supporting mHealth interventions for chronic musculoskeletal pain and assess their effectiveness in mHealth apps for chronic pain management. Concretely, we aim to answer the following research question:

RQ1 Which motivational design features are preferred by employees in an intervention supporting their chronic musculoskeletal pain, and why?

RQ2 Does this preferences differ between employees (intervention receivers) and health coaches (intervention providers)?

Through in-depth focus groups with 23 participants in total (from the perspective of 14 employees as well as 9 health coaches), we extract design goals related to implementing motivational features in chronic pain mHealth interventions to steer future work.

2   Related Work

We first discuss recent literature on mHealth interventions and adherence outcomes, followed by different gamification frameworks and techniques that support mHealth adherence.

2.1   mHealth Interventions and Adherence

mHealth interventions address challenges faced by those with chronic musculoskeletal pain by offering convenience and increased accessibility to treatment resources. Self-monitoring tools that allow users to log pain levels, activity, and medication usage can empower patients and aid healthcare providers in identifying patterns for improved management plans [9]. Additionally, mHealth apps often deliver educational resources on pain management, stress-reduction techniques, and appropriate exercises, making relevant information readily available. Studies also highlight the benefits of integrated remote coaching and online support groups within mHealth platforms. This access to professional guidance and peer support combats feelings of isolation and has demonstrated the ability to boost adherence to treatment plans.

However, while mHealth interventions have shown positive outcomes, there is a mixed level of success [33], with one of the main reasons being high attrition rates. A recent study showed that in both controlled RCT settings, as well as real world interventions, the average drop-out rate tends to be 40% (95% CI 16–63) and 49% (95% CI 27–70) respectively [25], showing a need for additional understanding to increase retention rates.

2.2   Motivational Techniques

Motivational features have often been studied as a tool to increase adherence, taking on the form of gamification, behaviour change techniques or other persuasive design strategies [13]. Gamification for example is defined by Deterding as the use of game-like elements in non-game contexts [8]. These gamification elements comprise of small components built with a single purpose (i.e. leaderboards for social comparison, badges and streaks for incentives, etc.) - which differ from full-fledged and immersive game experiences as in serious games [35] - and can be used in mHealth interventions to improve adherence and engagement, support behaviour change, or improve self-management and health knowledge. Another valuable approach lies in the use of nudges and reminders. Nudges - subtle cues within an interface that guide user behaviour - can be highly effective in promoting positive actions [2]. Reminders, whether push notifications or in-app messages, can help keep users on track with treatment plans and encourage logging of important health data.

Studies have shown that some mHealth interventions incorporating motivational features lead to improved patient engagement, higher treatment satisfaction, and increased treatment adherence compared to traditional, non-gamified approaches [19,29]. Additionally, these techniques stimulate behavioural change by playing on both extrinsic and intrinsic motivation, supporting long-term health behaviour adherence [3]. However, surveys also show that when motivational features are implemented without careful consideration, their effectiveness decreases and can even result in adverse outcomes [32,35]. This is due to a lack of standardisation or frameworks that guide which gamification techniques should be selected [24], as well as a lack of generalisability across different subdomains within mHealth interventions [20]. While the subdomain of chronic pain interventions has received increasing attention from the gamification community [1,18,19,26], it also lacks any formal overview regarding which motivational features are preferred and which are not - a gap that this work aims to address (Fig. 1).

3   Experimental Design

In this section, we will outline the design of our experiment, including the motivational techniques evaluated, as well as the study methodology.

3.1   Motivational Technique Design

We aim to evaluate which motivational features are preferred by both patients experiencing chronic pain, as well as health coaches specialising in guiding said patients in order to ensure medical validity. The limitation with previous work on implementing motivational features to support chronic illness or pain interventions boil down to either randomly selecting a few techniques without rigorous guidelines, or even lacking mention of the exact gamification techniques used. Using prior work of Geuens et al. [13] on motivational features, we list the 24 techniques (Table 1), across 6 categories, that we design and aim to evaluate in this study together with employees as well as health coaches. We refer to https://lensesofmotivationaldesign.com/ for a thorough description of all features.

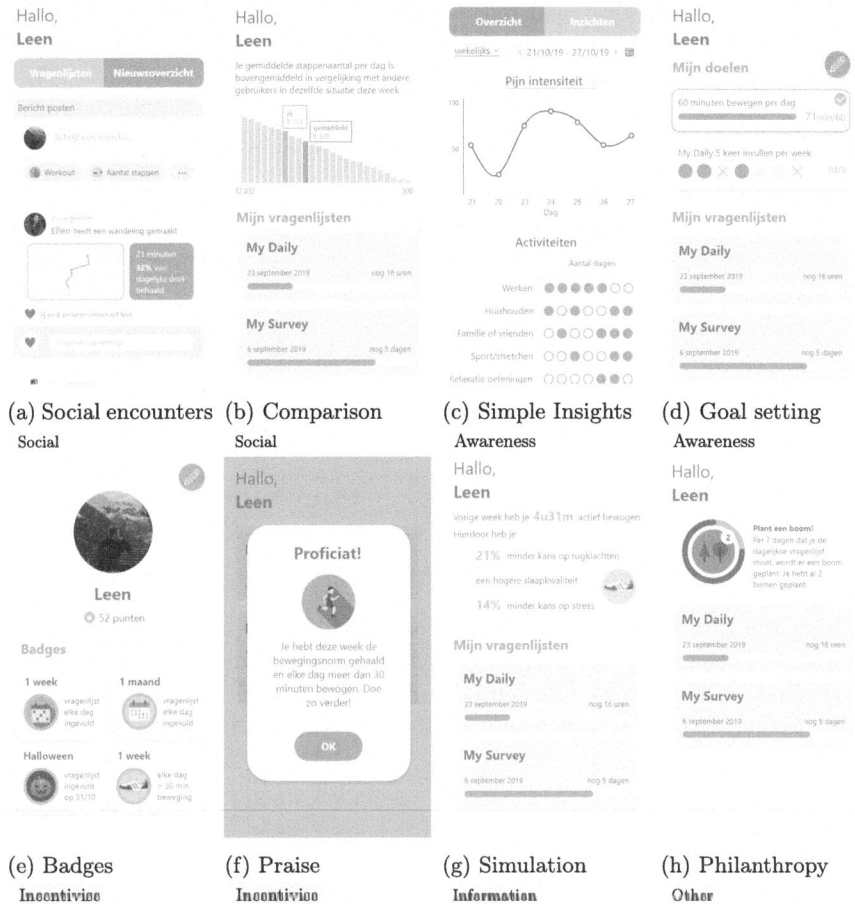

Fig. 1. Few examples of designs showcasing gamification techniques within a chronic pain coaching and monitoring app

3.2 Study Design

To gain feedback on our proposed motivational feature designs and spark insightful discussions, we organised five focus groups with a total of 23 participants (G_1: 5 health coaches, G_2: 4 health coaches, G_3: 7 employees, G_4: 3 employees, G_5: 4 employees). First, each motivational design was discussed (Table 1) and users were asked to individually rate each motivational design on a 7-point Likert scale, ranging from $---$ (-3, not preferable) to $+++$ ($+3$, highly preferable), with 0 being a neutral score (indifferent). After explaining and rating each design (approx. 20 min), we transitioned to a group discussion elaborating each design and elaborating why each participant assigned their respective rating (approx. 80 min).

Table 1. Overview of motivational designs and their means as rated by health coaches (μ_{HC}) and employees (μ_E) in range $[-3; 3]$

Category	Motivational techn.	μ_E	μ_{HC}	Description
Awareness	Insights (Simple)	2.50	2.78	Visualises single questionnaire variables with line graphs
Awareness	Goal Setting	2.07	2.11	Allows users to set daily / weekly goals and tick them off
Awareness	Insights (Complex)	1.93	2.44	Visualises multiple questionnaire variables with line graphs to show trends
Awareness	Logging	0.86	3.00	Allowing user to log variables and track app use information
Information	General Info & Tips	1.86	2.33	Receiving daily relevant short messages relevant to the coaching trajectory
Information	Simulation	1.71	1.78	Simulates how logged activities decrease risk factors by $x\%$
Information	Random Rewards / Info	0.86	1.56	I.e. a random relevant "fun fact of the day" displayed on the start screen or other places
Incentivise	Praise	2.14	2.44	Modals praising consistent / improving behaviour (i.e. activities, mood logging)
Incentivise	Points & Badges	0.71	0.67	Collecting points and badges after completing tasks (consecutively)
Incentivise	Streak	0.71	0.56	Rewards consistent behaviour by keeping score of consecutive days a task was finished
Incentivise	Time pressure	0.07	0.78	Using a timer bar and colours to indicate the remaining time left to fill in questionnaires
Reminders	Reminder (Consistency)	1.07	2.11	"Start your daily coaching, two more times to reach your 5-day coaching streak goal"
Reminders	Reminder (Authority)	0.79	1.11	"Your health coach advises you to fill in your questionnaire to get personalised tips"
Reminders	Reminder (Consensus)	-0.21	1.00	"Start your daily coaching, like 37 other users already have done today"
Reminders	Reminder (Scarcity)	-0.50	-0.44	"Today's a unique day to start your questionnaire and gain more health insights"
Social	Comparison	1.57	1.67	Comparison with their friends / colleagues (i.e. weekly steps)
Social	Cooperation	0.50	1.00	Allows users to form groups and check off goals collectively (i.e. walking group)
Social	Social Encounters	-0.36	0.44	A social feed that allows users to share their activities (i.e. walks, goals, etc.)
Social	Recognition	-0.57	0.22	Allows users to share completed goals on other social networks
Social	Competition	-0.36	0.00	Leaderboard comparing steps taken or amount of questionnaires filled in
Other	Philanthropist	1.11	1.44	Plants a tree for every week that a questionnaire was filled in daily
Other	Personalisation	1.92	0.78	Changes app theme, colours and other personalisable aspects
Other	Avatar	0.64	1.33	Allows users to create a customisable cartoon avatar
Other	Easter Eggs	0.50	0.22	Random unlocks, badges and surprises across app (i.e. opening app on Halloween)

Using the ratings, as well as the transcripts from the group discussion, we were then able to rank the feasibility of each motivational design, extract related themes, and describe general design take-aways regarding the use of these techniques in chronic pain mHealth interventions from both a patient as well as a therapist perspective.

4 Results

We will give an overview of the scores given by participants as an indicator (with μ_E and μ_{HC} representing the mean score given by employees and health coaches respectively), and explain them using transcripts from the focus groups.

4.1 Awareness and Personal Insights

Motivational features regarding awareness and personal insights were favoured by most (simple insights: $\mu_E = 2.50$, $\mu_{HC} = 2.78$, complex insights: $\mu_E = 1.93$, $\mu_{HC} = 2.44$), with HC_3 describing this as "the core functionality of the app". These results highlight the importance of self-monitoring and data-driven insights in mHealth for chronic pain management. Visualizations and goal-setting tools appear to provide tangible benefits, fostering a sense of understanding and control ($\mu_E = 2.07$, $\mu_{HC} = 2.11$). Interestingly, the higher preference for logging among health coaches ($\mu_E = 0.86$, $\mu_{HC} = 3.0$) suggests that such features might be particularly valuable for enabling communication and targeted coaching during sessions. However, qualitative feedback raised important concerns about the potential for catastrophising if negative results are presented without careful framing. Future mHealth design should prioritize framing insights in ways that foster understanding and self-efficacy, potentially incorporating guidance from health coaches within this process.

4.2 Reminders

While reminders were seen as 'an integral part of most health apps', participants placed a big emphasis on how those reminders should be worded. Reminders emphasizing consistency (e.g., "Start your daily coaching two more times to complete your 5-day coaching streak") received the highest average ratings from both groups ($\mu_E = 1.07$, $\mu_{HC} = 2.11$). Reminders framed with an authoritative tone (e.g., "Your health coach advises you to ...") were moderately preferred, while scarcity-based reminders (e.g., "Today's a unique day to finish ...") were the least favoured by both participants groups ($\mu_E = -0.5$, $\mu_{HC} = 0.0$). This indicates a preference for emphasising the achievement of small goals, whilst avoiding playing in on negative feelings (i.e. pressure) to remind users of their coaching.

4.3 Information

Motivational features focussing on providing relevant information were positively regarded by users. General information and tips were the most preferred by employees and health coaches alike ($\mu_E = 1.86$, $\mu_{HC} = 2.33$). However, HC_7 warned against potential information overload, saying: "Some apps share tips every 5 min. It could be our pitfall that we want to stuff all our knowledge into this app.". Simulation - showing how user progression and activity positively impacts their health outcomes based on scientific results - was also generally positively received ($\mu_E = 1.71$, $\mu_{HC} = 1.78$). However, health coaches remarked on their real-world applicability. Some employees emphasised that these numbers should be communicated as population averages, not personal simulations, with E_2 stating: "If it says there's a 20% lower chance for cardiovascular diseases, then I'd find that more believable because you know that is true on a global scale. However, if it says that [for my complaints specifically], no, because my complaints are unpredictable". Random information was the least preferred out of all three ($\mu_E = 0.86$, $\mu_{HC} = 1.56$). While HC_4 mentions that a "random tip of the day could motivate users to open their app daily", others, such as HC_7, warned against a potential "information fatigue".

4.4 Incentivising

Praise was seen as the most beneficial incentivising technique ($\mu_E = 2.14$, $\mu_{HC} = 2.44$), with HC_8 noting its potential to "stimulate behavioural change from a positive psychological approach". However, all focus groups cautioned against excessive use of praise - i.e. after filling in a questionnaire or every single walk logged, as their effectiveness could diminish. This is in line with guidelines for using badges by Zichermann et al. [36], suggesting that badges should not be over-congratulatory or reward rote tasks. Instead, as suggested by HC_3, reward mechanisms such as praises should hold "greater meaning by supporting personal, user-defined goals within the application". Points and badges received lukewarm reactions ($\mu_E = 0.71$, $\mu_{HC} = 0.67$), with HC_5 expressing the need for the badges to "be relevant and related to health", and E_1 saying: "It's positive, a nice extra, but not the reason I would use the app for".

Streaks ($\mu_E = 0.71$, $\mu_{HC} = 0.56$) and time pressure ($\mu_E = 0.07$, $\mu_{HC} = 0.78$), while potentially useful according to 14 participants, were seen as more divisive techniques, mainly due to their pressuring nature. HC_4 mentions these techniques "take away user autonomy". Whilst the functionality of i.e. time pressure was generally seen as, participants cautioned against the use of pressuring elements such as red colours or warning signs, with E_{12} mentioning: "If I have a bad day coping [with my pain], having this app give me additional anxiety would make me reluctant to use it".

4.5   Social Interactions

Generally, social interactions were the least preferred amongst participants, seen as a feasible feature by only 62% of health coaches, and 42% of the employees. Whilst some agreed that social interactions can help foster motivation, most raised at least one concern. 7 Participants addressed their lack of need for comparison and competition, with E_7 saying: "Going through your chronic pain journey is so personal, how could you even try to compete that", resulting in relatively low scores for competition ($\mu_E = -0.36$, $\mu_{HC} = 0.0$). About 5 participants were also concerned with the ethical and privacy side of social features, as "free and unmoderated input might potentially be dangerous" (E_7). Another privacy concern related to social platform updates during i.e. someone's sick leave, with E_5 mentioning: "If someone is able to take 10.000 steps daily, a colleague might go to their boss to say 'If he is able to take this many steps, does he really have chronic pain?' ". Interestingly, comparison

4.6   Other Features

The philanthropist feature was generally seen as a positive addition ($\mu_E = 1.14$, $\mu_{HC} = 1.44$), with E_1 mentioning: "I would be more engaged if it's for a good cause, compared to when I would do it for myself. Something external". However, health coaches note that it could also create resistance, with HC_2 mentioning that "there is a lot of negative press recently regarding [good causes]", and whether they actually come to fruition. HC_1 suggests "... maybe we can allow users to choose their good cause, that would work better". Personalisation scored relatively positive - with a slight favour towards employees ($\mu_E = 1.02$, $\mu_{HC} = 0.78$) - and received additional suggestions, such as "the ability to change font size or [other aspects] for people with disabilities" (HC_4). Avatars on the other hand, were more preferred by health coaches ($\mu_E = 0.64$, $\mu_{HC} = 1.33$). However, while health coaches suggested that linking the avatar to other functionalities - such as buying styles with earned points (HC_5) or unlocking clothes through badges

(HC_4) - could be beneficial, employees warned that this might shift the focus of the intervention, with E_3 and E_4 summarising this respectively as: "This would remind me too much of elementary school" and "we would only be preoccupied with that, earning clothes". Finally, easter eggs received a more neutral score ($\mu_E = 0.50$, $\mu_{HC} = 0.22$). While employee E_1 mentions: "It's fun, something positive and unexpected", E_2 adds to this: "It's not something necessary, but also not something bad".

5   Discussion

We will now answer the research question regarding which motivational features are preferred by employees for an intervention supporting chronic musculoskeletal pain, and whether this preference differs between employees and health coaches. Afterwards, we try to summarise them in two concrete design goals to help guide future work.

5.1   (RQ1) Which Motivational Design Features are Preferred by Employees in an Intervention Supporting their Chronic Musculoskeletal Pain, and Why?

Overall, there was a general preference for motivational features that emphasised positive reinforcement for chronic pain management. For example, praises, reminders emphasising consistent behaviour, or philanthropic nudges were unanimously considered as welcome additions, whereas competition leaderboards, scarcity reminders and time pressures playing in on negative emotions (i.e. through pressure or the sense of competition) sparked considerable amounts of discussion during the focus groups. While previous work categorised gamification on how these techniques were integrated (structural vs. content gamification - [11,30]), which target-user they tailor to (achievers, explorers, killers or socialisers - [10,28]) or the type of motivation they target the techniques to (internal vs. external gamification - [4]), recent work highlighted a delineation on the type of emotions these motivational techniques play on - with white hat techniques focusing on rewarding good behaviour and playing in on positive emotions, whereas black hat techniques play on the sense of urgency or anxiety to incentivise users [12]. In our work, we noticed that these so-called black-hat techniques sparked a considerable amount of negative feelings for users coping with chronic pain, leading to discomfort and distrust. This finding suggests that designers implementing motivational features in mHealth interventions should be particularly mindful of the emotional impact of black-hat motivational features, especially for vulnerable populations.

5.2   (RQ2) Does this Preference Differ Between Employees and Health Coaches?

While generally, the scoring and feedback coming from health coaches overlapped with that of employees, we do notice one noticeable emerging difference: health coaches place a strong emphasis on logging data, and features that strive for consistency in doing so. Health coaches deemed data logging as an essential part of any health intervention in order to provide accurate feedback and support, and change intervention needs when necessary. Consequently, features that support consistently logging and checking in on the intervention were also seen as more preferable by health coaches compared to employees, such as consistency reminders and time pressure. Employees on the other hand found logging to be more tedious, and emphasised the burden of daily tracking through questionnaires. Thus, whilst health coaches highlighted the need for consistent logging in order to support personalised interventions, we need to carefully consider the timeliness and frequency, and not [overdo it with the pressure to not burden the user].

5.3   Design Goal 1 - Adapt Communication to Minimise Negative Impact

Worsening conditions are detrimental across all types of chronic disease management. However, whereas with diabetes monitoring or chronic cardiac conditions a sense of urgency is imperative, this might not always be the case for people coping with chronic pain due to the condition being characterised by a lack of immediate relief. This lead to participants emphasising the need for different, less confrontational ways of communicating insights - for example, while insights and goal setting were among the most preferred techniques score-wise, participants denoted that it might have adverse effects for users experiencing prolonged periods of chronic pain. This was - according to participants - to avoid their tendency to catastrophise, a common phenomenon amongst people coping with chronic pain [21].

This theme of avoiding negative information extended beyond wording - as certain graphical elements also sparked anxiety and discomfort during focus groups. Previous work emphasises the use of colour feedback due to its ability to shape a person's mood and feelings, therefore playing a role in shaping attitudes [31], leading to its use in previous mHealth interventions [3]. However, participants in our study expressed caution in the use of alarming colours, such as using red to indicate time pressure or missed goals, as they could cause additional anxiety in moments where users already struggle to cope or experience pressure.

Therefore, it is essential to be mindful about how motivational features might promote negative patterns that could instigate catastrophising thinking. Designers should prioritise techniques that help users understand their progress and support their sense of self-efficacy. This might involve careful framing of information, incorporating tailored guidance from health coaches, and avoiding elements that cause pressure or anxiety, especially for users that are prone to catastrophising. However, we do want to mention that some users preferred seeing a sense of urgency or pressure to instigate motivation. Based on previous mHealth research we assume that the need to avoid negative information likely depends on the type of end user, i.e. the often used 'Warrior vs. Worrier' distinction [15], and users that are less likely to catastrophise (warriors) would have lesser need to avoid negative information in order to make more informative decisions. Therefore, the ability to personalise or tailor communication towards the type of end user would prove to be beneficial in future work.

5.4 Design Goal 2 - Prioritise Privacy and Individuality in Social Features

Participants also showed resistance towards social implementations of motivational features by denoting that chronic pain is a personal process that does not lend itself to comparing or competing. Leaderboards and competitive features might therefore be demotivating. Subsequently, factors related to prolonged chronic pain might make participants especially prone to upwards social comparison [34], leading to adverse effectiveness of social encounters, social competition and sharing achievements on social networks (recognition). Additionally, several ethical and privacy concerns were raised, such as social updates during sick leaves, causing reluctance to engage with the intervention in fear of being scrutinised. This contrasts previous works stating that social motivational features are the second most often used across mHealth interventions [35], and competition tends to be well-received [3]. Therefore, given the personal trajectory of chronic pain management, along with privacy and ethical concerns, we recommend limiting social interactions within the intervention, or at least ensuring strong moderation, to best support chronic pain management.

5.5 Ethical Considerations in Motivational Feature Design

As shown in this paper, the use of motivational features in mHealth interventions for pain management raises important ethical considerations. While these features can enhance engagement and adherence, they also have the potential to cause harm if not implemented thoughtfully. Our findings highlighted several key ethical concerns:

- Certain motivational features, such as time pressure, scarcity reminders, and competition leaderboards, can induce stress and anxiety in users. This is particularly concerning for individuals with prolonged or severe chronic pain, who may already be experiencing heightened stress levels.
- Excessive use of external rewards, such as points and badges, may undermine intrinsic motivation for behaviour change. It is crucial to strike a balance between extrinsic and intrinsic motivators to foster long-term adherence.
- Social features, while potentially supportive, raise concerns about privacy and data security. Users may be hesitant to share personal health information in a public forum, and there is a risk of data being misused or misinterpreted.
- Some motivational features, such as those that highlight negative health outcomes or compare users to others, may exacerbate catastrophising tendencies in individuals with chronic pain. This can lead to increased anxiety and a sense of hopelessness.

– It is important to consider the digital divide and ensure that motivational features are accessible to all users, regardless of their technological literacy or socioeconomic status.

To address these ethical concerns, we argue to focus on motivational features that emphasise positive reinforcement, such as praise, goal setting, and social support. Avoid features that induce pressure, anxiety, or negative social comparison. Use external rewards judiciously and ensure that they complement, rather than replace, intrinsic motivation for behaviour change. Implement robust privacy safeguards for social features and ensure that users have control over their data. Consider individual differences in pain experiences, coping mechanisms, and preferences when designing motivational features. Offer personalised options and allow users to customise their experience. Finally, design motivational features that are accessible to all users, regardless of their technological literacy or socioeconomic status. By carefully considering these ethical implications, designers can create mHealth interventions that not only promote engagement and adherence but also prioritise the well-being and autonomy of individuals with chronic pain.

6 Conclusion and Future Work

In this work, we set out to design an extensive list of 24 motivational features that could aid chronic pain employees in adhering to an mHealth intervention. Through 5 focus groups with health coaches and employees, we inquired about the needs for the different techniques through preference rankings and think-aloud discussions. These studies highlighted the promise of incorporating such motivational features for chronic pain management within mHealth interventions, while emphasising the vital importance of an ethically designed and user-centred approach. Our focus groups revealed a strong preference for white-hat motivational techniques that leverage positive reinforcement and avoid elements that could spark anxiety or discomfort. Designers must be particularly cautious with competitive elements like leaderboards, as they may lead to social comparison, exacerbate catastrophising tendencies, and raise ethical concerns about privacy and vulnerability.

Whilst this work gave extensive insights in how motivational features should be applied for supporting employees in a chronic musculoskeletal pain intervention, we want to note in order to generalise these results, future work should also consider the broad range of techniques and assess them with end users in their respective subdomain.

Acknowledgments. We would like to thank all participants for their time and valuable insights. This research is part of the research projects Personal Health Empowerment (PHE) with project number HBC.2018.2012, and has been ethically approved by the Ethics Committee Research UZ / KU Leuven (EC Research) with application number S-65610.

References

1. AlMarshedi, A., Wills, G., Ranchhod, A.: Guidelines for the Gamification of Self-Management of Chronic illnesses: Multimethod Study. JMIR Serious Games **5**(2), e12 (2017). https://doi.org/10.2196/games.7472
2. Caraban, A., Karapanos, E., Gonçalves, D., Campos, P.: 23 ways to nudge: a review of technology-mediated nudging in human-computer interaction. In: Proceedings of the 2019 CHI Conference on Human Factors in Computing Systems, pp. 1–15. ACM, Glasgow Scotland Uk (May 2019). https://doi.org/10.1145/3290605.3300733
3. Carvalho, R., Machado, D., Brandao, P.: Gamification, mHealth and user adherence. In: 2020 IEEE Symposium on Computers and Communications (ISCC), pp. 1–6. IEEE, Rennes, France (Jul 2020). https://doi.org/10.1109/ISCC50000.2020.9219674
4. Chen, J., Liang, M.: Play hard, study hard? The influence of gamification on students' study engagement. Front. Psychol. **13**, 994700 (Oct 2022). https://doi.org/10.3389/fpsyg.2022.994700
5. De Croon, R., Geuens, J., Verbert, K., Vanden Abeele, V.: A systematic review of the effect of gamification on adherence across disciplines. In: International Conference on Human-computer Interaction, pp. 168–184. Springer (2021)
6. De Croon, R., Wildemeersch, D., Wille, J., Verbert, K., Abeele, V.V.: Gamification and serious games in a healthcare informatics context. In: 2018 IEEE International Conference on Healthcare Informatics (ICHI), pp. 53–63. IEEE (2018)
7. De Kok, J., et al.: Work-related musculoskeletal disorders: prevalence, costs and demographics in the eu. In: European agency for safety and health at work, vol. 1 (2019)
8. Deterding, S., Dixon, D., Khaled, R., Nacke, L.: From game design elements to gamefulness: Defining "gamification". In: Proceedings of the 15th International Academic MindTrek Conference: Envisioning Future Media Environments, pp. 9–15. ACM, Tampere Finland (Sep 2011). https://doi.org/10.1145/2181037.2181040
9. Fan, K., Zhao, Y.: Mobile health technology: a novel tool in chronic disease management. Intell. Med. **2**(1), 41–47 (2022). https://doi.org/10.1016/j.imed.2021.06.003
10. Fuß, C., Steuer, T., Noll, K., Miede, A.: Teaching the Achiever, Explorer, Socializer, and Killer – Gamification in University Education. In: Hutchison, D., Kanade, T., Kittler, J., Kleinberg, J.M., Mattern, F., Mitchell, J.C., Naor, M., Nierstrasz, O., Pandu Rangan, C., Steffen, B., Sudan, M., Terzopoulos, D., Tygar, D., Vardi, M.Y., Weikum, G., Göbel, S., Wiemeyer, J. (eds.) Games for Training, Education, Health and Sports, vol. 8395, pp. 92–99. Springer International Publishing, Cham (2014). https://doi.org/10.1007/978-3-319-05972-3_11
11. Garone, P., Nesteriuk, S.: Gamification and learning: a comparative study of design frameworks. In: Duffy, V.G. (ed.) Digital Human Modeling and Applications in Health, Safety, Ergonomics and Risk Management. Healthcare Applications, vol. 11582, pp. 473–487. Springer International Publishing, Cham (2019). https://doi.org/10.1007/978-3-030-22219-2_35
12. Gellner, C., Buchem, I., Müller, J.: Application of the octalysis framework to gamification designs for the elderly. In: Proceedings of the 15th European Conference on Games-Based Learning, pp. 260–267. Academic Conferences Limited Reading, UK, Academic Conferences Limited Reading, UK, Reading, Berkshire, UK (2021). https://doi.org/10.34190/GBL.21.022

13. Geuens, J., Geurts, L., Gerling, K., Croon, R.D., Abeele, V.V.: A dyad of lenses for the motivational design of mhealth: bridging the gap between health theory and app design. In: 2019 IEEE International Conference on Healthcare Informatics (ICHI), pp. 1–12. IEEE, Xi'an, China (Jun 2019). https://doi.org/10.1109/ICHI.2019.8904839

14. Geuens, J., Geurts, L., Swinnen, T.W., Westhovens, R., Vanden Abeele, V.: Mobile Health Features Supporting Self-Management Behavior in Patients With Chronic Arthritis: Mixed-Methods Approach on Patient Preferences. JMIR Mhealth Uhealth **7**(3), e12535 (2019). https://doi.org/10.2196/12535

15. Geuens, J., Swinnen, T., Geurts, L., Westhovens, R., De Croon, R., Vanden Abeele, V.: Worriers versus Warriors: Tailoring mHealth to Address Differences in Patients with Chronic Arthritis. In: 2020 IEEE International Conference on Healthcare Informatics (ICHI), pp. 1–12. IEEE, Oldenburg, Germany (Nov 2020). https://doi.org/10.1109/ICHI48887.2020.9374322

16. Geuens, J., Swinnen, T.W., Westhovens, R., De Vlam, K., Geurts, L., Vanden Abeele, V.: A review of persuasive principles in mobile apps for chronic arthritis patients: opportunities for improvement. JMIR Mhealth Uhealth **4**(4), e118 (2016). https://doi.org/10.2196/mhealth.6286

17. Gouveia, R., Karapanos, E., Hassenzahl, M.: How do we engage with activity trackers?: A longitudinal study of Habito. In: Proceedings of the 2015 ACM International Joint Conference on Pervasive and Ubiquitous Computing, pp. 1305–1316. ACM, Osaka Japan (Sep 2015). https://doi.org/10.1145/2750858.2804290

18. Hoffmann, A., Faust-Christmann, C.A., Zolynski, G., Bleser, G.: Toward gamified pain management apps: mobile application rating scale-based quality assessment of pain-mentor's first prototype through an expert study. JMIR Form. Res. **4**(5), e13170 (2020). https://doi.org/10.2196/13170

19. Huang, X., Xiang, X., Liu, Y., Wang, Z., Jiang, Z., Huang, L.: the use of gamification in the self-management of patients with chronic diseases: scoping review. JMIR Serious Games **11**, e39019 (Dec 2023). https://doi.org/10.2196/39019

20. Johnson, D., Deterding, S., Kuhn, K.A., Staneva, A., Stoyanov, S., Hides, L.: Gamification for health and wellbeing: a systematic review of the literature. Internet Interv. **6**, 89–106 (2016). https://doi.org/10.1016/j.invent.2016.10.002

21. Keyaerts, S., Godderis, L., Delvaux, E., Daenen, L.: The association between work-related physical and psychosocial factors and musculoskeletal disorders in healthcare workers: Moderating role of fear of movement. J. Occup. Health **64**(1), e12314 (2022). https://doi.org/10.1002/1348-9585.12314

22. Kim, M., Kim, B., Park, S.: Social support, ehealth literacy, and mhealth use in older adults with diabetes: Moderated mediating effect of the perceived importance of app design. CIN: Comput., Inform., Nurs. **42**(2), 136-143 (Dec 2023). https://doi.org/10.1097/cin.0000000000001081, http://dx.doi.org/10.1097/CIN.0000000000001081

23. Klonoff, D.C.: The current status of mHealth for diabetes: will it be the next big thing? J. Diabetes Sci. Technol. **7**(3), 749–758 (2013). https://doi.org/10.1177/193229681300700321

24. Lister, C., West, J.H., Cannon, B., Sax, T., Brodegard, D.: Just a fad? gamification in health and fitness apps. JMIR Serious Games **2**(2), e9 (2014). https://doi.org/10.2196/games.3413

25. Meyerowitz-Katz, G., Ravi, S., Arnolda, L., Feng, X., Maberly, G., Astell-Burt, T.: Rates of attrition and dropout in app-based interventions for chronic disease: systematic review and meta-analysis. J. Med. Internet Res. **22**(9), e20283 (2020). https://doi.org/10.2196/20283

26. Miller, A.S., Cafazzo, J.A., Seto, E.: A game plan: gamification design principles in mHealth applications for chronic disease management. Health Inform. J. **22**(2), 184–193 (2016). https://doi.org/10.1177/1460458214537511
27. Moreno-Ligero, M., Moral-Munoz, J.A., Salazar, A., Failde, I.: mHealth intervention for improving pain, quality of life, and functional disability in patients with chronic pain: systematic review. JMIR Mhealth Uhealth **11**, e40844 (2023). https://doi.org/10.2196/40844
28. Park, S., Min, K., Kim, S.: Differences in learning motivation among bartle's player types and measures for the delivery of sustainable gameful experiences. Sustainability **13**(16), 9121 (2021). https://doi.org/10.3390/su13169121
29. Sañudo, B., et al.: A randomized controlled mHealth trial that evaluates social comparison-oriented gamification to improve physical activity, sleep quantity, and quality of life in young adults. Psychol. Sport Exer. **72**, 102590 (May 2024). https://doi.org/10.1016/j.psychsport.2024.102590
30. Seaborn, K., Fels, D.I.: Gamification in theory and action: a survey. Int. J. Human-Comput. Stud. **74**, 14–31 (Feb 2015). https://doi.org/10.1016/j.ijhcs.2014.09.006
31. Singh, S.: Impact of color on marketing. Manag. Decis. **44**(6), 783–789 (2006). https://doi.org/10.1108/00251740610673332
32. Six, S.G., Byrne, K.A., Tibbett, T.P., Pericot-Valverde, I.: Examining the effectiveness of gamification in mental health apps for depression: systematic review and meta-analysis. JMIR Mental Health **8**(11), e32199 (2021). https://doi.org/10.2196/32199
33. Stowell, E., et al.: Designing and Evaluating mHealth Interventions for Vulnerable Populations: A Systematic Review. In: Proceedings of the 2018 CHI Conference on Human Factors in Computing Systems, pp. 1–17. ACM, Montreal QC Canada (Apr 2018). https://doi.org/10.1145/3173574.3173589
34. Wang, J.L., Wang, H.Z., Gaskin, J., Hawk, S.: The mediating roles of upward social comparison and self-esteem and the moderating role of social comparison orientation in the association between social networking site usage and subjective well-being. Front. Psychol. **8**, 771 (May 2017). https://doi.org/10.3389/fpsyg.2017.00771
35. Xu, L., et al.: The effects of mhealth-based gamification interventions on participation in physical activity: systematic review. JMIR Mhealth Uhealth **10**(2), e27794 (2022). https://doi.org/10.2196/27794
36. Zichermann, G., Cunningham, C.: Gamification by Design: Implementing Game Mechanics in Web and Mobile Apps. O'Reilly Media, Inc., 1st edn. (2011)

Evaluation of Level System Structures on the Engagement of Participants in mHealth Applications

Lorenzo J James[1](✉) (iD), Laura Genga[1], Raoul Nuijten[1], Barbara Montagne[2], Muriel M Hagenaars[3], and Pieter ME Van Gorp[1]

[1] Eindhoven University of Technology, Eindhoven, The Netherlands
L.J.James@tue.nl
[2] Center for Mental Health Care, Amersfoort, The Netherlands
[3] Utrecht University, Utrecht, The Netherlands

Abstract. Mobile health apps offer a promising approach to promoting holistic healthy behavior change, in the increasing shift toward preventive measures against lifestyle diseases. In this study, we explore the impact of level system structures on the engagement of participants in mHealth apps. Two level-system structures were designed to promote healthy behaviors across physical, mental, and social dimensions. The research used a mixed-method design consisting of a two-arm within-subject crossover experiment, surveys, and interviews. University students and staff members (n=73) were randomly assigned to receive goals in either a single-stream or multi-stream level structure. Participants given the multi-stream level structure were in multiple levels simultaneously, while the single-stream level structure contained one level at a time. The results showed that while participants preferred the multi-stream level structure, there was no significant difference in engagement between the two-level structures. The results also indicated that the preferred configuration of multi-stream level structures did not incentivize participants to engage in goals across all holistic health dimensions. Future research should explore alternative configurations of multi-stream level structures to increase participant engagement.

Keywords: mHealth · health intervention · gamification · levels · level system · holistic health · Non Communicable diseases

1 Introduction

Nowadays, advancements in medicine and improved living conditions have improved the protection against communicable diseases, which are illnesses transmitted from person to person [3,33]. However, today non-communicable

H. Kondylakis and A. Triantafyllidis (Eds.): PervasiveHealth 2024, LNICST 612, pp. 104–120, 2025.
https://doi.org/10.1007/978-3-031-85575-7_6

diseases, or lifestyle diseases such as diabetes, cardiovascular, and respiratory diseases, are chronic diseases that account for up to 70% of all deaths world-wide [34]. Lifestyle diseases are partially a result of a combination of genetic and physiological factors but primarily stem from unhealthy behaviors such as bad food habits and physical inactivity [28,34].

The risk of developing lifestyle diseases could be prevented through healthy behaviors and lifestyle habits [30]. Prevention can be promoted by holistically improving health. Health is defined as a state of complete physical, mental, and social well-being [22]. Improving health holistically can be done physically through behaviors such as regular physical activity or healthy food habits, mentally by addressing conditions such as depression or anxiety, and socially by increasing social engagement [21,30,37]. As the world population ages and life expectancy increases, there is a heightened risk of developing lifestyle diseases, emphasizing the importance of preventive measures [5]. However, the process of preventing lifestyle diseases through health behavior change is difficult and is often marked by lapses and relapses into unhealthy behaviors [15]. A key element to fostering behavior change is to create goals using goal setting [11]. Following well-defined goals (i.e., Walk the 1 km track around the park three times a week) is associated with better shorter and longer-term healthy behavior change [25].

In recent years, mHealth apps have gained prevalence as a tool to promote healthy behavior change, by empowering individuals and health professionals with systems to track and monitor goal progression [12,19]. However, a major issue with mHealth apps is the low retention rate and faltering engagement of individuals using the apps [20]. The use of game design elements in apps, also referred to as gamification, has been shown to improve individuals' intrinsic motivation leading to continued use of mHealth apps resulting in higher engagement and a higher chance of achieving their goals [9,20]. Previous research has pointed out that when individuals using gamified mHealth apps are given goals, they experience more stress when the difficulty of the goal is higher than their current skill level [14]. The stress is potentially caused due to the participants not experiencing Flow [7,14]. Flow is a state of mind in which an individual is fully immersed in an activity [7]. Game elements can be designed to increase Flow, particularly the concept of level systems as they are designed to provide challenges that match the skill level of individuals using the app, thus facilitating Flow [16,26]. However, currently, there is a gap in the literature regarding the impact of level system structures on the engagement of participants in mHealth interventions.

Research on mHealth gamification has shown that configuring goals in unified and non-unified gamification structures can significantly impact participants' experiences in achieving health goals [27]. In non-unified gamification structures, participants are promoted and rewarded to achieve goals in each health dimension. In contrast, a unified gamification structure promotes and rewards participants for completing goals of all health dimensions in a combined structure [27]. These gamification structure variants can be configured in the form of a level system designed to promote holistic health goals. The level structure variants used in this paper are referred to as single-stream and multi-stream level structures, where a stream represents a series of progressively higher levels. A multi-stream level structure contains multiple (i.e., non-unified) levels simultaneously. A single-stream level structure contains one (i.e., unified) level at a time.

This study aimed to research which of the level structures is most engaging in mHealth apps. We expected that multi-stream level structures would intrinsically motivate individuals to people more than single-stream levels, due to the design giving participants increased autonomy to complete goals within the health domain of their choosing. Thus resulting in participants being more engaged with the mHealth app. Our hypothesis is as follows: 'When participants are given goals in a multi-stream level structure, they will be more engaged with the mHealth app.'. In this paper, we tested the hypothesis by evaluating the effects of a multi-stream level structure on the engagement of participants in a health intervention using a gamified mHealth app.

2   Theoretical Background

2.1   Behavior Change

The concept of engagement in the context of this paper, refers to an individual's behavior leading to interactions with the mHealth app. To incentivize these interactions, the mHealth app used in this study makes use of behavior-change concepts. Behavior change in individuals requires capability, encompassing both psychological and physical abilities to execute the targeted behavior, along with the opportunity facilitated by external factors enabling the behavior, and the motivation to enact the behavior [18]. mHealth apps particularly have the potential to enhance the motivational aspect. Motivation can be categorized into extrinsic and intrinsic motivation, with extrinsic stemming from external factors and intrinsic from personal interest [8]. Intrinsic motivation tends to endure longer because it fulfills the three internal needs of the individual: competence, the need to feel capable of the behavior; autonomy, the need for self-control; and relatedness, the need for connection with behaviors and social support [8]. mHealth apps can target intrinsic motivation by incorporating features that appeal to the three needs for promoting intrinsic motivation, leading to higher engagement [10].

2.2   Levels

Gamification has increasingly been utilized in mHealth apps to increase participant engagement in interventions across various health domains, including mental health, physical health, and general promotion of healthy behavior change [6] [10,35]. The concept of levels in the context of games is a space available to a player during the completion of an objective [26]. Levels are generally sequential, with each level having progressively difficult objectives to complete [17,26]. The increasing difficulty generally matches the player's skill progression throughout completing the levels [26]. Players can progress in multiple levels simultaneously, and each level has its own set of objectives to complete to advance to the next [17]. In some configurations, players can revert to the previous level due to rules such as, not completing a level on time or failing to complete all objectives within a game session. The structure of difficulty progression present in level systems can be mapped to the skill and difficulty concepts of the Flow theory [7]. The difficulty levels have directly been linked to affecting the Flow state of individuals [36]. By structuring the difficulty of the level objectives optimally, participants may be prompted to experience Flow. Levels have also been used to incentivize engagement in games, by using progression locking, which locks certain areas of the apps until certain conditions are met, and progression blocking features which block all progression within the app until conditions are met [24,31]. The progress principle is a theory from the business management literature that states that individuals are more productive and perform better when they have the feeling of making progress toward their goals [2]. Gaining small wins increases this feeling of progression. Game levels have been linked to the progress principle as they are designed to invoke feelings of progression and achievement of small objectives (i.e., goals) [2,26]. Therefore the goals in the level structures should be small enough for participants to gain small wins with an increasing difficulty to keep participants in Flow [2,7].

3   Methods

3.1   Study Design

The study was conducted using a mixed-method research design. Quantitative data was measured using a two-arm within-subject crossover experiment and surveys. Qualitative data was gathered using interviews and surveys (i.e., created goals). This study took place over five weeks and consisted of two intervention periods, each consisting of fifteen days, separated by a one-week break. An overview of the study design can be seen in Fig. 1. In the pre-intervention stage of the study, participants were randomly grouped into the study arm first receiving goals displayed in a single-stream level structure (SS-MS), or in the study arm first receiving goals displayed in a multi-stream level structure (MS-SS). In the intervention phase of the study, participants received health goals displayed in the respective level structure. After the break period, participants would serve as their control group and receive the other level structure for the second intervention period. Thus participants were exposed to both level structures. Before the intervention phase of the study, participants signed a paper-based informed consent form in person. All study procedures and data protection were reviewed and approved by the Ethical Review Board of the Eindhoven University of Technology (Experiment Reference: ERB2023ID547).

3.2   Recruitment

For this study, a pool of healthy lifestyle goals was created using participant input. During the preparation stage of the study, 18 students from a university in the Netherlands were recruited using convenience sampling [29]. Students were recruited at the sports center of the university through direct invitations by the researchers. They were given a survey requesting to create three increasingly difficult goals that they relate to, for each health dimension. The students who took part in the preparation stage of this study did not take part in the following stages. To recruit participants for the intervention stage of the study, convenience sampling was also employed [29]. Participants eligible to take part in this study had to be eighteen or older. They also had to be enrolled as either a student or a staff member of a university in the Netherlands at the time of the study. Participants were recruited at a university in the Netherlands and recruitment was carried out via flyers and direct invitations to potential participants. Upon being approached, individuals received supplementary information about the study in the form of an information document, which included the overall goal of the study, its duration, and what a participant could expect to do during the study. Participants were also informed that all active participants had a chance of winning a reward at the end of the study.

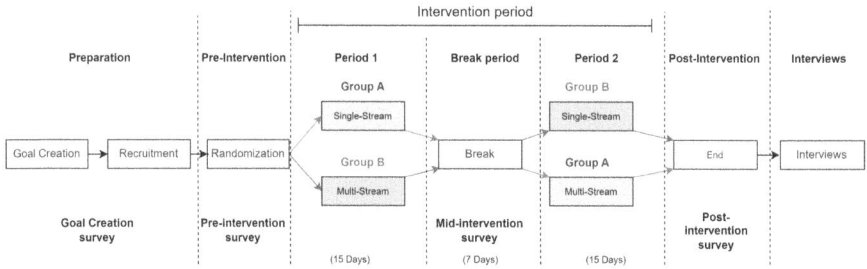

Fig. 1. This figure shows the mixed method research design used for this study, displaying the preparation phase, the intervention period, when which survey was conducted, and when the interviews were held.

3.3   Intervention Context

GameBus. GameBus is a configurable gamification platform that enables research on health interventions through the rapid prototyping of digital health apps, designed to promote participant engagement with lifestyle goals [32]. We used a custom configuration of GameBus as an mHealth app. The configuration built for the study was a multi-platform and cross-browser web app. In the app, participants were challenged to complete goals that improve their holistic health by promoting mental, social, and physical health goals. The app had three main pages: score points, leaderboards, and the levels page. The score points page displayed all available goals within the current level the participant was in. On this page, participants could also submit self-reports on the completion of the goals. Additionally, participants could optionally also describe how they completed the goal or attach photographic evidence of the goal being completed.

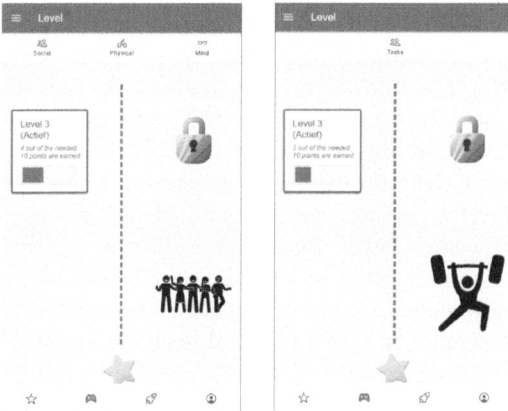

Fig. 2. The figure on the left displays a screenshot of the level system with a multi-stream level structure in the mHealth application. The figure on the right displays the level system with a single-stream level structure in the mHealth application.

For each self-report registered, participants got points towards the level system and progression bars. The progression bar feature was implemented to promote the concept of small wins. The leaderboard page displayed the total amount of points a participant has scored and the average amount of points scored by all participants. The levels page shown in Fig. 2, displayed the total levels available within each dimension a participant is active in. This page also displayed how many points were needed to advance to the next level.

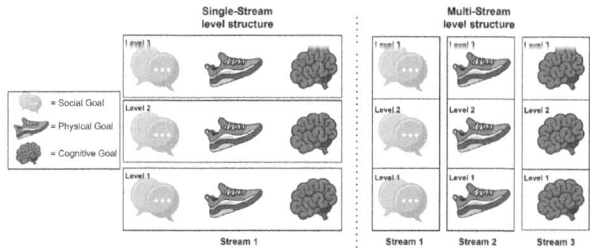

Fig. 3. The figure on the left displays the single-stream level structure where participants needed to complete goals of all health dimensions to proceed to the next level. The figure on the right showcases the multi-stream level structure where participants can level up within multiple streams concurrently and individually of each other. Each stream in the multi-stream level structure consists of levels containing goals specific to a health dimension.

Level System. For this study, we designed, implemented, and compared two different level system structures: 1) single-stream, and 2) multi-stream level structures. During the study, the mHealth app only displayed one of the two, level structures at a given time. We defined a stream of levels as a sequence of levels wherein players could advance or regress. As seen in Fig. 3[1] [2] [3], the single-stream level structure used in this study supported only one stream of levels, with each level containing goals of all health dimensions. However, in the multi-stream level structure, three single-stream levels exist in parallel. In the multi-stream level structure, each stream of levels consists of levels containing goals of a specific health dimension. Additionally, in the multi-stream level structure, participants could independently advance or regress within each stream without interference from other streams. Meaning participants could be in level two of the stream containing physical health goals, while simultaneously being in level three of the stream containing cognitive health goals. In both level structures, there were streams of three levels consisting of three goals per health dimension, resulting in an equal workload. At the start of the intervention, each participant began at level one. Both level structures had a total of nine unique goals. Each goal could be completed multiple times and consecutively, with a maximum amount of times based on the goal's frequency setting. Participants scored points by completing goals available within a level. Once a participant scored enough points within a level, they proceeded to the next level. The amount of points earned from completing a goal depended on the difficulty of the goal. The overall goal of the participants was to complete all the levels available to them. Once participants completed level three, no more goals were displayed in the app. Participants had fifteen days to complete all three levels before the phase of the intervention period ended. The system uses a form of progression blocking, when participants fail to complete level one within five days, level two within ten days, or level three within fifteen days, the system would reset and the participant would regress to the preceding level.

The goals used in the intervention phase of the study were aggregated versions of the goals created by the students during the preparation phase of the study. During the goal-creation phase, the students were asked to report how frequently they wanted to engage in certain activities before considering a goal to be completed. An example of a goal used during the intervention is the following: Level 1 - "Talk to an (old) family member or friend" 3x in five days. Level 2 - "Plan an activity with another person" 3x in five days. Level 3 - "Talk to a new person today" 3x in five days. To promote participant Flow, we reduced the difficulty of the lower levels by lowering the frequency required to advance to the next level. As a result, participants in level one needed to complete the goals once before advancing to level two. Level two required participants to complete the level two goal twice before progressing to level three. Level three required participants to complete the level 3 goal at the participant-reported frequency.

---

[1] https://shorturl.at/aeixT.

[2] https://shorturl.at/emLNY.

[3] https://shorturl.at/bAX34.

3.4   Measurements

The objective quantitative engagement of the participants, as measured by the mHealth app, was categorized into two types: active and passive engagement. Active engagement was quantified by the number of goals performed by a participant, while passive engagement was determined by the number of navigational click-throughs made by a participant. Throughout the study, one survey was conducted to collect demographic information, and the Intrinsic Motivation Inventory (IMI) survey was conducted before, during, and after the intervention period to collect the perceived intrinsic motivation of the participants throughout the intervention. The IMI evaluates self-reported perceived intrinsic motivation through a 5-point Likert scale [23]. Following the intervention period of the study, semi-structured interviews were carried out to gather qualitative data in the form of subjective participant opinions on the level structures, perceived engagement, and feedback on areas of improvement. The interviews were recorded using a smartphone and one of the researchers made notes on any points of significance.

3.5   Data Analysis

A statistical comparison was conducted on the quantitative engagement measured between the two study arms to evaluate the impact of multi-stream levels on participant engagement. Before conducting the analysis, the system data was preprocessed by removing outliers and premature dropouts (i.e., participants who did not take part in both intervention phases), and calculating the mean engagement of each participant. The data was subjected to Shapiro-Wilk and Anderson-Darling tests to evaluate their conformity to a normal distribution. The interquartile range was calculated to remove outliers. Furthermore, independent t-tests were conducted to determine the statistical significance between the groups, using a significance level of $p = 0.05$. Additionally, a statistical analysis was carried out between the two groups across each intervention period to examine the perceived intrinsic motivation of participants. Before conducting the analysis, the survey data was preprocessed equally to the engagement data. The group means were calculated for each IMI measurement period. Subsequently, a one-way ANOVA test was employed to ascertain the statistical significance between the two groups, using a significance level of $p = 0.05$. Lastly, thematic analysis was conducted on the interview data. Thematic analysis is a method to systematically organize and interpret the text to uncover themes relevant to the research aim [4]. For thematic analysis, the interviews were automatically transcribed using two AI transcription tools: 1) Google Cloud's Chirp model[4] and 2) Amazon Web Service's Automatic Speech Recognition service[5]. A copy of the raw data of the AI-generated interview transcripts can be found on Figshare [13]. The AI-generated transcription data was cross-checked with the researcher's notes to verify the validity, and transcription mistakes were

---

[4] https://cloud.google.com/speech-to-text/v2/docs/chirp-model.

[5] https://aws.amazon.com/transcribe/.

changed. The transcriptions were read by one of the researchers to find any patterns, themes, and key points of significance present in the transcription data. The thematic analysis was done by hand and the notes were coded by grouping similar answers and comments from the participants together. The coded groups were grouped into themes and revised iteratively. Finally, the results were reported in a thematic analysis.

4   Results

4.1   Participants

For this study, 73 participants were recruited, of which 39 participants actively participated in the intervention phase of the study. Participants were considered active when they had completed one or more goals in both phases of the intervention. Out of the active participants, 20 were in the SS-MS study arm, and 19 participants were in the MS-SS study arm. All 39 participants filled in the first demographics and IMI survey, 22 completed the second IMI survey and 19 completed the last IMI survey. Lastly, 15 participants took part in the interviews.

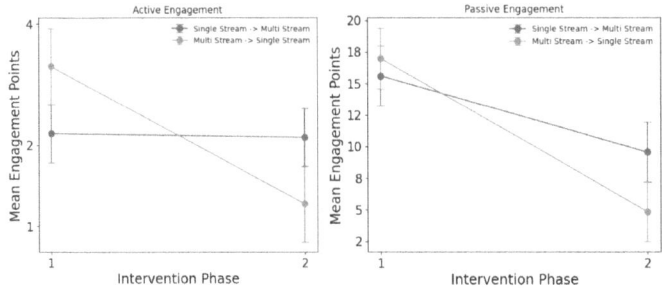

Fig. 4. The graph on the left displays the active engagement measured of participants in both groups over the two intervention periods. The graph on the right displays the passive engagement measured.

4.2   Engagement Data

Active Engagement. The total number of goals registered in the mHealth app by participants in the SS-MS study arm was 184, of which 99 were registered in the first phase of the intervention period and 85 were registered in the second intervention period. The total number of goals performed by participants in the MS-SS study arm was 172, of which 123 were before the break period and 49 were after the break period. Although the active engagement of participants of both study arms dropped, the over-time engagement of participants in the SS-MS study arm was higher when comparing group means. Additionally, when comparing means, the drop in active engagement over time was also lower in the SS-MS study arm as seen in Fig. 4. However, the analysis conducted on the active engagement between the two groups during the first phase of the intervention resulted in a p-value of 0.68, and a p-value of 0.26 during the second phase of the intervention. Indicating no statistical significance between the two groups.

Passive Engagement. The total number of navigational interactions participants made in the mHealth app by participants in the SS-MS study arm was 1098. In the first phase of the intervention, participants made 689 navigational interactions within the app, and 408 navigational interactions in the second phase of the intervention. The total number of navigational interactions performed by participants in the MS-SS study arm was 690. In the first phase, there were 233 navigational interactions and after the break period, there were 49 navigational interactions. When comparing the mean passive engagement, participants in the MS-SS study arm initially had a higher engagement. However, as seen in Fig. 4 their engagement dropped sharper than the participants in the SS-MS study arm. The analysis conducted on the passive engagement between the two study arms in the first phase of the intervention resulted in a p-value of 0.80 and a p-value of 0.17 in the second phase of the intervention. The results indicated that there was no statistically significant difference between the two groups.

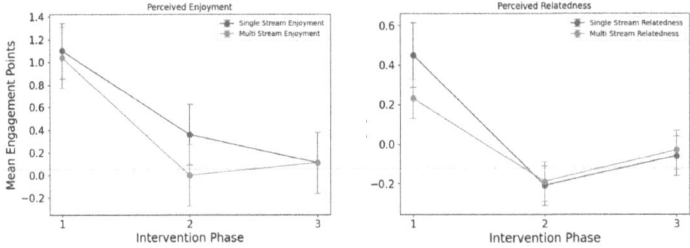

Fig. 5. The graph on the left displays the perceived mean enjoyment measured of participants in both groups over all three measurement periods. The graph on the right displays the perceived mean relatedness.

4.3   Perceived Motivation Data

In the pre-intervention phase of the study, all 73 participants completed the IMI survey. During the break period, 22 participants completed the second IMI survey, and in the post-intervention phase of the study, 19 participants completed the IMI survey.

The perceived enjoyment of participants in both study arms steadily dropped over the three IMI measurement phases. However, the perceived enjoyment of the participants in the MS-SS study arm dropped lower than the perceived enjoyment of the participants in the SS-MS study arm. Although the perceived enjoyment of the participants in the MS-SS study arm measured in the post-intervention phase increased when compared to the perceived enjoyment of this group during the break period. The results of the statistical analysis conducted

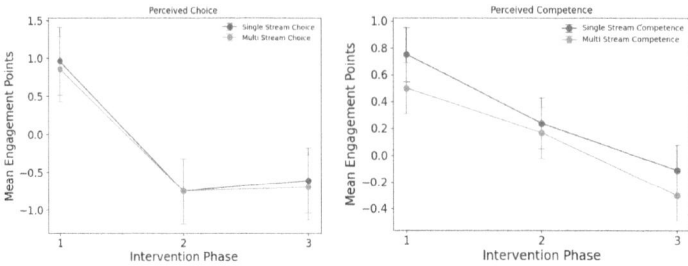

Fig. 6. The graph on the left displays the perceived mean choice measured of participants in both groups over all three measurement periods. The graph on the right displays the perceived mean competence.

on the perceived enjoyment of both study arms show that there was no statistical significance between the two groups, with a p-value of 0.77.

The perceived competence of participants in both study arms steadily dropped throughout the three measurement phases. As seen in Fig. 6, the participants in the SS-MS study arm scored slightly higher in perceived competence during all measurement phases. The results may indicate that participants over time felt less confident in their ability to complete the goals given to them once using the app. The results of the statistical analysis conducted on the perceived competence between the two study arms indicate that there was no statistical significance between the groups, with a p-value of 0.64.

The perceived relatedness of participants in both study arms dropped sharply between the measurement in the pre-intervention phase and the break period, as seen in Fig. 5. This may indicate that after participants used the mHealth app, the app may have not met their expectations regarding how related they would feel to the app. However, in both study arms, the perceived relatedness slightly increased between the break period and the post-intervention phase of the study. Initially, in the pre-intervention phase, the participants in the SS-MS study arm scored higher in perceived relatedness, but lower in the subsequent break period and post-intervention phase. This may indicate that participants may have slightly more relatedness with a multi-stream level structure. The statistical analysis conducted on the perceived relatedness of the participants in both study arms resulted in a p-value of 0.82, indicating that there was no statistical significance between the two groups.

The perceived choice of participants in both study arms dropped sharply between the measurement in the pre-intervention phase and the break period. In both study arms, however, the perceived choice increased slightly between the break period and the post-intervention phase. However, in both the break period and post-intervention measurement, the mean perceived choice score scored below 0. This may indicate that before the intervention, participants in both groups equally perceived they had much choice in the mHealth app, however, once they used the mHealth apps they perceived limited autonomy in their choices. The results of the statistical analysis conducted between the two study arms resulted in a p-value of 0.94, indicating no statistical significance between the two groups.

4.4   Interview Data

The thematic analysis of the interview transcripts resulted in the 3 following themes: difficulty level, social comparison, and level structure preferences.

Participants stated that advancing through the level structures was a difficult experience with Participant 1 stating that "this first stage is a little bit hard to do" due to the goals being too "generic". Participant 5 echoed this by indicating that some goals "were difficult" and "the difficulty level was hard to achieve. It was as if the [app] was too difficult.". Additionally, Participant 13 noted a tendency to register goals near the level system's reset time, stating "Apparently, I always go to other activities the very last day before everything got reset" indicating frustration with the lack of clarity regarding reset timings. Despite the frustration, they remained open to the timer concept by stating "I'm not against it [the timer] per see". These insights may indicate a need to reduce the size of the goals, provide more variety of goals in each level stream, and reduce the difficulty level in the earlier levels, in both level structures.

Participants indicated that the level system should be integrated with a social comparison feature outside the social goals, with Participant 2 stating "I could not see how well [other participants] were doing" and highlighting "I couldn't compare myself to other people ... So what does my Level 3 mean, for example, right.". The sentiment is echoed by Participant 4 affirming that the app felt "lonely". Both Participant 5 and Participant 7 matched that sentiment by respectively stating "I did not see how I could compare myself" and "I wish that I could uh see also more things maybe about the levels, [the] average level that people are or some more details about other participants". The insights of the participants strongly indicate that despite the leaderboard function participants lack ways to compare their progress with others.

Participants unanimously have a preference for receiving goals in a multi-stream level structure. Participant 7 stated, "I think maybe the level system in each category would be better fit for me because maybe at some point, I don't want to focus on physical activities but want to focus on socializing" Participant 9 expressed that the advantage of the multi-steam level system is the ability to focus on specific activities rather than having to sustain engagement across all dimensions to progress, stating, "sometimes [I don't want] to sustain every type of activity, I just want to strengthen the physical exercise". This was echoed by Participant 6, saying, "From my perspective, I would always choose the [multi-stream level] option since I just believe that if we have one activity, we have to completely concentrate on that activity to be on a good level.". Indicating that participants related to the multi-stream level structure. However, Participant 2 noted a drop in engagement with certain goals over time, stating "So I just like [registered] the [goals in the one dimension] I always do and the other two I just kind of ignored.". Participant 4 shared this experience by expressing "There were three objectives that were being prompted to me and I think I vibed with

two of them like I could feel that I had something to share with two of them.".
The results indicate that participants purposely ignored the goals in certain
health dimensions. A few participants did favor the single-stream level system.
Participant 5 expressed "On one hand, [I did not like it], but on the other hand,
maybe that's good because then you develop your weak spots." This was echoed
by Participant 13, noting that despite the challenges "[single-stream] forces you
to do those [other goals]." Indicating that a few participants saw the need to
achieve goals within health dimensions they normally do not work on. However,
some reasons why participants had reservations about single-stream levels were
as Participant 14 stated "[It is] kind of demotivating. If you have to do all of
them, go to the next level. I think the [multi-stream level system], you still
see progress in at least one of the categories." Participant 11 shared a similar
sentiment, indicating "I already mentioned that I didn't like that [in the single
stream level system], your points also counted toward the other categories.".
While some participants appreciated the focus on weaknesses provided by single-
stream levels, most participants found the requirement to complete tasks across
all categories demotivating.

Outside of the themes analyzed, participants gave feedback on how to improve
the level structures. Participant 10 proposed adding an additional player level
system comparable to Massive Multiplayer Online Role Playing Games where
"You [have multiple] different categories of what you could level up [and an] overarching combat level.". Participant 11 indicated that there should be more levels
and would have liked seeing "your progress within the levels", something Participant 5 lacked, stating "I did not know if I was progressin". Overall participants
wanted the level system to display more player progression.

5   Discussion

5.1   Main Findings

The multi-stream level structure may be less holistic and healthy than the
single-stream level structure. In the interviews, many participants indicated a
lack of interest in one or more dimensions present in the mHealth app. This
indicates that the multi-stream level structure may incentivize participants to
solely achieve the goals within the health dimensions they are comfortable with,
neglecting goals in the other dimensions that contribute to their holistic health.
Despite multi-stream level structures possibly being less healthy holistically, participants unanimously preferred it over the single-stream level structure. Participants were slightly more engaged when given a multi-stream level structure.

Although participants subjectively preferred the multi-stream level structure
and the objective data states that there was more passive and active engagement
when both groups of participants were given goals in the multi-stream level structure, the difference between the objectively measured engagement of the groups
was not significant. This implies no significant difference in engagement when
participants are given the less-preferred and possibly healthier single-stream level
structure. Single-stream level structures are therefore not inferior to multi-stream

level structures for incentivizing engagement, resulting in our hypothesis being incorrect. The subjective views of participants on the level structures may not have a statistically significant impact on engagement. This opens the possibilities for experimentation with level structures to promote health, with minimal potential impact on participant engagement. The results may also indicate that the content of the levels has a bigger impact on engagement than the structure in which it is presented.

Interestingly, during the interviews participants indicated that the goals were challenging despite the difficulty of the goals being lowered to a level lower than the perceived skill of the participants. This may indicate that to keep players in Flow, the difficulty of goals present in earlier levels should be significantly easier than the perceived skilled level of the participants [7]. This result may also suggest that the goals were not small enough for participants to feel progression through small wins [2].

5.2   Limitations

This study had several limitations, including a study population limited to only students and staff members of a Dutch university. As a result, the results cannot be generalized beyond this context. In this context, participants may have introduced a potential bias, as multiple participants indicated that their primary motivation for continued participation in the intervention was to provide sufficient data for the researchers. Another potential bias may have been introduced by informing participants that there was a chance to win a reward for actively participating in the study. Moreover, the sample size of the study was too small to have large power in the quantitative analysis using engagement data.

The scope of this study was solely to evaluate the engagement of participants in mHealth apps and not the effectiveness of level structures on health outcomes. Additionally, it was also out of the scope of this study to measure the Flow participants experienced during the use of the mHealth app.

Finally, the current configurations of the level system could be expanded. Participants are currently limited to three levels in each level stream. Additionally, each stream in the multi-stream level structure contained goals from a specific dimension. However, the structure of the level stream could be adjusted to include goals from multiple dimensions per level. This adjustment could potentially maintain the sense of autonomy of participants in making their own choices while encouraging them to pursue goals across various dimensions.

5.3   Future Work

In future research, conducting a larger study with more participants will be necessary to increase statistical power for analysis. The results of this study lack generalizability. Replicating the study in diverse contexts, involving participants beyond a university setting needs to be conducted to obtain more generalizable results.

A possible future configuration to consider is the use of progression locking where progression in a level stream can be locked until the participant also progresses to the other level streams. This locking feature could possibly incentivize participants to work on all streams simultaneously. This configuration may have a negative impact on participant engagement as it may restrict the autonomy of participants. However, the results indicate that the structure of the levels may not have such a statistically significant impact on the engagement of participants.

Furthermore, there should be further experimentation with different configurations of the level system to benefit holistic health. The level system could be extended by experimenting with a multi-stream structure that incorporates a mix of health dimension goals within the levels of each stream. Additionally, there should be experimentation with an overarching level system, such as player-level systems in role-playing games that track the player's progress independently of the current goal-based level system [1]. Moreover, future studies should consider incorporating more than three levels per stream. Lastly, adding elements of social comparison of the level system should be considered to improve participant-relatedness with the mHealth app.

6   Conclusion

In this paper, we evaluated the impact of level system structures on the engagement of participants in mHealth apps. The results indicated that despite the participants unanimously preferring a multi-stream level structure, there is no significant impact on engagement when participants are given a multi-stream level structure compared to a single-stream level structure. The results also possibly indicate that the structure of a level system may not have a big impact on the engagement of participants in mHealth apps. Moreover, the findings suggest that a multi-stream level structure configured with streams of levels consisting of goals of only one health dimension incentivizes participants to solely achieve goals within the health dimensions they are comfortable in. This results in participants not achieving goals that holistically improve their health. Using a single-stream level structure in mHealth apps may be healthier for participants, as it incentivizes them to work on all health dimensions. However, more experimentation with different configurations of multi-stream level structures should be done such as goals of multiple dimensions within each stream, progression locking, and social comparisons of level systems.

References

1. Adams, E.: Fundamentals of Role-Playing Game Design. New Riders (2014)
2. Amabile, T., Kramer, S.: The progress principle: Using small wins to ignite joy, engagement, and creativity at work. Harvard Business Press (2011)
3. Balwan, W.K., Kour, S., et al.: Lifestyle diseases: the link between modern lifestyle and threat to public health. Saudi J. Med. Pharm. Sci. **7**(4), 179–84 (2021)
4. Braun, V., Clarke, V.: Thematic analysis. American Psychological Association (2012)

5. Byass, P.: Correlation between noncommunicable disease mortality in people aged 30–69 years and those aged 70–89 years. Bull. World Health Organ. **97**(9), 589 (2019)

6. Cheng, V.W.S.: Recommendations for implementing gamification for mental health and wellbeing. Front. Psychol. **11**, 586379 (2020)

7. Csikszentmihalyi, M., Csikzentmihaly, M.: Flow: The psychology of optimal experience, vol. 1990. Harper & Row New York (1990)

8. Deci, E.L., Ryan, R.M.: Self-determination theory. Handbook of Theories of Social Psychology **1**(20), 416–436 (2012)

9. Deterding, S., Sicart, M., Nacke, L., O'Hara, K., Dixon, D.: Gamification. using game-design elements in non-gaming contexts. In: CHI'11 Extended Abstracts on Human Factors in Computing Systems, pp. 2425–2428 (2011)

10. Dugas, M., Gao, G., Agarwal, R.: Unpacking mhealth interventions: a systematic review of behavior change techniques used in randomized controlled trials assessing mhealth effectiveness. Digital Health **6**, 2055207620905411 (2020)

11. Epton, T., Currie, S., Armitage, C.J.: Unique effects of setting goals on behavior change: Systematic review and meta-analysis. J. Consult. Clin. Psychol. **85**(12), 1182 (2017)

12. Jakob, R.: Factors influencing adherence to mhealth apps for prevention or management of noncommunicable diseases: systematic review. J. Med. Internet Res. **24**(5), e35371 (2022)

13. James, L.: Transcription files (5 2024). https://doi.org/10.6084/m9.figshare.25738086.v1

14. James, L.J., et al.: Evaluation of personalized treatment goals on engagement of smi patients with an mhealth app. In: 2022 IEEE International Conference on Bioinformatics and Biomedicine (BIBM), pp. 1568–1573. IEEE (2022)

15. Kelly, M.P., Barker, M.: Why is changing health-related behaviour so difficult? Public Health **136**, 109–116 (2016)

16. Klarkowski, M., Johnson, D., Wyeth, P., Smith, S., Phillips, C.: Operationalising and measuring flow in video games. In: Proceedings of the Annual Meeting of the Australian Special Interest Group for Computer Human Interaction, pp. 114–118 (2015)

17. McGuire, M., Jenkins, O.C.: Creating games: Mechanics, content, and technology. CRC Press (2008)

18. Michie, S., Van Stralen, M.M., West, R.: The behaviour change wheel: a new method for characterising and designing behaviour change interventions. Implement. Sci. **6**, 1–12 (2011)

19. Milne-Ives, M., Lam, C., De Cock, C., Van Velthoven, M.H., Meinert, E., et al.: Mobile apps for health behavior change in physical activity, diet, drug and alcohol use, and mental health: systematic review. JMIR Mhealth Uhealth **8**(3), e17046 (2020)

20. Mustafa, A.S., Ali, N., Dhillon, J.S., Alkawsi, G., Baashar, Y.: User engagement and abandonment of mhealth: a cross-sectional survey. In: Healthcare, vol. 10, p. 221. MDPI (2022)

21. Nimrod, G., Ben-Shem, I.: Successful aging as a lifelong process. Educ. Gerontol. **41**(11), 814–824 (2015)

22. Organization, W.H., et al.: Health is a state of complete physical, mental and social well-being and not merely the absence of disease or infirmity. In: International Health Conference, New York, pp. 19–22 (1946)

23. Reynolds, J.L.: Intrinsic Motivation Inventory (IMI) Scale (DUTCH). Handbook of Research on Electronic Surveys and Measurements, pp. 1–6 (2006)

24. Riekki, J.: Free-to-play games: what are gamers paying for? B.S. thesis, J. Riekki (2016)
25. Samdal, G.B., Eide, G.E., Barth, T., Williams, G., Meland, E.: Effective behaviour change techniques for physical activity and healthy eating in overweight and obese adults; systematic review and meta-regression analyses. Int. J. Behav. Nutr. Phys. Act. **14**, 1–14 (2017)
26. Schell, J.: The Art of Game Design: A book of lenses. CRC press (2008)
27. Shahrestani, A., Van Gorp, P., Le Blanc, P., Greidanus, F., de Groot, K., Leermakers, J.: Unified health gamification can significantly improve well-being in corporate environments. In: 2017 39th Annual International Conference of the IEEE Engineering in Medicine and Biology Society (EMBC), pp. 4507–4511. IEEE (2017)
28. Sharma, M., Majumdar, P.: Occupational lifestyle diseases: an emerging issue. Indian J. Occup. Environ. Med. **13**(3), 109–112 (2009)
29. Stratton, S.J.: Population research: convenience sampling strategies. Prehosp. Disaster Med. **36**(4), 373–374 (2021)
30. Tabish, S., et al.: Lifestyle diseases: consequences, characteristics, causes and control. J. Cardiol. Curr. Res. **9**(3), 00326 (2017)
31. Ten Velde, G., Plasqui, G., Willeboordse, M., Winkens, B., Vreugdenhil, A., et al.: Feasibility and effect of the exergame boosth introduced to improve physical activity and health in children: Protocol for a randomized controlled trial. JMIR Res. Protocols **9**(12), e24035 (2020)
32. Van Gorp, P., Nuijten, R.: 8-year evaluation of gamebus: Status quo in aiming for an open access platform to prototype and test digital health apps. Proc. ACM Human-Comput. Interact. **7**(EICS), 1–24 (2023)
33. Webber, R.: Communicable diseases: A global perspective. Cabi (2019)
34. World Health Organization: Noncommunicable diseases (ncds) - fact sheet. https://www.who.int/news-room/fact-sheets/detail/noncommunicable-diseases (2023). Accessed 22 April 2024
35. Xu, L., et al.: The effects of mhealth-based gamification interventions on participation in physical activity: systematic review. JMIR Mhealth Uhealth **10**(2), e27794 (2022)
36. Yu, D., et al.: Research on user experience of the video game difficulty based on flow theory and fnirs. Behav. Inform. Technol. **42**(6), 789–805 (2023)
37. Zheng, S., et al.: Effectiveness of holistic mobile health interventions on diet, and physical, and mental health outcomes: a systematic review and meta-analysis. E Clin. Med. **66** (2023)

Perspectives on Contextual Information in Dutch Cardiac Rehab: Implications for Holistic Telemonitoring

Irina Bianca Șerban[1(✉)], Steven Houben[1], Sara Colombo[2],
and Aarnout Brombacher[1]

[1] Eindhoven University of Technology, Eindhoven, The Netherlands
i.b.serban@tue.nl
[2] Delft University of Technology, Delft, The Netherlands

Abstract. Cardiac telerehabilitation (CTR) relies heavily on telemonitoring, predominantly gathering automated biophysical or survey data for clinical decision-making. However, lifestyle change during and after cardiac rehabilitation (CR) outside hospitals is impacted by many contextual factors, including mental well-being or social support. Failure to acknowledge these factors in remote cardiac care could result in healthcare professionals (HCPs) offering standardized recommendations that hinder health management. To gain insights into the utilization of contextual information in clinical decision-making in Dutch CR, we conducted semi-structured interviews with seven HCPs and CR experts. Our data analysis highlights the importance of routine, physical, and psychosocial information during holistic clinical decision-making. We argue for a transition towards a holistic approach to telemonitoring in CTR, discussing implications for more inclusive and contextual data-gathering practices.

Keywords: cardiac rehabilitation · contextual information · holistic care · telemonitoring · qualitative study

1 Introduction

Cardiovascular disease (CVD) ranks among Europe's top mortality causes [101]. Lifestyle interventions, like *cardiac rehabilitation* (CR), significantly enhance CVD prognosis by targeting the improvements of behavioral risk factors such as insufficient physical activity, unhealthy dietary habits, prolonged stress, and smoking [88,101]. Post-COVID-19, cardiac telerehabilitation (CTR) is gaining traction globally, notably in the Netherlands [25,79]. By leveraging communication and telemonitoring technologies (e.g., mobile and sensor-based devices), CTR facilitates *the transmission of information* between patients who undergo

© ICST Institute for Computer Sciences, Social Informatics and Telecommunications Engineering 2025
Published by Springer Nature Switzerland AG 2025. All Rights Reserved
H. Kondylakis and A. Triantafyllidis (Eds.): PervasiveHealth 2024, LNICST 612, pp. 121–147, 2025.
https://doi.org/10.1007/978-3-031-85575-7_7

the CR program in the home environment and healthcare professionals (HCPs) who use that information to check lifestyle advice adherence and provide feedback and recommendations [43]. Nonetheless, the required monitoring information related to CR-targeted behaviors varies across systems and lacks a clear definition in human-computer interaction (HCI) research. Patients typically adhere to clinical recommendations independently, tracking data such as physical activity levels, consumed foods, and stress levels via self-reported surveys or wearable sensors for HCPs to use as metrics in their clinical decision-making process [27,63,97]. However, changing one's behavior *outside the controlled hospital environment* can be influenced by many *personal, contextual factors*, such as work, family, and morale, currently not captured by telemonitoring technologies [44,59]. Although *holistic care* principles are implemented in co-located CR, enabling HCPs to gather comprehensive insights into the physical, mental, spiritual, and contextual aspects of the patient's experience, thereby facilitating personalized rehabilitation approaches [99], this is rarely the case in CTR. Despite telemonitoring's pervasive role in remote cardiac care and the patient's everyday life [55], its design often prioritizes gathering behavior-descriptive data (e.g., step count, sleep quality score), neglecting the patient's situational and experiential context.

Recent research in HCI demonstrates the value of juxtaposing wearable sensor data with patient-generated contextual information, such as motivation and personal experiences with lifestyle change, for clinical decision-making [95]. Failing to monitor a patient's ever-changing context alongside quantified behaviors can lead to the depersonalization of behavior data, rendering it unactionable for HCPs [95]. This can result in standardized recommendations for patients in remote environments, potentially hindering long-term health outcomes [11,94]. Although the need for combining objective behavior data with contextual insight in health tracking has been expressed [2,19,95], there is a lack of investigations into *what types of patient contextual information is relevant, and how it is utilized by CR HCPs in lifestyle coaching and counseling* as a first step towards more inclusive CTR telemonitoring practices. To address this gap, we explore multidisciplinary perspectives on using contextual information in CR practices. We engage with seven HCPs and CR specialists in the Netherlands area, where the adoption of telemonitoring in remote care is of growing interest [55]. We find that HCPs prioritize a deep understanding of the situational circumstances of behaviors like motivation and routines over detailed behavior descriptions such as physical activity or stress levels. We identify the composition of *contextual information* needed in CR and its use in clinical decision-making, propose an alternative holistic approach to telemonitoring, and discuss implications for the future design and development of telemonitoring technologies in CTR.

2 Background and Motivation

2.1 Multidisciplinary CR Teams, Holistic Care and Contextual Information

The Multidisciplinary Efforts in CR. Cardiac rehabilitation (CR) is considered essential for long-term recovery and patient management [32], addressing the crucial CVD risk factor: unhealthy lifestyle [77,85]. CR, a complex model of care, involves multidisciplinary teams of CR-trained HCPs, including *nurses, dietitians, physiotherapists, cardiologists, psychologists, and sports physicians* [93]. As a main part of CR programs, HCPs conduct educational and training sessions addressing healthy behaviors (also called "core components") like physical activity, diet, emotional recovery, and coping [50]. Each professional is assigned a distinct core rehabilitation component [34], or assumes the overall responsibility of overseeing the patient's rehabilitation trajectory [93]. The nurse typically acts as the case manager, offering ongoing phone consultations and addressing patient queries, while physicians and psychologists provide periodic consultations or address issues as flagged by the nurse. The HCP network engages in collaborative assessment of behavioral factors and patient adherence to recommendations, coordinating care to address various aspects of patient well-being [10]. Following program reassessment, HCPs guide individual self-management [16], emphasizing the implementation and maintenance of healthy behaviors at home [32,88].

Holistic Care Principles in CR. From a patient's perspective, being diagnosed with a heart condition and facing significant interventions, along with a flood of information and lifestyle changes, can be profoundly challenging. This process is much more complex than merely following recommendations on exercise and healthy eating [67,94]. By embracing *holistic care principles*, HCPs collaborate to provide goal oriented care tailored to the patient's needs *beyond illness* by looking at the patient as a whole, specifically, as the unity of *body, mind, spirit, and surrounding systems* [99]. In co-located CR, HCPs gather patient information on core components, adapting goals based on individual insights for improved outcomes [10,66,93]. For instance, family narratives are documented next to the objective assessment of physical improvements for goal and advice adaptation [50,69]. Nonetheless, the type of information these narratives contain and the strategies HCPs use to obtain information contextualizing healthy behaviors from patients are unknown. Although plenty of clinical studies investigate patients' experiences with CR programs [29,31,41] and barriers and facilitators of patient participation [1,58], adherence [35,68], completion [73], and self-management post-program [22,83], these insights are mainly used to suggest improvements of CR procedures. They are not discussed in the context of clinical decision-making. Armed with the knowledge that utilizing insights into patient barriers, facilitators, and overall context in clinical decisions during CR significantly correlates with shortened recovery time post-cardiac event [54,59], we aim to outline initial categories of contextual information used in clinical decision-making in CR from the perspective of a multidisciplinary group of HCPs. These insights may inform the development of a CTR system that integrates comprehensive principles from co-located CR practices.

2.2   Telemonitoring Practices and Data Needs in C(T)R.

Current Telemonitoring in Remote Cardiac Care. Cardiac telerehabilitation (CTR) technologies emerge as solutions to enhance CR participation by overcoming barriers such as program awareness, transportation issues, and low social support, compounded by increased risk factors post-in-clinic phase [12,63,64,103]. CTR often employs telemonitoring (e.g., wearable sensors or self-reporting automated surveys) and communication tools (e.g., texting, videoconferencing) for patient-clinician information and feedback exchange to ensure adherence to lifestyle recommendations [17,56]. After analyzing recent systematic reviews of CTR systems, we have found a consistent trend: this exchange heavily relies on quantifying core CR components (i.e., behaviors), particularly physical activity [17,43,49,56,61,65,71,84]. For instance, Zhang et al. [105] utilize a wearable activity tracker to monitor physical activity levels (i.e., through acceleration and steps) between hospitalization and CR, providing data for nurses to offer online feedback. Similarly, Herkert et al. [52] track exercise progress through in-app surveys and activity sensors, measuring post-session exertion and daily activities. Although less common, other telemonitoring systems extend beyond physical activity, including self-reporting cigarette consumption via in-app surveys, uploading meal images, logging weight changes, self-evaluating sleep quality, and measuring sleep efficiency with wearable sensors [18,28,37,46,80,92,100]. While a detailed examination of data collected by CTR systems warrants further investigation, our focus lies elsewhere. Instead, we highlight the prevailing emphasis on *quantifying behavior* in current CR lifestyle telemonitoring and the oversight of *contextual information* like perceived self-efficacy, habits, and family obligations crucial for understanding human behavior in home settings [73]. Notably, while evaluating their CTR system, Herkert et al. [52] highlight the inability to proactively prevent decreased exercise adherence due to the lack of information on patients' physical complaints and motivators. As telemonitoring advances, designers must acknowledge the challenge of expecting *diverse patients with various circumstances* to conform to standardized feedback solely based on biophysical data and automated surveys [94]. Recent HCI research underscores the importance of individualized design for cardiac technologies [33,94], as neglecting this may lead to misalignment with the patient's "normality" [96], poor engagement, adherence, and effectiveness in behavior change [51].

Data Requirements in Telerehabilitation. Due to the intricate network of HCPs and complex targeted behavioral components, defining data requirements for lifestyle monitoring in CTR is challenging. Examples of collected data vary from system to system. In exercise-based CTR, Shimbo et al. [70] suggest measuring activity intensity parameters and participant condition indicators in exercise. In a comprehensive CTR portal, Goevaerts et al. [46] classify self-reported data such as physical activity, sedentary behavior, alcohol, nutrition intake, and stress to detect and assess risk behaviors. Nonetheless, within recent HCI and Computer-Supported Cooperative Work (CSCW) research, there is a suggestion that the data needs of HCPs in CTR are more intricate than what current systems provide. In a study on telemonitored data supporting CR, Tadas et al. [95] highlight the concept of "situated objectivity", which integrates standardized, automated data with contextual understanding [78]. They emphasize the importance of periodically sampling personal experiences alongside objective data like physical activity levels to contextualize them effectively. The transition from *data* to *information* can assist HCPs in understanding patients' challenges in meeting recommended targets. These conclusions find support in other telemonitoring interventions. Caldeira et al. [26] highlight HCPs' reliance on patients' subjective input for interpreting telemonitored data in stroke telerehabilitation. Similarly, Amorim et al. [3] note the need for patient subjective input in HCPs' decision-making for musculoskeletal conditions telerehabilitation. Andersen et al. [4] emphasize the importance of the patient's own data interpretation in collaborative ICD data analysis. Akinsiku et al. [2] stress the significance of telemonitoring information tied to the patient's context in stroke physical rehabilitation, categorizing it into areas like motivation, mental health, and caregiver assessment. There is a lack of similar studies delineating the contextual information needed in CTR; we expand on existing work and define similar information categories within CR. While Akinsiku et al. [2] term this information "experiential", we will use the term "contextual information". This distinction arises from the differing focus between stroke and cardiac rehabilitation; the latter involves a more complex recovery process, with patients undertaking long-term behavioral changes influenced by various contextual everyday life factors extending beyond mere task execution.

3   Study Design and Method

Acknowledging that behavior-descriptive data gathered in CTR is not enough for holistic clinical decision-making, we aim to understand *what types of patient contextual information is relevant, and how it is utilized by CR HCPs in lifestyle coaching and counseling* as a first step towards holistic telemonitoring.

Participant recruitment was done through snowball sampling from a teaching hospital in the Netherlands, a CR center in North Belgium (Noord Brabant area), and two Universities in the Netherlands. CR programs in North Belgium are very similar to the Dutch programs. We selected at least one participant for each CR behavioral component (2 psychologists – CP1 and CP2, one dietitian – DT, one physiotherapist – PT, one sports physician – SP) and two CR experts (one project manager – PM, one specialized nurse practitioner – NP) (Appendix A.2).[1] We conducted individual semi-structured interviews, lasting 45 to 90 min each. Four interviews were in person, while three were held online via Microsoft

---

[1] In this paper, participants to this study are also referred to as 'HCPs' or 'clinicians'.

Teams due to COVID-19. All interviews were audio recorded, with online ones also video recorded with participants' consent.

Before the study, an interview guide and a visual Miro board were developed to guide the conversation. The board contained patient barriers and facilitators of attendance, adherence, and completion of CR identified from a representative corpus of literature (Appendix A.1). After being introduced to the context and aim of the research, participants were given 10 min to review the Miro board. Questions addressed the types of information related to the patient's context participants use in lifestyle coaching and counseling, methods of collecting such information, and their link to addressing CR-targeted behaviors. Participants used the Miro board to define categories of information starting from the collection on the board. Recordings were transcribed verbatim. Semantic and descriptive thematic analysis was employed to identify recurring themes containing contextual information [30]. Transcriptions were segmented into distinct meaning units related to contextual factors (e.g., work and routines), each assigned a consecutive code to maintain context [40]. These meaning units and Miro visualizations were used to identify recurring themes representing broader categories of contextual information (e.g., everyday normality).

4   Results

4.1   Various and Subjective Ways of Collecting Contextual Information

Our findings emphasize the crucial role of *patient contextual information* in clinical decision-making within CR, essential for understanding patients and guiding their rehabilitation journey. HCPs rely on personal and situational context to grasp the reasons behind patient behaviors. While lifestyle behavior data (e.g., self-reported physical activity levels, physiotherapy session metrics, self-reported smoking habits) is a starting point, contextual insights (e.g., busy family life) help elucidate underlying reasons for why patients behave in a certain way. HCPs follow *holistic care* principles, interviewing patients and asking open-ended questions. During intake appointments, case managers collect comprehensive information on patients' well-being and surrounding systems. Other HCPs might use issues with adherence (e.g., low physical activity) as triggers for delving further into a patient's personal situation. The information is recorded in the patient's medical file and becomes available to the rest of the multidisciplinary team. Important contextual information for CR coaching includes details about the patient's *everyday normality, social environment, psychological and physical well-being*, and *ability to leverage knowledge.*

Participants come from different expertise and specializations, each an important puzzle piece during CR. We observe different approaches in which they extract and document contextual information based on the different degrees of closeness with the patient, as well as with administrative versus clinical perspectives. For instance, the nurse practitioner (NP) has the most personal relationship with the patients and views them as a complex ecosystem of factors, not as a clinical subject defined by one's condition. They use the intake appointment at the beginning of CR as an essential opportunity to establish a comprehensive patient profile. Subsequently, during consultations or therapy sessions (e.g., psychotherapy or physiotherapy), all HCPs try to get to know the patient personally to gain trust and adapt their advice to the individual. However, there are friction points regarding how holistic these consultations are since the level of intimacy of the conversation, even though deemed important, is not standardized. For instance, the project manager (PM) argues that the textbook procedure of CR intake appointments is not personal enough: *"it's [the intake appointment] not really focused on the more difficult things to grasp - like their needs, wishes, past experiences, and expectations. [...] I think it's really important to really understand the patient more than just the numbers that are attached to them - my age is 59, my weight is 120 kg and my physical activity behavior is low".* All our participants, however, unanimously agree that CR is a personalized journey shaped by the patient's unique circumstances. Specialists, for instance, employ subjective interpretation and professional intuition to navigate the complexities of personal situations, stratifying patients into appropriate treatment strategies. The psychologist (CP2) assists patients with minimal social support and mood disorders such as anxiety or depression. The sports physician (SP) identifies physical restrictions based on the patient's well-being and explores personal exercise possibilities by targeting trainable aspects according to daily routines, physical capabilities, and mental well-being. Conversely, the dietitian (DT) might try to understand the patient according to a structured procedure, beginning with background factors such as lifestyle and comorbidities, then inquiring into personal factors like social support and confidence, and ultimately focusing on existing dietary knowledge and beliefs regarding illness and treatment.

Although of different types, the entanglement among the contextual information HCPs use for clinical decision-making is significant. For instance, a patient's *social framework and support* directly influence their *routines and obligations* in the home environment, while their *comorbidities and physical limitations* can negatively affect their *motivation and health beliefs*. Similarly, *depression and anxiety* can limit a patient's *ability to leverage CR knowledge* about healthy behaviors in their everyday life. HCPs use entanglements and dependencies to extract the right contextual information and identify root problems in a patient's rehabilitation to provide personalized strategies. At the same time, we observe that behavioral data can become contextual information when identifying issues with other behaviors. For instance, data about physical activity levels is utilized as context for dietary problems, whereas information on the patient's smoking behavior can be used to contextualize a decline in exercise capacity.

4.2 Contextual Information About the Everyday Normality

Creating an initial profile based on the patient's *everyday normality* is essential for pinpointing practical barriers and customizing the care pathway accordingly. This information is regularly updated with follow-up questions throughout CR to assess how patients are adjusting their normality to rehabilitation goals and whether these goals align with their habitual lives. By gathering this data, HCPs aim to establish a personal connection with the patient, fostering trust and gaining insights into their individual needs. NP exemplifies: *"I always ask: 'what kind of work did you do before?' just to get to know them. I do not identify the patient because of a heart attack – it could happen to anyone – but because I know which patient I'm talking to"*.

Existing Lifestyle, Work, Routines, and Obligations. Before initiating any lifestyle changes, the patient's existing lifestyle is evaluated using standardized questionnaires like the International Physical Activity Questionnaire [98] supplemented by open-ended discussions. DT underlines: *"You first need to know what the current behaviors are before you can assess where changes need to be made"*. Lifestyle information, including existing physical activity levels, dietary habits, and stress patterns, is registered and becomes available to the multidisciplinary HCP team through the electronic patient record, as it can significantly affect patient progress. Patients with healthy habits may adapt more easily to recommendations and reach goals faster, so the pace of change can be personalized. Additionally, DT emphasizes the importance of prior lifestyle in tailoring education, highlighting the need for insights into the necessity for new health behaviors, especially for patients with limited awareness of their habits. However, participants note that patients' recall of their exercise routines and eating habits is not always accurate, posing challenges in setting appropriate goals.

Work patterns and routines are also considered when designing treatment plans, as they could often interfere with the new types of behavior patients need to learn. PM exemplifies: *"People who are used to cycle to work instead of taking the car, especially for physical activity behavior, that's really important. [...] But if you always took the car, it is difficult to start to cycle to work"*. Participants observe a trend among patients with demanding jobs and hectic schedules who struggle to find time and energy for exercise or counseling sessions. In such instances, HCPs must provide flexible counseling options and alternative training methods while offering stress management support. Understanding household and family responsibilities is also vital, as they influence patient priorities and adherence to recommendations. HCPs tailor suggestions to match the patient's priorities to enhance their overall quality of life. SP recalls about a young patient with children: *"if they [i.e., a patient] have to prioritize the things they have to do, they choose for their children, then physical fitness and then work [...] so we adapt the training [...]. First month of rehab focus on family, and then pick up pace in exercise"*.

Resources In and Around Home. Regarding more practical factors, participants highlight the impact of income status on therapy adherence and long-term self-management. While insurance companies in the Netherlands strongly support CR, higher-income patients may have easier access to healthier food resources and specialized trainers outside the hospital. HCPs consider a patient's financial situation to recommend affordable, nutritionally suitable food options aligning with cardiac restrictions. PM presents opportunities for suggesting alternative exercise options by using information about the patient's local environments, such as nearby parks or recreational facilities, for those unable to afford gym memberships or personal trainers.

4.3 Contextual Information About the Social Environment

All participants stressed the importance of understanding the patient's *social environment*, both in and outside the home. This information enables HCPs to anticipate or address challenges related to therapy adherence, such as a patient with family members exhibiting unhealthy eating habits. It also informs clinical decision-making, such as involving individuals from the patient's social network in treatment or engaging patients in peer groups.

Social Framework and Support. Participants concur that understanding the patient's social background, including marital status, cohabitants, friends, and children, is crucial for counseling and training across all lifestyle behaviors. As knowledge acquisition and application occur at home, the family can significantly impact the patient's progress, both actively and passively. While this isn't standard practice in CR and varies among practitioners, our participants conduct dyadic interviews and sometimes therapy sessions to address this. SP mentions: *"[. . .] if I see a patient and the partner next to them, I can treat them both, and it helps. But if you are alone, it's much more difficult"*. The patient and their informal caregiver are asked about lifestyle behaviors, family obligations, and tasks. This allows DT, for example, to provide dietary advice and information tailored not only to the patient but also to the family and caregivers. PT and NP illustrate instances where one family member must make lifestyle changes while another is responsible for cooking and grocery shopping. Participants also investigate the dynamics between patients and caregivers, including perceived support, recognizing that a lack thereof can impede therapy adherence or discourage participation in CR. On the other hand, excessive support can lead to over-protectiveness or anxiety. CP1 exemplifies: *"if the partner is anxious - the partner is checking 'Are you feeling okay? I think you are not feeling okay. Have you checked your pulse?' Well, that's not helping. Because then the patient doesn't get the trust they need to do things by themselves again"*. In such cases, professionals engage partners in consultations, provide structured guidance on supporting a family member with cardiac issues, and may even refer them to psychosocial therapy.

Connections with Peers. HCPs also appreciate gaining insight into the nature of peer support patients are receiving. Some participants encourage community building and bonding in their practice - in some cases, peer advice comes with a certain empathy and understanding the clinician cannot offer. Nonetheless, this approach is not standardized. CP1 describes: *"It depends on what your personal style is as a psychologist, I really try to get them talking to each other (in group sessions) because it can really be helpful. [...] They all have been through the same. There's a lot of understanding, and empathy, and understanding lowers stress. [...] it really can help you [the patient] be calmer, be safe. [...] They can really confront each other in an easier and better way than I would do that"*.

Professionals may suggest online communities or group sessions to patients who lack peer contact.

4.4   Contextual Information About Mental Well-Being

Information about *mental well-being* can help identify the roots of existing challenges such as low patient progress or adherence. Patients are screened for depressive disorders and anxiety using standardized questionnaires (e.g., Beck Depression Inventory [66]). Throughout rehabilitation, patients share their mental challenges through open-ended discussions with HCPs, who communicate them to the multidisciplinary team, leading to collaborative care adjustments.

Depression and Anxiety. HCPs prioritize investigating if patients have a predisposition to anxiety, depression, or mood problems, which can hinder confidence and self-efficacy. Patients with a history of these issues or with a type-D personality [62] characterized by negative affectivity and social inhibition may require special psychological attention. SP explains that addressing depressive symptoms first is crucial, as they can impede treatment progress and patient empowerment. Patients who have experienced a cardiac event before participating in CR may face worries about their future and the trauma of the heart attack. This trauma can lead to anxiety about being physically active again, resulting in inactivity, lack of motivation, and, ultimately, depression. CP1 recalls: *"I recently had a patient and he had a stroke, and he was somewhere far away from home. He's really scared to walk alone in the dark because he's so scared that it will happen again. And he's really having panic attacks as well, really hyper-alert".* Patients in need are referred to a clinical psychologist to address emotional challenges. Group sessions are recommended, while individual sessions and Eye Movement Desensitization and Reprocessing (EMDR) therapy [91] are offered to those dealing with trauma. It is important to note that this information may not always emerge at the onset of rehabilitation, as some patients may be hesitant to open up or discuss intimate thoughts and feelings. Rather, contextual information about psychological challenges is continuously collected, and most times, patients need to recognize these challenges themselves and ask for help. NP mentions that oftentimes, anxiety spikes after the program ends when the patient is left with little to no professional support at home.

Motivation and Health Beliefs. Participants document motivational levels during HCP-patient discussions, recognizing low motivation as a primary barrier to behavior change, program attendance, adherence, and completion. While pinpointing the exact causes for low determination is challenging, participants look at factors such as high anxiety, unhealthy coping mechanisms, low self-efficacy, and personality traits that contribute to low motivation. Professionals acknowledge that individuals with low self-efficacy for exercise need encouragement and reassurance of achievable progress. For instance, the sports physician (SP) empowers patients by forecasting their physical fitness post-program and demonstrating ongoing improvements, showing that exercise goals are achievable. They explain: *"If they [i.e., the patients] understand that they have a choice*

*either to have a lower life expectancy but also lower physical fitness with its conse-
quences or a possibility to gain this physical fitness, then most people will choose
the physical fitness. [...] But that's what patients don't realize themselves. They
have to be explained that that's possible".* By also altering treatment and treating various anxiety or mood problems, motivation can be positively influenced.
Furthermore, understanding patients' beliefs about their health situation is crucial contextual information. CP2 uses attribution theory [47] to grasp patients'
perceptions and attitudes about their condition, while DT focuses on influencing
negative beliefs about lifestyle changes by educating them on the consequences
of unhealthy nutrition: *"Most of the time they don't think they eat that unhealthy
or that it [i.e., unhealthy eating] has that much of an influence".* Negative health
beliefs can stem from difficulty accepting the diagnosis and viewing the body as
"failing". CP1 illustrates the challenge of emphasizing the importance of rest to
overly active patients who struggle to adjust their pace after a cardiac event.

4.5   Contextual Information About Physical Well-Being

Physical well-being is paramount in a patient's circumstances, as physical pains
and limitations can impede lifestyle improvements, particularly in enhancing
physical activity behavior. HCPs look into how comorbidities and the patient's
subjective perception of symptoms hinder progress and offer personalized tools
or suggestions.

Comorbidities and Limitations. Patients with CVD generally have other
long-term chronic conditions, such as diabetes or chronic obstructive pulmonary
disease (COPD), which can negatively affect the uptake of CR recommendations.
Participants stress that comorbidities can impact the patient's perception of the
severity of the cardiac condition and its implications for the future, thereby
affecting patient physical and mental progress. Additionally, the presence of
comorbidities like diabetes or cancer can diminish motivation and reduce the
energy and time available for CR. HCPs heed energy levels, health perception,
and life outlook related to comorbidities to comprehend why some patients lack
motivation to improve their health. Clinicians can suggest alternative physical
activity plans for patients with comorbidities like obesity, arthritis, or COPD
by considering physical limitations such as knee pain, fatigue, or breathing difficulties. The sports physician (SP) and physiotherapist (PT) adjust exercise
difficulty and the pace of lifestyle changes for these patients. SP highlights how
individuals with chronic conditions adapt their behavior to physical limitations:
*"There are people who have such bad lungs and still work full time. But they have
learned to work very slow. [...] And the people that accept their condition, they
walk maybe with a rollator [i.e., walker] or with an electric bicycle, they walk
more slowly and they take more time, they finish the physical activity and they
also take rest".*

Perceptions of Symptoms. Perceiving symptoms accurately in relation to the
cardiac condition is deemed crucial for patients to manage their health effectively.
Participants emphasize clinicians' duty to gather data on perceived symptoms

and educate patients on symptom recognition to ease anxiety from misinterpreta-
tions. CP1 highlights that post-cardiac event, patients often become hyperaware
and misinterpret symptoms, leading to stress, anxiety, and insecurity: *"After a
stroke, you feel the vulnerability of your body. [...] you monitor your body, and
that makes you feel a lot more aware of it. And that can lead to misinterpreta-
tion because, for example, you feel your heartbeat after you walk up the stairs.
Maybe it was the same before. But now they think 'Maybe it's a stroke' [...] They
get really anxious"*. Participants advocate for self-awareness, self-reflection, and
respecting the body's boundaries by prioritizing rest when necessary. CP2 and
PT underscore the importance of breaking a harmful cycle: misinterpreting bod-
ily signals leads to anxiety, which in turn instills fear of movement. Clinicians
aim to uncover the underlying causes of symptoms and complaints by inquiring
about physical discomfort, fears, and concerns.

4.6   Contextual Information About Leveraging Knowledge

Providing knowledge is central to CR programs, and understanding and applying
it is key to long-term behavior change. Patients receive extensive educational
materials during the program, but this diminishes after discharge. They are
educated about their diagnosis, rehabilitation procedures, and prognosis, with
each piece of information being significant. HCPs make efforts to document and
use information regarding patients' *ability to leverage knowledge* for therapy
improvement in their practice.

The Ability to Absorb Knowledge. During consultations, participants try
to adapt the difficulty of the educational materials to the level of understanding
of the patient. Even though they try to simplify clinical language, it is sometimes difficult to grasp whether a patient has understood the information. For
instance, SP describes that in some cases, patients who are not literate do not feel
safe enough to communicate their need for assistance in comprehending the provided information. Detecting early signs of this reluctance can be detrimental to
their health and progression. Patients receive information orally and in writing,
being allowed to express any uncertainties. HCPs also inquire about self-acquired
information sources to prevent patient misinformation. NP describes: *"I think it's
important to see how the patient gets their personal information. Is it by talking
with other patients who also had a heart attack? Or is it a professional or is it
on the Internet to see reviews from medication, for example, that are also clinical?"*. Participants express their struggle with helping patients filter through the
right information at home. Sometimes, patients base important decisions such as
stopping medication intake on self-found knowledge. Participants mention that
misinformation can also lead to a lack of interest in the program. HCPs stress the
importance of gathering patient feedback to enhance the relevance and usability of provided information, with the goal of improving patient knowledge and
understanding. PM recounts the impact of non-personalized educational sessions,
noting low engagement levels and the need for content alignment with individual experiences. They highlight the challenge of maintaining interest when the

content doesn't directly relate to the patient's condition, suggesting a need for tailored information delivery.

The Ability to Implement Knowledge. NP partly attributes the lack of motivation to the patients' low ability to use what they learn in the program in real-life situations. During consultations, clinicians may inquire about challenges patients face during the practical application of clinical recommendations to achieve set goals (e.g., eat less fatty foods) and suggest personalized adjustments or interventions accordingly. They utilize patient narratives to pinpoint obstacles like difficulty in adjusting daily schedules to rehabilitation activities or the lack of self-efficacy and confidence to maintain a behavior.

5   Discussion

Our research was motivated by the misalignment between current CTR practices and holistic, co-located CR approaches. While CTR relies on telemonitoring data that quantify CR behaviors for HCP decision-making in lifestyle coaching, co-located CR aims to understand the patient comprehensively, a sum of behavioral, spiritual, physical, and situational factors [99]. To improve the alignment between CTR monitoring practices and co-located CR care, we first need to understand the types of contextual information that HCPs consider in their decision-making process within specific hospitals. This study identifies five kinds of contextual information about patients' daily lives used in Dutch CR (i.e., everyday normality, social environment, mental and physical well-being and ability to leverage knowledge). While CTR offers accessible CR programs, its current design provides HCPs with information disconnected from the individual and fails to capture the dynamic nature of a patient's daily life. Although achieving this fully may be challenging, we argue that objective behavioral data should be complemented by a more sophisticated understanding of the patient's context through open data collection methods that capture information related to the five identified categories. We discuss implications for the design of more holistic CTR telemonitoring below.

5.1   Aligning with Co-located CR: from Objective to Situated Data

As Martinez et al. [33] mention in recent work on cardiac technologies, *"design work is and should always be context-specific"*. Although telemonitoring technologies have become pervasive in CR [36,55], they (1) present HCPs with data that quantify and characterize behaviors in isolation from the patient's situated context (e.g., [25,52]), and (2) lack the means to capture contextual information and present it in a meaningful and useful way to clinicians. Our study shows that the current telemonitoring paradigm in CTR does not align with current co-located CR practices.

Previous work on health technologies for rehabilitation emphasizes looking beyond automated data collection and quantification of behavior. Bhat et al. criticize the negative spaces in health datafication, underlying the omission of information from alternative subjective sources [19]. Tadas et al. [94] advocate for designing cardiac technologies that reflect patients' everyday lives and individual differences. In their later work on CTR, they stress the importance of combining *automated data with subjective patient experiences* [95], signaling a shift in clinical decision-making toward considering the *situated objectivity of data* [78]. With a similar motivation, Akinsiku et al. propose a paradigm reconceptualization for situated stroke telerehabilitation systems that capture the lived experiences of patients next to their movement data [2]. Driven by a missing comparable investigation in the context of CTR, we examine the information outlining the situatedness of patients' behavior in CR used by HCPs to make clinical decisions, and we urge designers of cardiac telemonitoring technologies to include *subjective and non-automated data collection methods* as a circumstantial completion of behavior data that can help clinicians provide tailored, holistic care (Fig. 1).

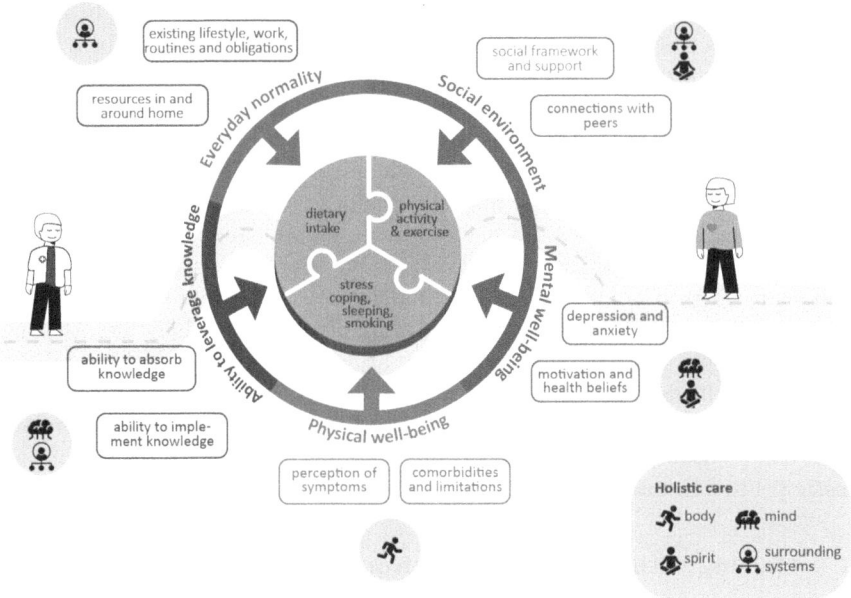

Fig. 1. Types of contextual information that could be captured by holistic CR telemonitoring aligned with holistic care principles [99].

Our investigation into co-located CR revealed that contextual information is gathered during periodical doctor-patient interviews, documented through open note-taking by clinicians, and serves as a shared knowledge base for the multidisciplinary team [13]. HCPs utilize contextual information to address barriers in patient adherence to CR components, with data collection methods relying on common sense, experience, and subjective perspectives. In CTR, a dynamic action-reaction process occurs, where clinicians observe red flags or negative trends in automatically collected data and respond accordingly [52]. In transitioning to a more nuanced approach to data-based decision-making, we advocate for a more *open approach to data collection*, which is backed by recent research findings [2,95]. Open approaches refer to less structured, *more spontaneous collection moments and alternative, expressive, and qualitative data-gathering methods* beyond standardized questionnaires and passive sensors. Examples can include functionalities that allow patients or clinicians to annotate behavior data through open text fields at any time, prompting impromptu questions to patients and incorporating more diverse data types such as audio or video recordings, pictures, or short diaries. One example is the recent design of Chromatize, a flexible, manual self-tracking application by Barker-Canler et al. [15]. These approaches can help avoid the de-personalization of CTR data and care [11]. While exploring open approaches to telemonitoring, designers must consider *HCPs' workflows and patient self-reporting burden* [57,81]. Involving clinicians and patients in designing data collection methods can mitigate workload and reporting overload [20]. This can be done, for example, by following Andersen et al.'s [6] conceptual guidelines for addressing divergent patient-clinician concerns and designing data collection and representation features in line with key characteristics of physician's progress notes (e.g., [13]). For instance, Seals et al. [89] recommend visually connecting objective data with clinical goals and patient narratives for efficient access to important information. Contextual information within CTR can serve as a semantic layer to behavior data, providing "details on demand". Moreover, our insights, supported by previous work [4,48,89], highlight the importance of *patient-clinician relationships, discussions, and shared reflections*, indicating that data visualizations should support patient-clinician conversations, accommodate low levels of data literacy, effectively convey progress or trends, and illustrate clinician explanations effectively. Lastly, it is worth noting that objective data can sometimes evolve into contextual information [2]. For example, details about a patient's diet can help a sports physician explain a decrease in energy affecting overall functional capacity. To achieve this, telemonitoring interventions should be able to collect a comprehensive dataset covering all key CR components. As emphasized in the recent study of Goevaerts et al. [46], such solutions are infrequent and need further development and exploration.

5.2   Implications for Collecting Contextual Information

Our research argues that telemonitoring systems should capture diverse patient contextual information through open data-collection methods to help clinicians personalize therapies, and align patient goals with health goals and recommended lifestyle changes [33,96]. Our findings align with Akinsiku et al. [2] on the experiential information needed in stroke rehabilitation, such as mental and physical health, motivations, and fears. We add to this by addressing the complexities of the CR context, including nuanced needs regarding knowledge absorption, patient lifestyles, and social dynamics. We offer recommendations on how to capture such information in CTR.

The Everyday Normality. We find that understanding the patient's health habits, work patterns, routines, and home resources is crucial for HCP's collaborative goal-setting, problem-solving, calibrating clinical objectives, and adjusting therapies, as it contextualizes behaviors in the patient's lived environment. CTR telemonitoring technologies should:

- prompt questions about a patient's everyday normality at program onset, creating a shared database for the multidisciplinary team to make collaborative and individual treatment decisions – e.g., knowing a patient's routines aids in tailoring training intensity, pace of change, and recommended schedules, such as whether they walk or drive to work or if they have a dog to walk each morning.
- prompt patients to periodically, throughout the program document significant changes in their everyday normality, allowing for customized therapy adaptations (as illustrated in Tadas et al.'s intervention [95]) – e.g., economic issues, family obligations, or work priorities can impact patient adherence to CR adherence, and lacking this contextual information can lead to high drop-out rates and hinder behavior maintenance [51].

The Social Environment.   Information on social support, family dynamics, and peer interaction is vital for HCPs. Although previous research underscores the pervasive role of family and informal caregivers in long-term lifestyle change [83], remote cardiac care falls short in addressing the transitional dynamics of a patient's social relationships [72]. CTR telemonitoring technologies should:

- collect comprehensive information on stakeholders involved in long-term lifestyle changes at home, including family status and levels of social support in various activities (e.g., exercising with friends, cooking with a spouse) at program onset. This aids in deciding on family involvement or individual interventions for caregivers, as partner distress or noncooperation can adversely affect patient well-being and adherence in CR [24].
- formalize family or informal caregivers' roles in telemonitoring (e.g., by enabling them to participate in data collection). This can provide insights into the patient's and family's lifestyle changes and coping mechanisms. Family-centered remote care interfaces and caregiver input options are essential [2,8,39,90,104] but still underexplored in interface design.
- enable patients to express social challenges and needs they might hesitate to voice during in-person consultations, facilitating support for family obstacles and connecting with other cardiac patients for community support.

The Mental Well-Being. HCPs extensively utilize information about the patient's depression, anxiety, motivation, and health beliefs to build profiles, prioritize clinical goals, recommend suitable therapies, and intervene during low morale. CTR telemonitoring technologies should:

- enable mental health assessment using validated questionnaires (e.g., the Beck Depression Inventory [66]) before, during, and after the program. CTR systems often lack mental health tracking [51,65] – one existing example is the LifeStyleScore app that periodically assesses perceived stress [46].

- enable and empower periodic self-reflection by allowing patients to augment objective data overviews with other mental factors (e.g., motivation, health beliefs, psychological struggles) and insights from their decision-making processes. Such data is essential to clinicians but is overlooked, although its absence has been proven to hinder proactive CTR dropout prevention [52].

The Physical Well-Being. Participants also rely on information about the patient's other chronic conditions, physical pains, symptoms, and side effects during consultations, physiotherapy sessions, or patient calls to provide tailored therapy recommendations. CTR telemonitoring technologies should:

- record the range of comorbidities at program onset and enable periodical logging of physical complaints (e.g., [53,75]). Pain, its timing, medication side effects affecting physical well-being, and complaints due to comorbidities can significantly contribute to program dropout if not addressed in time [52].
- prompt the patient's subjective perception of symptoms alongside commonly monitored vital signs such as blood pressure and heart rate [8,12] throughout the program. Overanalyzing body signals can lead to fear of movement and exercise. Sampling patients' subjective perception of felt symptoms has been encouraged before [5,7], as its clinical validation can create in-the-moment knowledge about recognizing one's body signals for patients [96].

The Ability to Leverage Knowledge. The patient's understanding of educational materials, information during consultations, and ability to implement recommendations in daily life are essential for successful CR adherence and long-term lifestyle change [93]. CTR telemonitoring technologies should:

- provide means for patients to express concerns and needs regarding overwhelming or confusing information. Patients should be able to provide open feedback electronically or comment on clinical recommendations and educational materials as an outlet for expressing a lack of understanding (e.g., Tadas et al.'s weekly open questionnaire [95]) or inform clinicians about concerns arising from unreliable information sources (e.g., as supported in Ongwere et al.'s work [76]). This can help clinicians prevent misinformation and provide educational materials adapted to patients' understanding levels. Such adaptations have been explored in interventions like Gibson et al.'s tablet application for adults with mild intellectual disabilities [45].
- gather evidence not only on behavior change trends but also on the patient's self-efficacy and reasons behind challenges they face in practical knowledge implementation outside the hospital environment.

6   Conclusion

This study presents multiple perspectives on using patient contextual information in clinical decision-making in Dutch CR, defining its types and impact on lifestyle coaching and counseling. We discuss implications for holistic telemonitoring inspired by our results, including ways to gather and use identified contextual data in CTR. We advocate for a shift in designing telemonitoring systems that incorporate open, more flexible data collection approaches that support the "situated objectivity" of behavior data, making it meaningful for HCPs by closely aligning it with patients' individual identities. Enhanced telemonitoring can make data more actionable, but designers must consider trade-offs like clinician workload and patient self-reporting burden. While comprehensive data collection is challenging, emerging open data collection approaches (e.g., [15, 19]) offer potential. Future work should also raise multi-stakeholder awareness about the importance of considering patient context in CTR intervention design.[2]

A   Appendix

A.1   Patient Barriers and Facilitators in CR Presented on the Miro Board

Table 1. Barriers and facilitators of patient behavior in cardiac rehabilitation utilized to create the Miro board visualization used in the interview.

Category	Contextual factors
Socio-demographic	age, profession, educational level, income status, race, gender, family composition, relationship status, social support, family/home obligations, available free time, routines and habits, upbringing, previous lifestyle, geography around the home, living situation, insured/not insured, culture and religion
Practical and resource-related	transport to the center, distance to the center, endorsement by the HCP, length of the program, quality of the program, similar exercise opportunities around the home, safe environment in the program, amount of suggested changes, timing between hospitalization and the beginning of the program, timing of the information, support after the end of the program, inclusion of the partner in the program, personalization of the program, quality and quantity of the information, information provided to the partner, chosen goals
Psychological, cognitive, and personality-related	depression, anxiety, mood problems, anxiety to perform physical activity, self-efficacy, confidence, motivation, familiarity with one's body, trust in the efficiency of the program, ability to negotiate with oneself, self-control, ability to understand information, ability to self-reflect, ability to manage one's time, self-awareness, personality type, perception of symptoms, beliefs about the illness and treatment, perception of consequences of illness, coping mechanisms, resourcefulness, self-esteem
Clinical and physical	other comorbidities, physical fitness, physical activity levels, self-sufficiency, presence of symptoms

The list above identifies barriers and facilitators affecting patient behavior during and after CR. In the absence of studies documenting information used by clinicians in CR to guide lifestyle coaching and counseling, we select studies whose aim is to understand why patients face difficulties in completing CR programs in order to improve the programs. The review aimed to develop a supporting overview that could guide the conversation with the participants. The

[2] This work is supported by the ITEA 4 INNO4HEALTH 19008 Project.

list has been compiled by looking at (i) various behavioral models (e.g., biopsy-chosocial [23,44], socio-ecological [38,74], Com-B [102], trans-theoretical [82], and Fogg Behavior Model [42]) as well as (ii) a representative corpus of studies which explore diverse sources of barriers and facilitators in CR ranging from patient interviews to medical records (e.g., [29,68,103]), investigations into patient dropouts at different stages like CR uptake, adherence, completion or self-management (e.g., [14,21,64,87]), or barriers of specific sub-groups such as women or rural patients (e.g., [1,9,41,60]) (Tables 1 and 2).

A.2 Participants

Table 2. Participants; information about their role and expertise was gathered from the interviews, as well as public websites with the participants' consent

Participant ID and expertise	Experience and role
CP1 - Clinical psychologist at the Department of Clinical Psychology in a teaching hospital	They consult patients in cardiac rehabilitation, geriatrics, and oncology. Specialized in trauma treatment with EMDR (Eye Movement Desensitisation and Reprocessing) [91], they assess psychiatric and psychological problems (that were already present or developed after the cardiac event), supervise psycho-educational prevention modules (group sessions), and offer individual treatment of patients if necessary.
CP2 - Clinical psychologist, psychotherapist, and tobacco addiction specialist working in a CR clinic	With decades of experience, they hold a similar role to CP1. They also help patients during the smoking cessation process.
SP - Sports physician specializing in injury treatment, chronic conditions, and vascular problems, working in a teaching hospital	With decades of experience, they help patients with chronic conditions improve their physical fitness. They are nationally involved in developing exercise tests and training programs for patients with heart disease, lung disease, and cancer. They conduct cardiopulmonary exercise testing, formulate training recommendations, offer consultations for discussing test results and recommendations, supervise results of exercise stress tests [86].
NP - Nurse practitioner specialized in cardiac rehabilitation	With decades of experience, they hold the title of "case manager", i.e. patient advocate that supports, guides, and coordinates patient care. They conduct intake sessions for discussion of lifestyle behavior/changes and individual goals, perform assessments for risk for anxiety and depression, and end evaluation of the CR program.
DT - Dietitian and researcher in nutrition	With a Ph.D. in dietary assessment, they have practiced as a dietitian. They perform work on advancements in dietary assessment and the use of data for health behavior research. During the CR program, dietitians assist patients in making better dietary choices.
PT - Professor of physiotherapy and former physiotherapist in a cardiac rehabilitation center	With a Ph.D. in factors influencing rehabilitation outcomes they teach physiotherapy at the University. They have years of experience as a physiotherapist in a CR clinic. As a physiotherapist, they supervise the individually tailored exercise training program and are a supporter of a physically active lifestyle.
PM - Professor of behavioral change and former project manager in a cardiac rehabilitation hospital unit	With a Ph.D. specializing in cardiac telerehabilitation programs, they develop lifestyle interventions to prevent chronic conditions. Previously a hospital project manager in the CR unit, they were responsible for conducting research and developing efficient CR programs for patients together with clinicians.

References

1. Ades, P.A., Waldmann, M.L., Polk, D.M., Coflesky, J.T.: Referral patterns and exercise response in the rehabilitation of female coronary patients aged 62 years. Am. J. Cardiol. **69**, 1422–1425 (1992). https://doi.org/10.1016/0002-9149(92)90894-5

2. Akinsiku, A., Graham, Y., Avellino, I., Mentis, H.M.: It's not just the movement: experiential information needed for stroke tele rehabilitation. In: Conference on Human Factors in Computing Systems - Proceedings (2021). https://doi.org/10.1145/3411764.3445663

3. Amorim, P., Paiva, J., de Lima, J.S., da Fonseca, L.P., Martins, H., Silva, P.A.: Lessons learned from investigating patients' and physiotherapists' perspectives on the design of a telerehabilitation platform. Disabil. Rehabil. Assistive Technol. (2023). https://doi.org/10.1080/17483107.2023.2287160

4. Andersen, T., Bjørn, P., Kensing, F., Moll, J.: Designing for collaborative interpretation in telemonitoring: re-introducing patients as diagnostic agents. Int. J. Med. Inf. **80** (2011). https://doi.org/10.1016/J.IJMEDINF.2010.09.010

5. Andersen, T.O., Andersen, P.R.D., Kornum, A.C., Larsen, T.M.: Understanding patient experience: a deployment study in cardiac remote monitoring. In: Proceedings of the 11th EAI International Conference on Pervasive Computing Technologies for Healthcare (2017). https://doi.org/10.1145/3154862

6. Andersen, T.O., et al.: Aligning concerns in telecare: three concepts to guide the design of patient-centred e-health. Comput. Support. Coop. Work CSCW Int. J. **27**, 1181–1214 (2018). https://doi.org/10.1007/S10606-018-9309-1/FIGURES/8

7. Andersen, T.O., Fritsch, J., Matthiesen, S.: Patient data work with consumer self-tracking: exploring affective and temporal dimensions in chronic self-care. LNICST **488 LNICST**, 666–680 (2023). https://doi.org/10.1007/978-3-031-34586-9_44/COVER

8. Andersen, T.O., Langstrup, H., Lomborg, S.: Experiences with wearable activity data during self-care by chronic heart patients: qualitative study. J. Med. Internet Res. **22**(7), e15873 (2020). https://doi.org/10.2196/15873

9. Angelis, C.D., Bunker, S., Schoo, A.: Exploring the barriers and enablers to attendance at rural cardiac rehabilitation programs. Aust. J. Rural Health **16**, 137–142 (2008). https://doi.org/10.1111/J.1440-1584.2008.00963.X

10. Arena, R., et al.: Increasing referral and participation rates to outpatient cardiac rehabilitation: the valuable role of healthcare professionals in the inpatient and home health settings. Circulation **125**, 1321–1329 (2012). https://doi.org/10.1161/CIR.0B013E318246B1E5

11. Arnold, M., Kerridge, I.: Accelerating the de-personalization of medicine: the ethical toxicities of COVID-19. J. Bioethical Inquiry **17**, 815–821 (2020). https://doi.org/10.1007/S11673-020-10026-7/METRICS

12. Ashfaq, Z., et al.: A review of enabling technologies for internet of medical things (IoMT) ecosystem. Ain Shams Eng. J. **13**, 101660 (2022). https://doi.org/10.1016/J.ASEJ.2021.101660

13. Bansler, J., et al.: Physicians' progress notes. In: ECSCW 2013: Proceedings of the 13th European Conference on Computer Supported Cooperative Work, 21-25 September 2013, Paphos, Cyprus, pp. 123–142 (2013). https://doi.org/10.1007/978-1-4471-5346-7_7

14. Barber, K., Stommel, M., Kroll, J., Holmes-Rovner, M., McIntosh, B.: Cardiac rehabilitation for community-based patients with myocardial infarction: factors predicting discharge recommendation and participation. J. Clin. Epidemiol. **54**, 1025–1030 (2001). https://doi.org/10.1016/S0895-4356(01)00375-4

15. Barker-Canler, M., Gooch, D., van der Linden, J., Petre, M.: Flexible minimalist self-tracking to support individual reflection. ACM Trans. Comput.-Hum. Interact. (2022). https://doi.org/10.1145/3660339

16. Barlow, J., Wright, C., Sheasby, J., Turner, A., Hainsworth, J.: Self-management approaches for people with chronic conditions: a review. Patient Educ. Couns. **48**, 177–187 (2002). https://doi.org/10.1016/S0738-3991(02)00032-0

17. Batalik, L., Filakova, K., Batalikova, K., Dosbaba, F.: Remotely monitored telerehabilitation for cardiac patients: a review of the current situation. World J. Clin. Cases **8**, 1818 (2020). https://doi.org/10.12998/WJCC.V8.I10.1818

18. Beatty, A.L., Magnusson, S.L., Fortney, J.C., Sayre, G.G., Whooley, M.A.: VA FitHeart, a mobile app for cardiac rehabilitation: Usability study. JMIR Hum. Factors **5**(1), e8017 (2018). https://doi.org/10.2196/HUMANFACTORS.8017

19. Bhat, K.S., Kumar, N.: Sociocultural dimensions of tracking health and taking care. Proc. ACM Hum.-Comput. Interact. **4** (2020). https://doi.org/10.1145/3415200

20. Blandford, A., Gibbs, J., Newhouse, N., Perski, O., Singh, A., Murray, E.: Seven lessons for interdisciplinary research on interactive digital health interventions. Digital Health **4**, 205520761877032 (2018). https://doi.org/10.1177/2055207618770325

21. Bock, B.C., Carmona-Barros, R.E., Esler, J.L., Tilkemeier, P.L.: Program participation and physical activity maintenance after cardiac rehabilitation. Behav. Modif. **27**, 37–53 (2003). https://doi.org/10.1177/0145445502238692

22. Bock, B.C., Marcus, B.H., Pinto, B.M., Forsyth, L.H.: Maintenance of physical activity following an individualized motivationally tailored intervention. Ann. Behav. Med. **23**, 79–87 (2001). https://doi.org/10.1207/S15324796ABM2302_2

23. Borell-Carrió, F., Suchman, A.L., Epstein, R.M.: The biopsychosocial model 25 years later: principles, practice, and scientific inquiry. Ann. Fam. Med. **2**, 576 (2004). https://doi.org/10.1370/AFM.245

24. Bouchard, K., Gareau, A., McKee, K., Lalande, K., Greenman, P.S., Tulloch, H.: Dyadic patterns of mental health and quality of life change in partners and patients during three months of cardiac rehabilitation. J. Fam. Psychol. (2021). https://doi.org/10.1037/FAM0000898

25. Brouwers, R.W., et al.: Cardiac telerehabilitation as an alternative to centre-based cardiac rehabilitation. Neth. Heart J. **28**, 443–451 (2020). https://doi.org/10.1007/S12471-020-01432-Y/FIGURES/1

26. Caldeira, C., Figueiredo, M.C., Dodakian, L., Souza, C.R.D., Cramer, S.C., Chen, Y.: Towards supporting data-driven practices in stroke telerehabilitation technology. Proc. ACM Hum.-Comput. Interact. **5**, 33 (2021). https://doi.org/10.1145/3449099

27. Cannière, H.D., et al.: Wearable monitoring and interpretable machine learning can objectively track progression in patients during cardiac rehabilitation. Sensors **20**, 3601 (2020). https://doi.org/10.3390/S20123601

28. Chen, S.H., et al.: Patient perspectives on innovative telemonitoring enhanced care program for chronic heart failure (ITEC-CHF): usability study. JMIR Cardio **5**, e24611 (2021). https://doi.org/10.2196/24611

29. Clark, A.M., Whelan, H.K., Barbour, R., MacIntyre, P.D.: A realist study of the mechanisms of cardiac rehabilitation. J. Adv. Nurs. **52**, 362–371 (2005). https://doi.org/10.1111/J.1365-2648.2005.03601.X

30. Clarke, V., Braun, V., Hayfield, N.: Thematic analysis. In: Qualitative Psychology: A Practical Guide to Research Methods, vol. 222, p. 248 (2015)

31. Cooper, A.F., Jackson, G., Weinman, J., Horne, R.: A qualitative study investigating patients' beliefs about cardiac rehabilitation. Clin. Rehabil. **19**, 87–96 (2005). https://doi.org/10.1191/0269215505CR818OA

32. Corr, U., et al.: Secondary prevention through cardiac rehabilitation: physical activity counselling and exercise training: key components of the position paper from the cardiac rehabilitation section of the European association of cardiovascular prevention and rehabilitation. Eur. Heart J. **31** (2010). https://doi.org/10.1093/EURHEARTJ/EHQ236

33. Cruz-Martínez, R.R., Wentzel, J., Bente, B.E., Sanderman, R., Gemert-Pijnen, J.E.V.: Toward the value sensitive design of ehealth technologies to support self-management of cardiovascular diseases: content analysis (2021). https://doi.org/10.2196/31985

34. Dalal, H.M., Doherty, P., Taylor, R.S.: Cardiac rehabilitation. BMJ **351** (2015). https://doi.org/10.1136/BMJ.H5000

35. Daly, J., Sindone, A.P., Thompson, D.R., Hancock, K., Chang, E., Davidson, P.: Barriers to participation in and adherence to cardiac rehabilitation programs: a critical literature review. Prog. Cardiovas. Nurs. **17**, 8–17 (2002). https://doi.org/10.1111/J.0889-7204.2002.00614.X

36. Davis, M.M., Freeman, M., Kaye, J., Vuckovic, N., Buckley, D.I.: A systematic review of clinician and staff views on the acceptability of incorporating remote monitoring technology into primary care. Telemed. e-Health **20**, 428–438 (2014). https://www.liebertpub.com/doi/10.1089/tmj.2013.0166

37. Ding, H., et al.: The effects of telemonitoring on patient compliance with self-management recommendations and outcomes of the innovative telemonitoring enhanced care program for chronic heart failure: randomized controlled trial. J. Med. Internet Res. **22**, e17559 (2020). https://doi.org/10.2196/17559

38. Centers for Disease Control and Prevention: The social-ecological model: a framework for prevention (2022). https://www.cdc.gov/violenceprevention/about/social-ecologicalmodel.html

39. El-Dassouki, N., et al.: The value of technology to support dyadic caregiving for individuals living with heart failure: qualitative descriptive study. J. Med. Internet Res. **24**, e40108 (2022). https://doi.org/10.2196/40108

40. Elliott, R., Timulak, L.: Descriptive and interpretive approaches to qualitative research. In: A Handbook of Research Methods for Clinical and Health Psychology, pp. 147–159 (2005). https://doi.org/10.1093/med:psych/9780198527565.001.0001

41. Fletcher, S.M., Burley, M.B., Thomas, K.E., Mitchell, E.K.: Feeling supported and abandoned: mixed messages from attendance at a rural community cardiac rehabilitation program in Australia. J. Cardiopulm. Rehabil. Prev. **34**, 29–33 (2014). https://doi.org/10.1097/HCR.0B013E3182A52734

42. Fogg, B.: A behavior model for persuasive design. **350** (2009). https://doi.org/10.1145/1541948.1541999

43. Frederix, I., et al.: Increasing the medium-term clinical benefits of hospital-based cardiac rehabilitation by physical activity telemonitoring in coronary artery disease patients. Eur. J. Prev. Cardiol. **22**, 150–158 (2015). https://doi.org/10.1177/2047487313514018

44. Gatchel, R.J., Peng, Y.B., Peters, M.L., Fuchs, P.N., Turk, D.C.: The biopsychosocial approach to chronic pain: scientific advances and future directions. Psychol. Bull. **133**, 581–624 (2007). https://doi.org/10.1037/0033-2909.133.4.581

45. Gibson, R.C., Dunlop, M.D., Bouamrane, M.M., Nayar, R.: Designing clinical AAC tablet applications with adults who have mild intellectual disabilities. Assoc. Comput. Mach. (2020). https://doi.org/10.1145/3313831.3376159
46. Goevaerts, W.F., Limpt, N.C.T., Lu, Y., Kop, W.J., Kemps, H.M., Brouwers, R.W.: Evaluation of an application for the self-assessment of lifestyle behaviour in cardiac patients. Neth. Heart J. **32** (2024). https://doi.org/10.1007/S12471-023-01835-7
47. Graham, S.: An attributional theory of motivation. Contemp. Educ. Psychol. **61**, 101861 (2020). https://doi.org/10.1016/j.cedpsych.2020.101861
48. Gupta, A., Heng, T., Shaw, C., Gromala, D., Leese, J., Li, L.: Oh, I didn't do a good job: how objective data affects physiotherapist-patient conversations for arthritis patients, pp. 156–165. Association for Computing Machinery (2020). https://doi.org/10.1145/3421937.3421991
49. Hanlon, P., Daines, L., Campbell, C., Mckinstry, B., Weller, D., Pinnock, H.: Telehealth interventions to support self-management of long-term conditions: a systematic metareview of diabetes, heart failure, asthma, chronic obstructive pulmonary disease, and cancer. J. Med. Internet Res. **19** (2017). https://doi.org/10.2196/JMIR.6688
50. Hartstichting: Hartrevalidatie (2021). https://www.hartstichting.nl/hart-en-vaatziekten/behandelingen/hartrevalidatie
51. Heimer, M., et al.: ehealth for maintenance cardiovascular rehabilitation: a systematic review and meta-analysis. Eur. J. Prev. Cardiol. **30**, 1634–1651 (2023). https://doi.org/10.1093/EURJPC/ZWAD145
52. Herkert, C., Graat-Verboom, L., Gilsing-Fernhout, J., Schols, M., Kemps, H.M.C.: Home-based exercise program for patients with combined advanced chronic cardiac and pulmonary diseases: Exploratory study. JMIR Formative Res. **5**, e28634 (2021). https://doi.org/10.2196/28634
53. Herkert, C., Kraal, J.J., Spee, R.F., Serier, A., Graat-Verboom, L., Kemps, H.M.C.: Quality assessment of an integrated care pathway using telemonitoring in patients with chronic heart failure and chronic obstructive pulmonary disease: protocol for a quasi-experimental study. JMIR Res. Protocols **9**, e20571 (2020). https://doi.org/10.2196/20571
54. Holder, G.N., Young, W.C., Nadarajah, S.R., Berger, A.M.: Psychosocial experiences in the context of life-threatening illness: the cardiac rehabilitation patient. Palliat. Support. Care **13**, 749–756 (2015). https://doi.org/10.1017/S1478951514000583
55. Huygens, M.W.J., et al.: The uptake and use of telemonitoring in chronic care between 2014 and 2019: nationwide survey among patients and health care professionals in the netherlands. J. Med. Internet Res. **23**, e24908 (2021). https://doi.org/10.2196/24908
56. Hwang, R., Gane, E.M., Morris, N.R.: No transport? No worries! Cardiac telerehabilitation is a feasible and effective alternative to centre-based programs. Heart Fail. Rev. **1**, 1 (2023). https://doi.org/10.1007/S10741-023-10301-W
57. Iott, B., Caverly, T., Fishstrom, A., King, D., Meng, G., Flynn, A.: Clinician perspectives on the user experience, configuration, and scope of use of a patient reported outcomes (pro) dashboard. In: PervasiveHealth: Pervasive Computing Technologies for Healthcare, pp. 21–30 (2019). https://doi.org/10.1145/3329189.3329198
58. Jackson, L., Leclerc, J., Erskine, Y., Linden, W.: Getting the most out of cardiac rehabilitation: a review of referral and adherence predictors. Heart **91**, 10–14 (2005). https://doi.org/10.1136/hrt.2004.045559

59. Jeng, C., Braun, L.T.: Bandura's self-efficacy theory: a guide for cardiac rehabilitation nursing practice. J. Holis. Nurs. **12**, 425–436 (1994). https://doi.org/10.1177/089801019401200411

60. Johnson, J.E., Weinert, C., Richardson, J.K.: Rural residents' use of cardiac rehabilitation programs. Pub. Health Nurs. **15**, 288–296 (1998). https://doi.org/10.1111/J.1525-1446.1998.TB00352.X

61. Kakria, P., Tripathi, N.K., Kitipawang, P.: A real-time health monitoring system for remote cardiac patients using smartphone and wearable sensors. Int. J. Telemed. Appl. **2015**(1), 373474 (2015). https://doi.org/10.1155/2015/373474

62. Kim, S.R., Kim, S., Cho, B.H., Yu, S., Cho, K.H.: Influence of type D personality on health promoting behaviours and quality of life in stroke patients: a cross-sectional study in South Korea. J. Stroke Cerebrovasc. Dis. **30**(5), 105721 (2021). https://doi.org/10.1016/j.jstrokecerebrovasdis.2021.105721

63. Kinast, B., Lutz, M., Schreiweis, B.: Telemonitoring of real-world health data in cardiology: a systematic review. Int. J. Environ. Res. Pub. Health **18**, 9070 (2021). https://doi.org/10.3390/IJERPH18179070/S1

64. Knudsen, M.V., et al.: Lifestyle after cardiac rehabilitation: did the message come across, and was it feasible? An analysis of patients' narratives. Health **6**, 2641–2650 (2014). https://doi.org/10.4236/HEALTH.2014.619303

65. Kondratova, I., Fournier, H.: Virtual cardiac rehabilitation in a pandemic scenario: a review of HCI design features, user acceptance and barriers. LNCS (including subseries Lecture Notes in Artificial Intelligence and Lecture Notes in Bioinformatics) vol. 13330, pp. 485–499. Springer (2022). https://doi.org/10.1007/978-3-031-05581-2_34/TABLES/4

66. Kreikebaum, S., Guarneri, E., Talavera, G., Madanat, H., Smith, T.: Evaluation of a holistic cardiac rehabilitation in the reduction of biopsychosocial risk factors among patients with coronary heart disease. Psychol. Health Med. **16**, 276–290 (2011). https://doi.org/10.1080/13548506.2010.542170

67. Kristofferzon, M.L., Löfmark, R., Carlsson, M.: Striving for balance in daily life: experiences of Swedish women and men shortly after a myocardial infarction. J. Clin. Nurs. **16**, 391–401 (2007). https://doi.org/10.1111/J.1365-2702.2005.01518.X

68. Lane, D., Carroll, D., Ring, C., Beevers, D., Lip, G.Y.: Predictors of attendance at cardiac rehabilitation after myocardial infarction. J. Psychosom. Res. **51**(3), 497–501 (2001). https://doi.org/10.1016/S0022-3999(01)00225-2

69. Luijks, H., van Boven, K., olde Hartman, T., Uijen, A., van Weel, C., Schers, H.: Purposeful incorporation of patient narratives in the medical record in the Netherlands. J. Am. Board Fam. Med. **34**, 709–723 (2021). https://doi.org/10.3122/JABFM.2021.04.200609

70. Shimbo, M., Amiya, E., Komuro, I.: Telemonitoring during exercise training in cardiac telerehabilitation: a review. Rev. Cardiovasc. Med. **24**, 104 (2023). https://doi.org/10.31083/J.RCM2404104/2153-8174-24-4-104/FIG2.JPG

71. Morimoto, Y., et al.: Web portals for patients with chronic diseases: scoping review of the functional features and theoretical frameworks of telerehabilitation platforms. J. Med. Internet Res. **24**(1), e27759 (2022). https://doi.org/10.2196/27759

72. Murnane, E.L., Walker, T.G., Tench, B., Voida, S., Snyder, J.: Personal informatics in interpersonal contexts. Proc. ACM Hum.-Comput. Interact. **2** (2018). https://doi.org/10.1145/3274396

73. Murray, J., Craigs, C.L., Hill, K.M., Honey, S., House, A.: A systematic review of patient reported factors associated with uptake and completion of cardiovascular

lifestyle behaviour change. BMC Cardiovas. Disord. **12**, 1–12 (2012). https://doi.org/10.1186/1471-2261-12-120/TABLES/8

74. NIH, N.I.o.H.: Principles of Community Engagement - Second Edition. National Institutes of Health (U.S.). Centers for Disease Control and Prevention (U.S.) (2011)

75. O'Connor, C.M., et al.: Efficacy and safety of exercise training in patients with chronic heart failure: Hf-action randomized controlled trial. JAMA **301**, 1439 (2009). https://doi.org/10.1001/JAMA.2009.454

76. Ongwere, T., Cantor, G.S., Clawson, J., Shih, P.C., Connelly, K.: Design and care for discordant chronic comorbidities: a comparison of healthcare providers' perspectives. In: PervasiveHealth: Pervasive Computing Technologies for Healthcare, pp. 133–145 (2020). https://doi.org/10.1145/3421937.3422013

77. Organization, W.H.: Cardiovascular diseases (CVDS) (2021). https://www.who.int/news-room/fact-sheets/detail/cardiovascular-diseases-(cvds)

78. Pantzar, M., Ruckenstein, M.: Living the metrics: self-tracking and situated objectivity. Digital Health **3**, 205520761771259 (2017). https://doi.org/10.1177/2055207617712590

79. Peretti, A., Amenta, F., Tayebati, S.K., Nittari, G., Mahdi, S.S.: Telerehabilitation: review of the state-of-the-art and areas of application. JMIR Rehabil. Assist. Technol. **4**, e7 (2017). https://doi.org/10.2196/rehab.7511

80. Piera-Jiménez, J., et al.: Changing the health behavior of patients with cardiovascular disease through an electronic health intervention in three different countries: cost-effectiveness study in the do cardiac health: advanced new generation ecosystem (do change) 2 randomized controlled trial. J. Med. Internet Res. **22**, e17351 (2020). https://doi.org/10.2196/17351

81. Pine, K.H., et al.: Data work in healthcare: challenges for patients, clinicians and administrators. In: Proceedings of the ACM Conference on Computer Supported Cooperative Work, CSCW, pp. 433–439 (2018). https://doi.org/10.1145/3272973.3273017

82. Prochaska, J.O., Velicer, W.F.: The transtheoretical model of health behavior change. A JHP **12**, 38–48 (1997). https://doi.org/10.4278/0890-1171-12.1.38

83. Pryor, T., Page, K., Patsamanis, H., Jolly, K.A.: Investigating support needs for people living with heart disease. J. Clin. Nurs. **23**, 166–172 (2014). https://doi.org/10.1111/JOCN.12165

84. Quazi, S., Malik, J.A.: A systematic review of personalized health applications through human-computer interactions (HCI) on cardiovascular health optimization. J. Cardiovasc. Develop. Dis. **9**, 273 (2022). https://doi.org/10.3390/JCDD9080273

85. Riegel, B., et al.: Self-care for the prevention and management of cardiovascular disease and stroke: a scientific statement for healthcare professionals from the American heart association. J. Am. Heart Assoc. Cardiovasc. Cerebrovasc. Dis. **6** (2017). https://doi.org/10.1161/JAHA.117.006997

86. Saba, M.A., Goharpey, S., Moghadam, B.A., Salehi, R., Nejatian, M.: Correlation between the 6-min walk test and exercise tolerance test in cardiac rehabilitation after coronary artery bypass grafting: a cross-sectional study. Cardiol. Therapy **10**, 201–209 (2021). https://doi.org/10.1007/S40119-021-00210-0/FIGURES/1

87. Scholz, U., Knoll, N., Sniehotta, F.F., Schwarzer, R.: Physical activity and depressive symptoms in cardiac rehabilitation: long-term effects of a self-management intervention. Soc. Sci. Med. **62**(12), 3109–3120 (2006). https://doi.org/10.1016/j.socscimed.2005.11.035

88. EACPR Committee for Science Guidelines, et al.: Secondary prevention through cardiac rehabilitation: physical activity counselling and exercise training: key components of the position paper from the cardiac rehabilitation section of the European association of cardiovascular prevention and rehabilitation. Euro. Heart J. **31**(16), 1967–1974 (2010)

89. Seals, A., et al.: Are they doing better in the clinic or at home?: understanding clinicians' needs when visualizing wearable sensor data used in remote Gait assessments for people with multiple sclerosis. In: Conference on Human Factors in Computing Systems - Proceedings (2022). https://doi.org/10.1145/3491102.3501989

90. Seo, K., Ryu, H., Kim, J., Jang, S.: RehabMasterTM: a pervasive Rehabilitation-platform for stroke patients and Theircaregivers (2014). https://doi.org/10.1007/978-1-4471-6413-5_6

91. Shapiro, F.: EMDR, adaptive information processing, and case conceptualization. J. EMDR Pract. Res. **1**(2), 68–87 (2007). https://doi.org/10.1891/1933-3196.1.2.68

92. Sookrah, R., Dhowtal, J.D., Devi Nagowah, S.: A dash diet recommendation system for hypertensive patients using machine learning. In: 2019 7th International Conference on Information and Communication Technology (ICoICT), pp. 1–6 (2019). https://doi.org/10.1109/ICoICT.2019.8835323

93. Supervia, M., et al.: Nature of cardiac rehabilitation around the globe. EClinicalMedicine **13**, 46–56 (2019). https://doi.org/10.1016/j.eclinm.2019.06.006

94. Tadas, S., Coyle, D.: Barriers to and facilitators of technology in cardiac rehabilitation and self-management: systematic qualitative grounded theory review. J. Med. Internet Res. **22** (2020). https://doi.org/10.2196/18025

95. Tadas, S., Dickson, J., Coyle, D.: Using patient-generated data to support cardiac rehabilitation and the transition to self-care. In: Conference on Human Factors in Computing Systems - Proceedings, p. 16 (2023). https://doi.org/10.1145/3544548.3580822

96. Tadas, S., Pretorius, C., Foster, E.J., Gorely, T., Leslie, S.J., Coyle, D.: Transitions in technology-mediated cardiac rehabilitation and self-management: qualitative study using the theoretical domains framework. JMIR Cardio **5**(2), e30428 (2021). https://doi.org/10.2196/30428

97. Thijs, I., Fresiello, L., Oosterlinck, W., Sinnaeve, P., Rega, F.: Assessment of physical activity by wearable technology during rehabilitation after cardiac surgery: explorative prospective monocentric observational cohort study. JMIR Mhealth Uhealth **7**, e9865 (2019). https://doi.org/10.2196/mhealth.9865

98. Vandelanotte, C., Bourdeaudhuij, I.D., Philippaerts, R., Sjöström, M., Sallis, J.: Reliability and validity of a computerized and Dutch version of the international physical activity questionnaire (IPAQ). J. Phys. Act. Health **2**(1), 63–75 (2005). https://doi.org/10.1123/jpah.2.1.63

99. Ventegodt, S., Kandel, I., Ervin, D.A., Merrick, J.: Concepts of holistic care. In: Health Care for People with Intellectual and Developmental Disabilities Across the Lifespan, pp. 1935–1941 (2016). https://doi.org/10.1007/978-3-319-18096-0_148/FIGURES/1

100. Ware, P., Ross, H.J., Cafazzo, J.A., Boodoo, C., Munnery, M., Seto, E.: Outcomes of a heart failure telemonitoring program implemented as the standard of care in an outpatient heart function clinic: pretest-posttest pragmatic study. J. Med. Internet Res. **22**, e16538 (2020). https://doi.org/10.2196/16538

101. Wilkins, E., Wilson, L., Wickramasinghe, K., Bhatnagar, P., Leal, J., Luengo-Fernandez, R., Burns, R., Rayner, M., Townsend, N.: European Cardiovascular Disease Statistics 2017. European Heart Network, Belgium (2017)

102. Willmott, T.J., Pang, B., Rundle-Thiele, S.: Capability, opportunity, and motivation: an across contexts empirical examination of the COM-B model. BMC Pub. Health **21**, 1–17 (2021). https://doi.org/10.1186/S12889-021-11019-W

103. Worcester, M.U.C., Stojcevski, Z., Murphy, B., Goble, A.J.: Factors associated with non-attendance at a secondary prevention clinic for cardiac patients. Eur. J. Cardiovasc. Nurs. J. Working Group Cardiovasc. Nurs. Eur. Soc. Cardiol. **2**, 151–157 (2003). https://doi.org/10.1016/S1474-5151(03)00031-8

104. Yang, W., et al.: Effectiveness of a family customised online FOCUS programme aimed on building resiliency in dyad relationship to support dyadic illness management in persons with heart failure and their informal caregiver: a randomised clinical trial protocol. BMJ Open **12**, e061405 (2022). https://doi.org/10.1136/BMJOPEN-2022-061405

105. Zhang, C., Soliman-Hamad, M., Robijns, R., Verberkmoes, N., Verstappen, F., IJsselsteijn, W.A.: Promoting physical activity with self-tracking and mobile-based coaching for cardiac surgery patients during the discharge-rehabilitation gap: protocol for a randomized controlled trial. JMIR Res. Protocols **9**, e16737 (2020). https://doi.org/10.2196/16737

3rd IOT-HR: Workshop on Internet of Things in Health Research

Enhancing In Vitro Fertilization with Environment Optimization Utilizing Artificial Intelligence (EIVF-AI)

Reza Khoshkangini[1]([⊠]), Elisabeth Mangrio[1], and Magnus Johnsson[2]

[1] Internet of Things and People Research Center, Department of Computer Science
and Media Technology, Malmö University, Malmö, Sweden
{reza.khoshkangini,elisabeth.mangrio}@mau.se
[2] Kristianstad University, Kristianstad, Sweden
magnus.johansson@mau.se

Abstract. In vitro fertilization (IVF) is of great aid to couples who are struggling to conceive. The IVF clinics, where couples undergo fertility treatments, require a carefully controlled environment to ensure the effectiveness of the procedures. In recent years, IVF has seen significant progress, thanks to new technologies and methods that improve success rates and expand options for infertile couples. One notable advancement involves combining pre-implantation genetic testing (PGT) with time-lapse imaging technology, which allows continuous monitoring of embryo development with minimal disturbance. This innovation improves the selection of healthy embryos for transfer, increasing success rates and reducing the risk of multiple pregnancies. However, maintaining a stable environment remains a key challenge. Fluctuations in temperature, humidity, air quality, and particulate matter can affect IVF success rates by disrupting the embryo's delicate environment and potentially causing implantation failure. We discuss in this position paper our approach to alleviate such environmental problems in our project EIVF-AI funded by the Swedish funding agency Vinnova.

Keywords: In vitro fertilization (IVF) · Machine Learning · Artificial intelligence · Optimization

1 Introduction

IVF clinics are essential for couples seeking fertility treatments, requiring a controlled and optimal environment to ensure the efficacy of the procedures. Recent advancements in IVF technology have significantly improved success rates and broadened options for couples facing infertility. Artificial Intelligence (AI) is now being utilized in IVF to enhance precision and efficacy, tailoring treatment plans to individual patient needs.

The IVF industry is characterized by rapid technological advancement, and AI is making significant inroads in several key areas such as embryo selection,

H. Kondylakis and A. Triantafyllidis (Eds.): PervasiveHealth 2024, LNICST 612, pp. 151–158, 2025.
https://doi.org/10.1007/978-3-031-85575-7_8

sperm sorting, and risk assessment [1–3]. AI technologies analyze factors including morphology, development, and genetics to evaluate embryo quality, identify viable embryos for transfer, and assess risks during IVF treatment. However, the laboratory environment's impact on IVF outcomes remains a crucial and underexplored area [4–6]. Factors like air quality, temperature, and light exposure within the laboratory can significantly influence embryo development and quality, ultimately affecting the success of IVF treatments.

We argue that the employment of vast yet underutilized data resources to enhance the efficacy of IVF procedures by leveraging AI and Machine Learning (ML) technologies can further improve IVF success rates, addressing critical global issues related to fertility, family planning, mental health, and socioeconomic equality. By analyzing and interpreting data on laboratory environmental factors, discerning their impact on pregnancy rates, and developing models to understand the efficiency of environmental conditions, we aim to identify actionable insights for various stakeholders involved in the process. In the remaining parts of this paper, we explore the EIVF-AI project, a collaborative effort between Malmö University (MAU), Kristianstad University (HKR), OpenLogger Systems AB, and Reproduktionsmedicinskt centrum (RMC). We do so by first priming the reader with some relevant background on the application of AI technology to IVF and embryology. Then we move on to a presentation of our particular approaches to apply AI to improve the understanding of laboratory environmental factors to enhance the efficacy of IVF procedures, and we finalize with a discussion and some conclusions.

2   AI Technology Applied to IVF and Embryology

Various kinds of AI technology have been applied in the context of IVF and embryology. This has been done with an emphasis on the evaluation of embryos, which in turn is important e.g. when deciding whether to implant an embryo or not. When it comes to evaluating embryos, it is important to keep track of its development over time, e.g. particular timings of cellular divisions and to detect various kinds of abnormal development. To aid in the automatization of this, automatic annotation of time-lapse microscopic photography of embryo development is of importance. Besides making the whole process more efficient it also makes it possible to avoid problems with intra- and interoperator variability associated with manual annotation. In particular, convolutional neural networks have been successfully employed for such automatic annotation of time-lapse photography of embryo development [6,7].

AI technology has been used in the context of embryo grading, focusing on blastocysts and their evaluation for implantation potential. As in the case of automatic annotation of time-lapse microscopic photography described above, there are similar challenges in human grading of embryos. A problem that AI algorithms can help alleviate [8,9].

There is an ongoing debate about using static images versus time-lapse microscopy videos for assessment, with AI systems showing promise in both scenarios. Efforts have been made to differentiate inner cell mass and trophectoderm using image segmentation and machine learning methods [10]. Studies demonstrate high accuracy in predicting blastocyst quality using AI models trained on embryo images [9]. Various statistical models and AI methods using morphokinetic parameters from time-lapse microscopy data have been developed to predict implantation potential at different stages of embryo development [11,12]. AI-based models have also been used to predict embryo implantation by analyzing embryo images or videos, although concerns exist regarding data imbalance and model validation [11,12]. Studies using AI on time-lapse microscopy data have shown promising results, with some models claiming improvements over embryologist grading. However, challenges such as unbalanced data sets and variability among laboratories need to be addressed for reliable AI predictions.

Another area important for IVF is embryo ploidy prediction. The use of invasive embryo biopsy techniques comes with its own challenges, and hence there are ongoing efforts to develop noninvasive methods. One such technique involves cell-free DNA analysis from spent embryo culture media [13], but AI-based analysis is also being explored. Studies have shown associations between embryo morphology, blastocyst grading, blastocyst scores, and embryo ploidy, with high-quality embryos more likely to be euploid [14,15]. Time-lapse microscopy studies have also linked embryo morphokinetics to ploidy status [16,17], although single aneuploidies may be difficult to predict through image analysis alone, whereas AI may identify complex aneuploidies more effectively. Nonetheless, neither noninvasive techniques nor preimplantation genetic testing for aneuploidy (PGT-A) can predict aneuploidies with 100% accuracy. Recent studies using AI and image analysis have shown promise in predicting ploidy status. For example, [18] utilized AI computer vision to predict embryo ploidy from a single blastocyst image with 70% accuracy, highlighting the potential of AI in noninvasive ploidy prediction, though the authors acknowledge the need for larger datasets to validate their algorithm.

Besides the employment for embryo grading and selection, and for embryo implantation success and ploidy prediction, AI technology has also been applied in some other, for IVF, relevant areas. For example, machine learning has been applied to assess and select competent oocytes [19], to analyze semen [20] and to evaluate sperm [21] and their genetic integrity [22]. One of the applicants for this grant has also been involved in the application of AI technology to predict the quality of semen based on environmental as well as lifestyle factors [23]. Other examples are the employment of AI technology and convolutional neural networks for miscarriage prediction and the employment of machine learning for ovary and uterus evaluation [24].

3 Proposed Statement

This position paper posits that implementing AI technologies to optimize laboratory environments in IVF clinics can significantly enhance success rates, providing substantial benefits for individuals and society. Thus, we explore the potential for applying AI technology to enhance the IVF success rate by aiding the understanding of various environmental parameters in and around the incubators. Through the implementation of AI technologies to optimize laboratory environments in IVF clinics, success rates can be significantly enhanced, which will provide substantial benefits for individuals and society. Below we present our approaches.

Modeling Temporal Dependencies in IVF Procedure Using Transformers. Using Transformers for time series data and prediction represents an advanced approach that leverages self-attention mechanisms to capture long-range dependencies within sequential data. In our approach, we analyze time series data featuring multiple features structured as a sequence, where each vector element corresponds to a timestamp. Each timestamp encompasses diverse features such as laboratory environmental data (e.g., temperature, humidity, particles) alongside embryo development parameters like morphokinetic timings and developmental stages. To analyze this data, we feed the sequence directly into a Transformer model after performing feature embedding. Feature embedding entails transforming raw or feature vectors into compact, meaningful representations using methods like learnable embeddings or linear projections. This transformation compresses each feature vector into a lower-dimensional space that captures essential information. Transformers leverage positional encoding such that these encodings provide the model with details about the order of features at each timestamp, effectively incorporating temporal information into the model. We utilize the Temporal Fusion Transformer (TFT) technique to train our multivariate time series data efficiently. TFT is specifically designed to handle such data, where each time step may contain multiple features or variables. To capture long-range dependencies within our integrated embryo development time series data synchronized with external variables, we will adapt attention layers in our transformers. The TFT's attention mechanism operates across both the time dimension (sequentially) and the feature dimension (across different variables like external and embryo development parameters). This capability allows the model to focus on specific features at specific time points based on learned dependencies, enabling accurate forecasting and pattern recognition. Furthermore, we aim to explore different approaches for building transformers based on our collected data to identify the most effective method or uncover any inherent trade-offs between them.

Data Efficient Learning Methods. A powerful strategy to address the challenge of a small training set in the IVF laboratory, involves leveraging synthetic data. Synthetic data has emerged as a promising solution to pre-train deep learning (DL) models, as it allows for effortless generation of labeled datasets using graphics engines. Generative DL models can play a crucial role in automatically synthesizing labeled datasets tailored to the specific learning task, with a content distribution that matches the data captured during IVF procedures, including factors such as development status and external laboratory environmental conditions like temperature, humidity, and particle levels. Currently, creating high-quality synthetic datasets often requires substantial time and expertise from qualified experts, particularly for tasks like generating driving scenes, controlling robots, or simulating indoor navigation. Therefore, there is a clear need to develop more efficient approaches. Techniques such as domain randomization and the use of generative adversarial networks (GANs) can be explored to adjust synthetic data distributions and make them more closely resemble the real-world data encountered in the IVF laboratory setting. These advancements will enhance the effectiveness of using synthetic data to augment limited training datasets in IVF research and development.

Learning from Multiple Sources Using Multimodal Learning. We explore how different sensor modalities can be utilized to make models by extracting complementary knowledge from data streams, which can vary in terms of their data type (e.g. humidity, temperature, particle levels, pH, VOC's and embryo development data), representation, sampling frequency, statistical properties, and noise levels, to name just a few. We have previously explored how to combine and model input from several modalities (see e.g. [10,11]). In the context of this project we draw on and extend this experience, but also investigate other approaches (see e.g. [13]) in an effort to obtain an improved and more accurate multimodal ML model that are more robust and less sensitive to a temporary lack of data from some of the data streams than the unimodal models. A multimodal learning approach will aid in utilizing all kinds of available data from sensors etc. to strengthen and make the ML models more robust, even though significant parts of the data may be unlabeled. This could be achieved by associating representations obtained through unsupervised training on unlabeled data [11]. We explore and compare the use of multimodal Boltzmann Machines [12] with sets of Associative Self-Organizing Map (A-SOM) [11] representations - one for each modality - that learn to associate their respective activity at the same time as they learn to represent the input space for their respective modality in a compressed manner. The learnt associations between the SOM representations for the various modalities enable the predictions of temporarily missing modalities. The multimodal representations are then used as input to a deep neural network structure. The overall idea is to obtain a more stable predictive model based on several of the available multimodal data streams including those with missing data whereas also utilizing unlabeled data.

Creating Trust Between IVF Procedure and EIVF-AI Using Explainable AI (XAI). XAI is a rapidly evolving field aimed at enhancing the transparency of AI systems, making them more interpretable to humans. As AI becomes increasingly integrated into various societal applications, particularly in domains like healthcare, XAI plays a critical role in ensuring responsible and ethical deployment of AI technologies. The application of XAI to analyze IVF time-series data holds significant potential for uncovering intricate relationships and improving our understanding of the factors influencing IVF success rates. This can lead to better patient outcomes and informed decision-making in reproductive medicine, including optimization of external environmental factors. We propose a novel approach utilizing transformer-based techniques such as BERT (Bidirectional Encoder Representations from Transformers) in conjunction with LIME (Local Interpretable Model-agnostic Explanations). BERT's capacity for processing sequential data will be leveraged by converting and tokenizing the time-series data into a format suitable for BERT. Each time point or sequence will be represented as a series of tokens for BERT's processing, capturing contextual information and dependencies between tokens. Next, LIME will be employed to generate local explanations for individual predictions. This involves perturbing the features of the selected instance while keeping other parts of the data constant. An interpretable model are then trained on this perturbed data, alongside corresponding predictions from the BERT model. The resulting model computes local feature importance scores, revealing the contribution of each feature (or time step) to BERT's predictions for the specific instance. The integration of BERT and LIME in this context offers complementary advantages, enabling both sequence-based representation learning and local interpretability of predictions for each embryo throughout the IVF procedure. Furthermore, we explore additional explainable techniques in combination with transformer-based approaches to identify the most effective solution for analyzing IVF and external data. This approach represents a cutting-edge application of XAI to address the challenges of interpreting complex time-series data in the context of IVF, with the goal of improving decision-making and patient outcomes in reproductive medicine.

4   Societal Benefits of Improved IVF Success Rates and Conclusion

Improving IVF success rates has profound implications for addressing societal issues such as declining birth rates and aging populations. The current variability in global IVF success rates, ranging from 30% to 50%, highlights inefficiencies in existing methodologies and the significant impact of external factors. By optimizing laboratory environments in IVF clinics through AI technologies, success rates can be significantly enhanced, providing substantial benefits to both individuals and society. The EIVF-AI project exemplifies how advanced AI techniques can improve IVF outcomes, thereby addressing critical global issues related to fertility and family planning. As society progresses towards sustainability and digital transformation, innovations in reproductive healthcare like these can shape a better future for all.

Acknowledgment. This study is supported by Enhancing In Vitro Fertilization with Environment Optimization Utilizing Artificial Intelligence (EIVF-AI)' project which was funded by Vinnova (Grant No. 2024-00088).

References

1. Letterie, G., MacDonald, A., Shi, Z.: An artificial intelligence platform to optimize workflow during ovarian stimulation and IVF: process improvement and outcome-based predictions. Reprod. Biomed. Online **44**(2), 254–260 (2022)
2. Fernandez, E.I., et al.: Artificial intelligence in the IVF laboratory: overview through the application of different types of algorithms for the classification of reproductive data. J. Assist. Reprod. Genet. **37**(10), 2359–2376 (2020)

3. Swain, J., VerMilyea, M.T., Meseguer, M., Ezcurra, D.: AI in the treatment of fertility: key considerations. J. Assist. Reprod. Genet. **37**(11), 2817–2824 (2020)

4. You, J.B., McCallum, C., Wang, Y., Riordon, J., Nosrati, R., Sinton, D.: Machine learning for sperm selection. Nat. Rev. Urol. **18**(7), 387–403 (2021)

5. Gardner, D.K., Kelley, R.L.: Impact of the IVF laboratory environment on human preimplantation embryo phenotype. J. Dev. Orig. Health Dis. **8**(4), 418–435 (2017)

6. Dirvanauskas, D., Maskeliunas, R., Raudonis, V., Damasevicius, R.: Embryo development stage prediction algorithm for automated time lapse incubators. Comput. Methods Programs Biomed. **177**, 161–174 (2019)

7. Malmsten, J., Zaninovic, N., Zhan, Q., Rosenwaks, Z., Shan, J.: Automated cell division classification in early mouse and human embryos using convolutional neural networks. Neural Comput. Appl. **33**, 2217–2228 (2021)

8. Richardson, A., et al.: A clinically useful simplified blastocyst grading system. Reprod. Biomed. Online **31**(4), 523–530 (2015)

9. Khosravi, P., et al.: Deep learning enables robust assessment and selection of human blastocysts after in vitro fertilization. NPJ Digit. Med. **2**(1), 21 (2019)

10. Saeedi, P., Yee, D., Jason, A., Havelock, J.: Automatic identification of human blastocyst components via texture. IEEE Trans. Biomed. Eng. **64**(12), 2968–2978 (2017)

11. Bodri, D., et al.: Predicting live birth by combining cleavage and blastocyst-stage time-lapse variables using a hierarchical and a data mining-based statistical model. Reprod. Biol. **18**(4), 355–360 (2018)

12. Milewski, R., Kuczyńska, A., Stankiewicz, B., Kuczyński, W.: How much information about embryo implantation potential is included in morphokinetic data? A prediction model based on artificial neural networks and principal component analysis. Adv. Med. Sci. **62**(1), 202–206 (2017)

13. Rubio, C., et al.: Multicenter prospective study of concordance between embryonic cell-free DNA and trophectoderm biopsies from 1301 human blastocysts. Am. J. Obstet. Gynecol. **223**(5), 751-e1 (2020)

14. Zhan, Q., Sierra, E.T., Malmsten, J., Ye, Z., Rosenwaks, Z., Zaninovic, N.: Blastocyst score, a blastocyst quality ranking tool, is a predictor of blastocyst ploidy and implantation potential. F&S Rep. **1**(2), 133–141 (2020)

15. Irani, M., et al.: Blastocyst development rate influences implantation and live birth rates of similarly graded euploid blastocysts. Fertil. Steril. **110**(1), 95–102 (2018)

16. Huang, T.T.F., Huang, D.H., Ahn, H.J., Arnett, C., Huang, C.T.F.: Early blastocyst expansion in euploid and aneuploid human embryos: evidence for a non-invasive and quantitative marker for embryo selection. Reprod. BioMed. Online **39**(1), 27–39 (2019)

17. Pennetta, F., Lagalla, C., Borini, A.: Embryo morphokinetic characteristics and euploidy. Curr. Opin. Obstet. Gynecol. **30**(3), 185–196 (2018)

18. Chavez-Badiola, A., Flores-Saiffe-Farías, A., Mendizabal-Ruiz, G., Drakeley, A.J., Cohen, J.: Embryo ranking intelligent classification algorithm (ERICA): artificial intelligence clinical assistant predicting embryo ploidy and implantation. Reprod. Biomed. Online **41**(4), 585–593 (2020)

19. Cavalera, F., et al.: A neural network-based identification of developmentally competent or incompetent mouse fully-grown oocytes. JoVE J. Visualized Exp. (133), e56668 (2018)

20. Agarwal, A., Henkel, R., Huang, C.-C., Lee, M.-S.: Automation of human semen analysis using a novel artificial intelligence optical microscopic technology. Andrologia **51**(11), e13440 (2019)

21. Javadi, S., Mirroshandel, S.A.: A novel deep learning method for automatic assessment of human sperm images. Comput. Biol. Med. **109**, 182–194 (2019)
22. McCallum, C., et al.: Deep learning-based selection of human sperm with high DNA integrity. Commun. Biol. **2**(1), 250 (2019)
23. Gil, D., Girela, J.L., De Juan, J., Gomez-Torres, M.J., Johnsson, M.: Predicting seminal quality with artificial intelligence methods. Expert Syst. Appl. **39**(16), 12564–12573 (2012)
24. Hariharan, R., et al.: Artificial intelligence assessment of time-lapse images can predict with 77% accuracy whether a human embryo capable of achieving a pregnancy will miscarry. Fertil. Steril. **112**(3), e38–e39 (2019)

Performing Audiometry Using Pupillometry: State-of-the-Market and Sensor Selection

Antonino Crivello[1], Davide La Rosa[1], Dimitri Belli[1], Mario Milazzo[2], and Filippo Palumbo[1(✉)]

[1] Institute of Information Science and Technologies "A. Faedo" National Research Council of Italy, 56124 Pisa, Italy
{antonino.crivello,davide.larosa,
dimitri.belli,filippo.palumbo}@isti.cnr.it
[2] Department of Civil and Industrial Engineering, University of Pisa, 56126 Pisa, Italy
mario.milazzo@unipi.it

Abstract. Hearing impairment poses a significant global health challenge, impacting millions of individuals across all age groups. Early detection and intervention are paramount, especially in infants and young children, to mitigate the adverse effects on speech, language, and cognitive development. Traditional audiometry methods, however, rely on subjective patient responses, rendering them unsuitable for non-collaborative individuals such as infants, newborns, and those with cognitive impairments. To address this limitation, the APURE (Audiometry with PUpil REsponse) project seeks to develop an objective audiometer leveraging pupillometry, the measurement of pupil size and reactivity. This paper presents a comprehensive state-of-the-market survey of eye-tracking systems, a crucial step in identifying the most suitable sensors for the APURE project.

Keywords: Pupillometry · Objective Audiometry · Eye-Tracking · Sensor Selection · Hearing Impairment

1 Introduction

Hearing impairment is a prevalent condition affecting millions of people worldwide [16]. Early detection and intervention are crucial for mitigating its impact on speech, language, and cognitive development, particularly in infants and young children. Traditional audiometry relies on subjective responses from patients, making it unsuitable for those unable to provide reliable feedback, such as infants, newborns, and individuals with cognitive impairments. This limitation necessitates the development of objective audiometry methods that can accurately assess hearing capabilities without requiring active participation from the patient.

© ICST Institute for Computer Sciences, Social Informatics and Telecommunications Engineering 2025
Published by Springer Nature Switzerland AG 2025. All Rights Reserved
H. Kondylakis and A. Triantafyllidis (Eds.): PervasiveHealth 2024, LNICST 612, pp. 159–169, 2025.
https://doi.org/10.1007/978-3-031-85575-7_9

Recent advancements in pupillometry, the measurement of pupil size and reactivity, have shown promise in the field of objective audiometry. Studies have demonstrated a correlation between Pupil Dilation Response (PDR) and auditory stimuli, suggesting that PDR could serve as a physiological indicator of sound detection and perception [1]. This non-invasive technique offers a potential solution for evaluating hearing thresholds in non-collaborative patients, as it does not rely on subjective reports or behavioral responses.

In this context, it is worth to remark the impact that the Internet of Things (IoT) has in eye tracking technology. As in many other applications of healthcare domain [4,5,11,14], eye tracking technology analyzes ocular movements and is a beneficiary of IoT advancements both in terms of enhanced connectivity and data processing capabilities. Conventional eye tracking systems, often constrained by standalone devices with limited computational and storage capacities, generally deployed in clinical settings, are nowadays transformed by IoT integration. This process facilitates connection to cloud services, increasing computational resources for instantaneous data analysis and implementation of machine learning algorithms. Consequently, this enhanced connectivity enables more sophisticated interpretation of ocular movement patterns, pupil response, gaze analysis and, in general, insights on human vision.

An important impact of IoT on eye tracking is the facilitation of real-time data acquisition and remote monitoring. In the healthcare domain, for instance, eye tracking serves as a valuable tool for monitoring patients with neurological conditions [3]. IoT-enabled eye trackers can continuously gather and transmit data to healthcare providers without delay. This capability enables early detection of anomalies and allows for timely interventions, ultimately improving patient outcomes. Similarly, in the marketing sphere, real-time data from IoT-integrated eye trackers provides immediate feedback on consumer behavior, enabling dynamic adjustments to advertising strategies.

In this context, the APURE (Audiometry with PUpil REsponse) project aims to leverage pupillometry to develop an objective audiometer that can be used in clinical settings. The project's primary objectives are to:

1. Develop an effective audiometry test for non-collaborative patients and validate it against gold-standard audiometry tests.
2. Provide an open biomedical solution for investigating the correlation between pupil response and focus on demanding tasks or emotional states.

To achieve these objectives, the APURE project will integrate expertise from various disciplines, including audiology, engineering, and computer science. The project will focus on developing a pupillometry system that can accurately measure pupil size and reactivity in response to auditory stimuli. The system will incorporate advanced signal processing and machine learning algorithms to analyze the collected data and correlate it with hearing thresholds. Preliminary results of the project and data collected in this first stage are available in [10]. In particular, the data collected in this work can be further analyzed to explore the correlation between physiological pupil responses to auditory stimuli and the emotional state of the user. The results could determine whether PDRs are a viable alternative or complement to traditional audiometric hearing tests in patients with limited responsiveness. They may also help to clarify how the visual and auditory systems work together to detect and localize external sounds.

The successful development and validation of an objective audiometer based on pupillometry would have a significant impact on the field of audiology. It would enable early detection and intervention for hearing impairments in populations that were previously difficult to assess, leading to improved outcomes for these individuals. Additionally, the open biomedical solution resulting from the project could contribute to research in other areas, such as cognitive science and psychology, where pupil response is used as an indicator of cognitive load or emotional state [6].

In this paper, we present a comprehensive survey of the eye-tracking sensor market, examining the strengths and weaknesses of various commercially available and open-source solutions. The survey will consider the specific requirements of the APURE project, with a particular emphasis on balancing performance, cost, and accessibility. By identifying the optimal sensor technology, we aim to pave the way for the development of an affordable, accurate, and user-friendly objective audiometer that can be readily deployed in clinical settings, ultimately improving the diagnosis and treatment of hearing impairments in diverse populations.

1.1   Sensor Selection Requirements

A comprehensive state-of-the-market survey is essential for identifying the most suitable sensors for the APURE project. The survey will target eye-tracking systems due to their non-invasive and convenient approach to measuring pupil response in real-world settings. The key characteristics to be evaluated include:

1. **Accuracy:** The accuracy of pupil size and reactivity measurements are critical for reliable audiometry results. The survey will assess the performance of different eye-tracking systems in terms of their ability to accurately track pupil movements and measure changes in pupil size. The range of accuracy has been set to $\leq 0.8°$.
2. **Sampling Rate:** The sampling rate of the eye-tracking system determines the temporal resolution of the pupil response data. A higher sampling rate allows for more detailed analysis of the PDR, which is crucial for identifying subtle changes in pupil size that may be indicative of hearing thresholds. The survey will evaluate the sampling rates of various eye-tracking systems and their suitability for capturing the dynamic nature of the PDR. The range of sampling rate has been set to $\geq 50\,\text{Hz}$.
3. **Field of View:** The Field of View (FOV) of the eye-tracking system refers to the angular extent of the observable area. A wider FOV allows for greater flexibility in head movements and gaze direction, which is important for ensuring the comfort and natural behavior of the patient during audiometry testing. The survey will compare the FOVs of different eye-tracking systems and their impact on user experience.

4. **Illumination:** The illumination conditions under which the eye-tracking system operates can significantly affect the quality of pupil measurements. Some systems may require controlled lighting environments, while others may be more robust to variations in ambient light. The survey will assess the performance of different eye-tracking systems under various illumination conditions to determine their suitability for clinical use.
5. **Data Processing and Analysis:** The ability to process and analyze the collected pupil response data is crucial for extracting meaningful information about hearing thresholds. The survey will evaluate the data processing capabilities of different eye-tracking systems, including their ability to filter noise, detect artifacts, and extract relevant features from the pupil response data.
6. **Cost and Accessibility:** The cost and accessibility of eye-tracking systems are important considerations for their widespread adoption in clinical settings. The survey will compare the prices of different systems and assess their availability to healthcare providers and researchers. The range of cost has been set to $\leq 15k€$.

By conducting a thorough state-of-the-market survey, the APURE project can identify the most appropriate eye-tracking sensors that meet the project's requirements in terms of accuracy, sampling rate, field of view, illumination, data processing, and cost. This will ensure that the developed audiometer is equipped with the best possible sensors for measuring pupil response and providing accurate and reliable audiometry results.

Due to space limitations, we present the most representative candidates from the available devices on the market, selected for their strong potential. Our selection is based on how well these devices meet the requirements outlined above and their key peculiarities, particularly those most useful for achieving the objectives of the APURE project.

2   State of the Market Survey

The state-of-the-art in eye-tracking technology is constantly evolving, with new systems and features emerging regularly. The following presents a comparative analysis of several prominent eye-tracking systems, considering the key characteristics relevant to the APURE project:

– **Pupil Labs Pupil Core**[1]: This open-source platform offers high accuracy $(0.6°)$ and a sampling rate of up to 200 Hz. Its 120-degree field of view allows for flexibility in head movements, and it is robust to varying light conditions. The open-source software provides extensive analysis tools, making it accessible and customizable for researchers and developers. Pupil Core has been used in various research studies, including investigations of cognitive processes and attentional mechanisms [12].

---

[1] https://pupil-labs.com/products/core.

- **Tobii Pro Glasses 3**[2]**:** This system offers high accuracy (0.6°) and a sampling rate of up to 100 Hz. Its 82-degree field of view is slightly narrower than Pupil Core, but it still allows for comfortable head movements. However, it requires controlled lighting conditions for optimal performance. The proprietary software provides advanced analysis features, making it suitable for research and commercial applications. Tobii Pro Glasses 3 have been used in studies on visual attention and social interaction [13].
- **SR Research EyeLink II**[3]**:** This high-end system offers exceptional accuracy (up to 0.01°) and a sampling rate of up to 500 Hz, making it the most precise option on the market. However, it requires controlled lighting and is very expensive, limiting its accessibility to well-funded research laboratories. EyeLink II has been extensively used in various research fields, including cognitive neuroscience, psychology, and linguistics [7].
- **ETVision Wearable Eye Tracker**[4]**:** This wearable eye tracking glasses offers high accuracy (0.5°) and a sampling rate of up to 180 Hz. The glasses can be equipped with an additional sun shield for very bright environments and a proprietary software is provided for data acquisition and analysis. The ETVision Wearable Eye Tracker can be used for gaze, pupillometry, saccade, and fixation data detection and has been used in children neuroscience studies [15].
- **EyeTech VT3 mini**[5]**:** This fixed compact and lightweight eye tracker offers good accuracy and a sampling rate of up to 200 Hz. Its wide field of view and robustness to varying light conditions make it suitable for real-world applications. The system comes with proprietary software for data analysis and visualization. EyeTech VT3 mini has been used in studies on reading and visual search [9].
- **Gazepoint GP3**[6]**:** This fixed affordable eye tracker offers decent accuracy and a sampling rate of up to 60 Hz. Its compact design and ease of use make it a popular choice for researchers and developers. The system comes with open-source software for data analysis and can be integrated with various programming languages. Gazepoint GP3 has been used in studies on human-computer interaction and usability [2].

As can be seen in Table 1, each system offers a unique combination of features and capabilities, catering to different needs and budgets. The Pupil Labs Pupil Core, with its open-source platform and affordability, is an attractive option for researchers and developers seeking flexibility and customization. The Tobii Pro Glasses 3, while more expensive, boasts advanced features and proprietary software that may be appealing to those requiring a comprehensive solution. The SR Research EyeLink II, with its exceptional accuracy and high sampling rate, is a top-tier choice for research laboratories with substantial funding. The ETVision

---

[2] https://www.tobii.com/products/eye-trackers/wearables/tobii-pro-glasses-3.
[3] https://www.sr-research.com/eyelink-ii.
[4] https://www.argusscience.com/ETVision.html.
[5] https://imotions.com/products/hardware/eyetech-vt3-mini.
[6] https://www.gazept.com/product/gazepoint-gp3-eye-tracker.

Table 1. Comparison of Eye-Tracking Systems

System	Accuracy	Sampling Rate	Field of View	Illumination	Data Processing and Analysis	Cost and Accessibility
Pupil Labs Pupil Core	High (0.6°)	Up to 200 Hz	120°	Robust to varying light conditions	Open-source software with extensive analysis tools	Relatively affordable, accessible to researchers and developers
Tobii Pro Glasses 3	High (0.6°)	Up to 100 Hz	82°	Requires controlled lighting	Proprietary software with advanced analysis features	Expensive, primarily targeted towards research and commercial applications
SR Research EyeLink II	Very high (0.01°)	Up to 500 Hz	Varies depending on model	Requires controlled lighting	Proprietary software with comprehensive analysis tools	Very expensive, primarily used in research laboratories
ETVision Wearable Eye Tracker	High (0.5°)	Up to 180 Hz	-	Sun shield provided for very bright environments	Proprietary software for data acquisition and analysis	Expensive, primarily used for research scopes
EyeTech VT3 mini	High (0.5°)	Up to 200 Hz	Wide	Robust to varying light conditions	Proprietary software for data analysis and visualization	Relatively affordable
Gazepoint GP3	Good (0.5° to 1°)	Up to 60 Hz	-	-	Open source software for data analysis, various programming languages supported	Affordable

Wearable Eye Tracker offers high flexibility and adaptability together with a proprietary software that allows extensive data analysis. The EyeTech VT3 mini is a compact and lightweight eye tracker suitable for real-world applications due to its wide field of view and robustness to varying light conditions. The Gazepoint GP3 is an affordable and user-friendly eye tracker with decent accuracy and open-source software, making it a popular choice for researchers and developers.

Ultimately, the selection of the optimal eye-tracking sensor for the APURE project will depend on a careful evaluation of these characteristics in light of the project's specific requirements and constraints. By considering the trade-offs between performance, cost, and accessibility, the project team can make an informed decision that will pave the way for the development of a successful objective audiometer.

3   Sensor Selection for the APURE Project

Given the project's objectives and constraints, we selected a set of requirements to be met during the device selection phase. As reported in Table 2, the eye tracker system should have an accuracy of at most 0.8° to ensure precise tracking and measurement and it should operate at a sampling rate of at least 50 Hz to capture rapid eye movements and provide smooth pupil data streams. Moreover, an accessible software API is necessary for seamless integration with various software platforms and to enable interfacing with customized software modules. Another requirement is the real-time wireless operation, essential for preserving the user mobility and reducing tethering constraints. An additional advisable feature is incorporating multiple IR cameras per eye, enhancing pupil detection accuracy by providing multiple viewpoints, reducing occlusion and improving robustness. Lastly, maintaining a total cost below 15,000€ ensures the system is economically viable for the project budget. It should be noted that the use of a threshold in Table 2 rather than a specific price for each product is justified by the fact that costs vary according to the sector requesting the product (public, private or academic). In addition, for devices with proprietary software, the cost of the licensing plan must be added to the initial price of the product. The latter is not fixed as each brand offers a range of plans to choose from.

Under all the above conditions, the Tobii Pro Glasses 3 emerges as the most suitable eye-tracking device for the APURE project while the Pupil Labs Pupil Core, could be considered as the second most appropriate choice. These wearable systems offer a compelling combination of accuracy, usability, and affordability, aligning with the project's goals of developing an objective audiometer that is both effective and accessible.

Table 2. Eye trackers requirements matching for the APURE project

Device	Requirement					
	Accuracy ≤0.8°	Sampling Rate ≥50 Hz	Software API	Real-time wireless operation	Multiple IR camera per eye	Cost ≤15k€
Pupil Labs Pupil Core	✓	✓	✓			✓
Tobii Pro Glasses 3	✓	✓	✓	✓	✓	✓
SR Research EyeLink II	✓	✓	✓			
ETVision Wearable Eye Tracker	✓	✓	✓	✓		
EyeTech VT3 mini	✓	✓	?			✓
Gazepoint GP3		✓	✓			✓

The Tobii Pro Glasses 3 with its high accuracy (up to 0.6°), offers high precision and a sampling rate of up to 100 Hz, which is sufficient for capturing the relevant aspects of the pupil dilation response. The system's wider field of view (82°) ensures user comfort and allows for natural head movements during audiometry testing. Although the Tobii Pro Glasses 3 requires controlled lighting conditions, this can be easily achieved in a clinical setting. The system's proprietary software provides advanced analysis features, which may be beneficial for in-depth investigation of the relationship between pupil response and auditory stimuli. The device, composed of the wearable glasses and a portable recording and wireless communicating unit, is shown in Fig. 1. The Tobii Pro Glasses 3 have been widely adopted in research and commercial applications due to their ease of use and robust performance. The provided web API easily allows to both capture the live streaming of the four eye cameras, the world camera and the pupil processed data, as shown in Fig. 2. For example, they have been used to study visual attention patterns in real-world scenarios, such as shopping behavior and driving performance [13]. The system's ability to capture natural eye movements in unconstrained environments makes it a valuable tool for understanding human behavior and cognition.

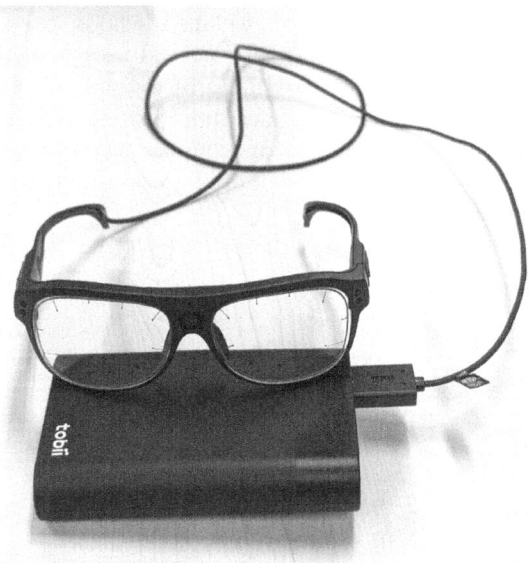

Fig. 1. The Tobii Pro Glasses 3 kit, composed of the wearable glasses unit connected to a portable computing unit that provides storage and connectivity.

The Pupil Labs Pupil Core, with its high accuracy (up to 0.6°) and sampling rate (up to 200 Hz), ensures precise and reliable measurement of pupil size and reactivity. This level of precision is crucial for capturing the subtle changes in pupil dilation that may be indicative of hearing thresholds. Additionally, the system's robustness to varying light conditions makes it suitable for use in diverse clinical settings, where lighting conditions may not always be perfectly controlled. The open-source nature of the Pupil Core platform further enhances its appeal, as it allows for customization and integration with other software tools, facilitating the development of a tailored solution for the APURE project. The only drawbacks of this system is the need to be connected through a USB cable to be operated and the fact that employs only one IR camera per eye. Overall, the versatility and adaptability of the Pupil Core have been demonstrated in various research applications. For instance, it has been successfully employed to investigate the effects of cognitive load on pupil dilation during complex tasks,

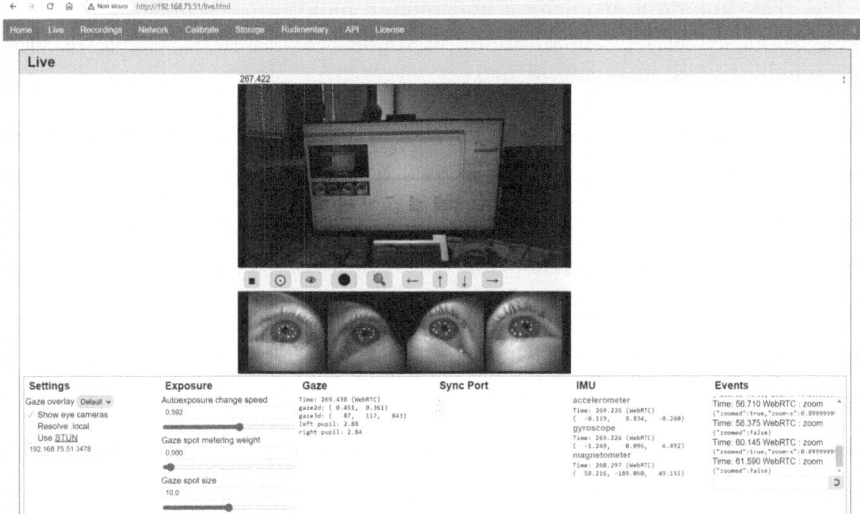

Fig. 2. Screenshot of the web API available through the glasses local WiFi hotspot providing real-time camera recording and sensors data streaming.

providing valuable insights into the relationship between cognitive processes and physiological responses [8]. Moreover, the Pupil Core's open-source nature has fostered a vibrant community of developers and researchers, contributing to a growing body of knowledge and resources for utilizing this technology in innovative ways.

While the SR Research EyeLink II boasts superior accuracy and sampling rate, its high cost and requirement for controlled lighting make it less suitable for the APURE project, which aims to develop an affordable and accessible audiometer for widespread clinical use. While the ETVision Wearable Eye Tracker might be interesting for the exposed features, its high cost make it not viable for the project. The EyeTech VT3 mini and Gazepoint GP3, while more affordable, do not offer the same level of accuracy and precision as the Pupil Core and Tobii Pro Glasses 3, which are essential for reliable audiometry results.

The choice between Tobii Pro Glasses 3 and Pupil Labs Pupil Core was guided by the specific priorities of the APURE project. Initially, we considered the Pupil Core for its cost effectiveness and open source flexibility. However, the advanced analysis functions and wider field of view of the Tobii Pro Glasses 3 were ultimately more critical to our analysis. Given the available funding, we decided to purchase and test the Tobii Pro Glasses 3.

4   Discussion and Conclusion

The convergence of IoT, ocular movement analysis and eye-tracking technology represents an interesting advancement, augmenting system capabilities and its applicability in different case study from healthcare to consumer behavior.

The real-time data acquisition and remote monitoring is facilitated by IoT enable responsiveness and adaptability in applications, in particular in the medical domain. Simultaneously, in market research, it allows for dynamic, data-driven strategy refinements.

In this paper we highlight the most promising eye tracker for clinical purpose available in the market. We try to highlight main features and characteristics of state-of-the-art technologies in this field, describing choices we made in our ongoing project. The Tobii Pro Glasses 3 and the Pupil Labs Pupil Core represent the most promising eye-tracking sensors for the APURE project. Their combination of accuracy, usability, and affordability aligns with the project's goals of developing an objective audiometer that is both effective and accessible. By leveraging these cutting-edge technologies, the APURE project can advance the field of audiology and improve the lives of individuals with hearing impairments.

Acknowledgements. This work was supported by the European Union - Next Generation EU through the Ministero dell'Università e della Ricerca, Italy, under the PRIN Grant 20222XCFA4, project A-Pure Audiometry with Pupil Response, Decreto Direttoriale n. 861.

References

1. Bala, A.D., Whitchurch, E.A., Takahashi, T.T.: Human auditory detection and discrimination measured with the pupil dilation response. J. Assoc. Res. Otolaryngol. **21**, 43–59 (2020)
2. Brand, J., Diamond, S.G., Thomas, N., Gilbert-Diamond, D.: Evaluating the data quality of the gazepoint GP3 low-cost eye tracker when used independently by study participants. Behav. Res. Methods **53**, 1502–1514 (2021)
3. Chiarion, G., et al.: e-pupil: IoT-based augmentative and alternative communication device exploiting the pupillary near-reflex. IEEE Access **10**, 130078–130088 (2022)
4. Crivello, A., La Rosa, D., Wilhelm, E., Palumbo, F.: A sensing platform to monitor sleep efficiency. In: Italian Forum of Ambient Assisted Living, pp. 335–345. Springer (2020)
5. Crivello, A., et al.: Experimental assessment of cuff pressures on the walls of a trachea-like model using force sensing resistors: insights for patient management in intensive care unit settings. Sensors **22**(2), 697 (2022)
6. Eckstein, M.K., Guerra-Carrillo, B., Singley, A.T.M., Bunge, S.A.: Beyond eye gaze: what else can eyetracking reveal about cognition and cognitive development? Dev. Cogn. Neurosci. **25**, 69–91 (2017)
7. Holmqvist, K., Nyström, M., Andersson, R., Dewhurst, R., Jarodzka, H., Van de Weijer, J.: Eye Tracking: A Comprehensive Guide to Methods and Measures. OUP Oxford (2011)
8. Hopstaken, J.F., Van Der Linden, D., Bakker, A.B., Kompier, M.A.: The window of my eyes: task disengagement and mental fatigue covary with pupil dynamics. Biol. Psychol. **110**, 100–106 (2015)
9. Jeelani, I., Albert, A., Han, K., Azevedo, R.: Are visual search patterns predictive of hazard recognition performance? Empirical investigation using eye-tracking technology. J. Constr. Eng. Manag. **145**(1), 04018115 (2019)

10. La Rosa, D., Bruschini, L., Tramonti Fantozzi, M.P., Orsini, P., Milazzo, M., Crivello, A.: Pupil data upon stimulation by auditory stimuli. Data **9**(3), 43 (2024)
11. Mallegni, N., et al.: Sensing devices for detecting and processing acoustic signals in healthcare. Biosensors **12**(10), 835 (2022)
12. Mathôt, S.: Pupillometry: psychology, physiology, and function. J. Cogn. **1**(1) (2018)
13. Onkhar, V., Dodou, D., De Winter, J.: Evaluating the tobii pro glasses 2 and 3 in static and dynamic conditions. Behav. Res. Methods 1–18 (2023)
14. Palumbo, F., et al.: "hi this is nestore, your personal assistant": design of an integrated IoT system for a personalized coach for healthy aging. Front. Digit. Health **2**, 545949 (2020)
15. Pinheiro, E.D., Sato, J.R., da Silva Soares Junior, R., Barreto, C., Oku, A.Y.A.: Eye-tracker and fNIRS: using neuroscientific tools to assess the learning experience during children's educational robotics activities. Trends Neurosci. Educ. 100234 (2024)
16. World Health Organization: Newborn and infant hearing screening: Current issues and guiding principles for action. WHO Reports (2010)

Multisensor Setup for Functional Capacity Testing: The Malisa Dataset

Dario Salvi[1(✉)], Carl Magnus Olsson[1], Hicham Lamrani Laghrib[2],
Kévin Merle[2], Noa Pothier[2], Selin Yildirim[2], Davide La Rosa[3],
and Filippo Palumbo[3]

[1] Internet of Things and People Research Center, Computer Science and Media
Technology (DVMT), Malmo University, Malmö, Sweden
`dario.salvi@mau.se`
[2] Polytech Clermont, Université Clermont Auvergne, Clermont-Ferrand, France
[3] Institute of Information Science and Technologies "A. Faedo", National Research
Council of Italy, 56124 Pisa, Italy

Abstract. Functional capacity testing is essential for assessing mobility changes, which can impact independence across various populations and health conditions. This study aims to implement instrumented function tests using a combination of affordable sensors, including sensorized mats, sensorized shoes, smartphones, and smartwatches. The goal is to provide objective, reliable, and detailed data on test outcomes, such as gait analysis. We have created a dataset from 6 participants of varying ages, each performing 5 standardized functional tests: Timed Up and Go, 30-Second Chair Rise, Locomo challenge, 10-meter walk, and 40-meter walk. Alongside the dataset, we have developed a tool for visualizing the sensor signals and marking key events to facilitate data analysis. This dataset is intended to support researchers in developing algorithms for extracting test-specific parameters, and for comparing sensors in terms of quality of the signals and ease of setup.

Keywords: Functional tests · Mobility tests · Wearable sensors · Sensorized mats · Sensorized shoes

1 Introduction

The changing demographics of the global population, with a growing number of individuals living with chronic conditions, poses significant challenges for healthcare systems worldwide. As more people require long-term care and support, there is a pressing need to ensure that individuals maintain optimal health to improve quality of life and reduce the burden on healthcare systems [5,9].

Mobility and physical function are key indicators of overall health and well-being, regardless of age. A variety of tests exist to assess physical function [9]. These tests focus on the capacity of the individual to accomplish specific tasks (e.g., activities from everyday living) or to measure physical performance (e.g. Timed Up and Go test and 6-Minute Walk Test) or muscle strength tests (e.g.

H. Kondylakis and A. Triantafyllidis (Eds.): PervasiveHealth 2024, LNICST 612, pp. 170–178, 2025.
https://doi.org/10.1007/978-3-031-85575-7_10

the hand grip strength test). The tests are designed to provide objective results taken in standardized conditions, while being sensitive to changes and capturing the real biology of complex and multi-domain functions and conditions. They have repeatedly shown predictive capacity for negative health outcomes, like hospitalizations or mortality, and they are therefore often used as general markers of well-being linked to chronic conditions in addition to simple parameters of mobility or strength [9].

Traditionally, these tests are conducted in clinics under the supervision of specialized health staff. The tests involve the measurement of a quantity such as duration to complete a test, walked distance or similar. For practical reasons, the test procedure is usually simple and conducted with simple instruments such as a stop watch. A certain level of subjectivity tends to leak into these tests, for example in terms of when exactly the test is considered started and completed, or how far a patient has actually walked, which introduces errors. Instrumented tests have been proposed with the use of digital technologies, particularly inertial sensors [1], smartphones [10], cameras [2] and wearables [8]. Through embedded sensors in such technologies, measurements can be made more reliable and objective, and may further be augmented with additional information, such as gait analysis, which contain meaningful indicators about the status of the tested person or even hold predictive powers of future health risks. For example, in the Timed Up and Go (TUG) test, the time to turn around [4] or the step length [12] have been found to be especially informative for assessing the status of patients.

Notwithstanding the rich literature in instrumented tests, and the presence of several technical solutions, limited works have compared these solutions in terms of benefits and trade-offs. Within this study, we therefore aim at comparing different types of sensors to be used within a number of functional tests. Our focus is particularly on devices that are commercially available or close to market, inexpensive and that could be used also in home environments, with the potential application of home monitoring. The immediate aim of this paper is not to provide a comparison of the solutions in terms of performances or costs, but rather to provide a dataset for the research community to use for the development of algorithms and for comparisons, created by the use of a large range of relevant solutions. The dataset includes raw sensors data which requires further processing in order to extract metrics and indicators that are clinically significant. A few datasets exist of data that can be used for the evaluation of function, such as gait analysis [3,6,11]. However, to the best of our knowledge, no dataset exists that includes raw information from multiple sensors collected while performing functional tests. This lack limits the ability to compare technical solutions in terms of reliability, signal quality, and other characteristics.

This paper is structured as follows: Sect. 2 describes the technical setup and the data collection procedures, Sect. 3 provides examples of the data that was collected and a tool for their analysis and Sect. 4 concludes the work and indicates future research directions.

2   Methods

For data collection purposes, six healthy volunteers were recruited to this study - three males and three females, aged between 36 and 63 (average 51.3). All subjects were researchers located at CNR, Pisa, Italy, and data was collected between 2023-10-27 and 2023-10-31. No ethical review was needed because we did not collect clinical or physiological data and because of the technical nature of the work. Consent was obtained from all participants.

Participants were instructed to perform a series of functional capacity tests:

– Timed Up and Go (TUG): the subject stands up from a chair, walks 3 m, turns around, walks back and sits down. The test was repeated 4 times, 2 at natural speed, and 2 at slow speed, using a metronome at 1 Hz to induce a cadence in the movement.
– 30-Second Chair Rise Test (30SCRT): the participant stands up and sits down on a chair repeatedly, as fast as possible, for 30 s. This task was executed once because it can be demanding for participants.
– Locomo challenge: the subject stands up from one chair, using only one leg and with the arms crossed so that these cannot aid the subject during the task. This task was also executed once.
– 10-meter walk test: participants are asked to walk on a pathway of 10 m, with additional 2 m at both ends, for acceleration and deceleration. Walking pace is assessed across the 10-meter distance. The test was repeated twice.
– 40-meter walk test: subjects walk at natural speed over a 20-meter corridor, back and forth. The test is similar to the 6-minute walk test, but shortened. Each participant repeated the test twice.

We acquired data from an ensemble of sensors simultaneously during the functional tests, in order to maximize comparability of data across the technologies used:

– SensingTex Sensing Mats[1]: are pressure sensorized mats with wireless connectivity and a spatial granularity of 2 square centimeters. We used 3 mats, one positioned over a chair, and two mats, 1.5 m long each, positioned to capture walking characteristics in the middle of the pathway. The mats covered the whole area of interest in the TUG, 30SCRT and Locomo challenge tests, but only a partial area in the 10 and 40-meter walk tests. The mats can capture detailed information about foot placement, pressure distribution, and temporal aspects of the gait cycle providing insights into balance, stride length, and the symmetry of gait, which are crucial for assessing mobility.
– Ki-Foot sensorized Shoes: equipped with inertial measurement units (IMUs) and five pressure sensors per shoe to gather comprehensive data on foot movement and pressure distribution [7]. The IMUs track movement and orientation, offering data on speed, acceleration, and directional changes, while pressure sensors across key points in the sole measure the distribution of force

---

[1] https://sensingtex.com.

throughout the gait cycle. This combination allows for a detailed analysis of foot-ground interactions, stride characteristics, and potential abnormalities in walking patterns.

- Smartphones: two smartphones were utilized, one attached to the lower back and the other held in the dominant hand, to record inertial sensor data, including acceleration, rotation rate and orientation. The smartphone placed on the lower back offers data reflective of the body core movements, while the smartphone held in the dominant hand can capture upper body dynamics and the coordination with the lower body during walking.
- Smartwatches: worn on the wrist to collect inertial sensor data and photoplethysmography (PPG). Two models were used: Sony mSafety[2] and BangleJS[3] [13]. Both devices were programmed with a custom firmware to stream raw sensors data. Worn on the arms, they can measure general activity levels, steps taken, and provide insights into the rhythm and pace of walking.
- Kinect: used to collect video with information about the position and pose. It can also be used as ground truth data for validating sensor readings.
- Polar H10 Heart rate sensor: is placed on the chest and computes heart rate and heart rate variability from electrocardiography. Useful as a reference for the (PPG), this sensor was only used in 3 tests.
- Polar Running Cadence[4] sensor: placed on a shoe, this determines the step rate and step distance of the person wearing it. It does not provide raw sensors data, but can be used as reference or to derive useful gait parameters.

These sensors were connected to 3 laptops either with USB connections (Kinect and sensorized mats) or wirelessly (smartwatches, sensorized shoes, heart rate and cadence sensors) to custom made applications. The smartphones run a web application, available at https://dariosalvi78.github.io/Malisa/, which gathered inertial sensor data and connected to the standard Bluetooth sensors for heart rate and cadence. The setup is visible in Fig. 1 and summarized in Table 1.

Devices that kept time, such as laptops, smartphones and watches, were synchronized at the beginning of each day by using network synchronization when available (laptops and smartphones) or manually (watches). Timestamping was done by those devices that kept time, i.e. laptops, smartphones and smartwatches. Timestamping was done both for data produced by the device itself, for example smartphones and smart watches, and for devices with no time keeping capability that were connected to them, for example via Bluetooth, timestamping was done at the receiving computer at the time the measurement was received. The source of timestamping is specifed in Table 1.

Participants started each test by pressing a button on the smartwatch held in the hand and completed the test by pressing the button again. The timestamps of those 2 events were used as official start and end times of each test.

---

[2] https://www.sonynetworkcom.com/msafety.

[3] https://banglejs.com.

[4] https://support.polar.com/en/cadence-sensor.

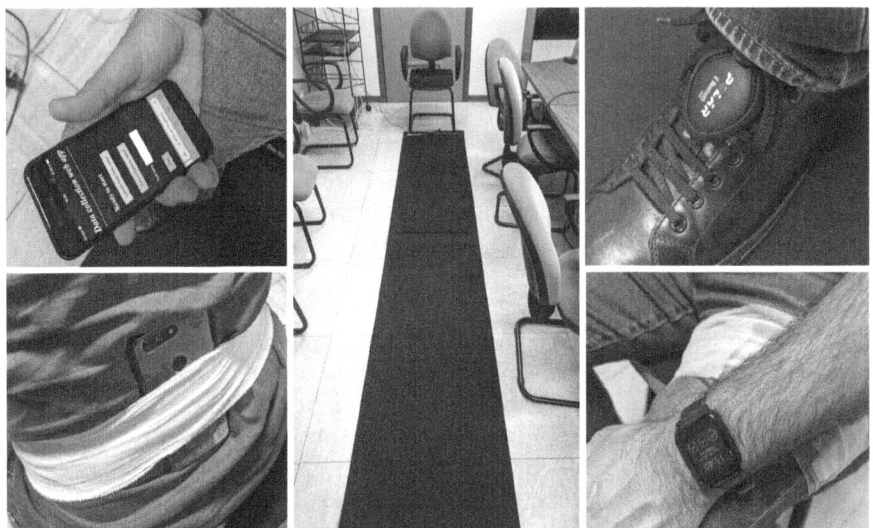

Fig. 1. The experimental test bed for gait analysis.

3   Results and Discussion

Data was collected using the dedicated software for each hardware. Each sensor was activated before the actual start of the test and was stopped after the end of the test. Start and end of each test was assumed to correspond to when the participant pressed the button on the hand-held phone. All collected signals were later post-processed to only include 5 s before the first press of the button to start the test, and 5 s after the second press of the button (signifying end of the test), to help in case of offsets between clocks among devices. In this way, all signals are "cut" around the same timestamps. All data was later stored in comma-separated format files, with a uniform format with all timestamps represented as Unix timestamps with decimals. The data repository is publicly available on: https://github.com/dariosalvi78/Malisa-Dataset.

In addition to pre-processing the data, we developed a software tool for the visualization of the signals, available at the same repository. The tool shows, for each participant and for each test, all signals acquired by all sensors (see Fig. 2) and allows to manually set markers on the plots. Markers can then be exported to a machine readable format, which allows researchers to conveniently use them in their analysis of the data. Markers can be used for identifying offsets between clocks, as they were not synchronized thoroughly during the experiments.

We present a qualitative analysis of the signals for a TUG for one subject to show how the phases of the tests can be identified in the data. The qualitative analysis could inspire the creation of algorithms that segment the data automatically. For instance, Fig. 3 shows the tri-axial rotation rate (gyroscope) signals of the smartphone positioned in the lower back during the TUG test.

Table 1. Summary of the employed devices with position, connection type, timestamping source and measured signals with sampling frequency.

Device	Position	Connection	Timestamps	Measured signals
SensingTex Sensing Mats	Chair and floor	USB	Connected laptop	Pressure @10 Hz
Ki-Foot sensorized Shoes	Feet	Bluetooth	Connected laptop	Pressure, acceleration, rotation, magnetic field @80 Hz
Smartphone	Hand, lower back	WiFi	On device	Acceleration, rotation, orientation @60 Hz
Sony mSafety	Wrist	CAT M1	On device	Acceleration @32 Hz, PPG @50 Hz
BangleJS	Wrist	Bluetooth	On device	Acceleration @12 Hz, magnetic field @ 12 Hz, HR @1 Hz, Step count
Kinect	Floor	USB	On device	Video and skeleton @30 Hz
Polar H10 heart rate sensor	Chest	Bluetooth	Connected smartphone	HR, HRV @1 Hz
Polar running cadence sensor	Shoe	Bluetooth	Connected smartphone	Step rate, step length, speed @1 Hz

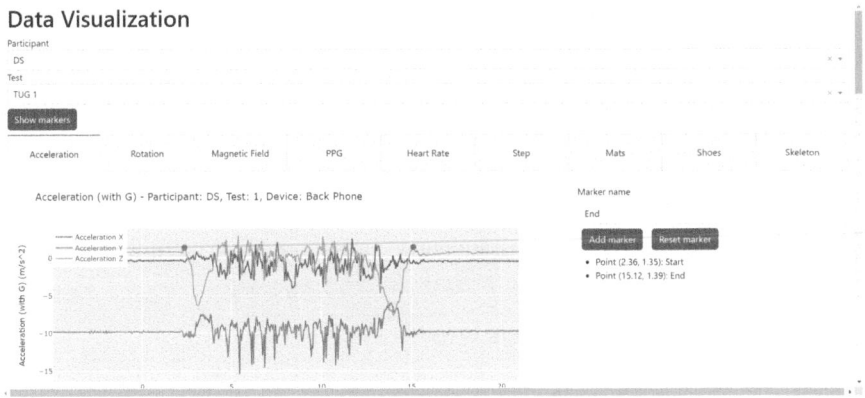

Fig. 2. Tool for visualizing the dataset. The acceleration gathered by the phone placed on the lower back is shown. A researcher can mark points on the signal and export them for later analysis.

While the subject is standing up, there is a rotation along the alpha axis corresponding to the participant leaning forward, followed by a counter rotation when the subject raises up their body. The walking phase is clearly visible from the regular, periodic rotations, followed by a pronounced rotation over the beta axis, corresponding to the turning around at the end of the 3 m path. A second segment with periodic, small rotations indicates the walk back and a second turning around over the beta axis corresponds to the final rotation before sitting down, indicated by the rotation along alpha which is similar to the earlier standing up phase.

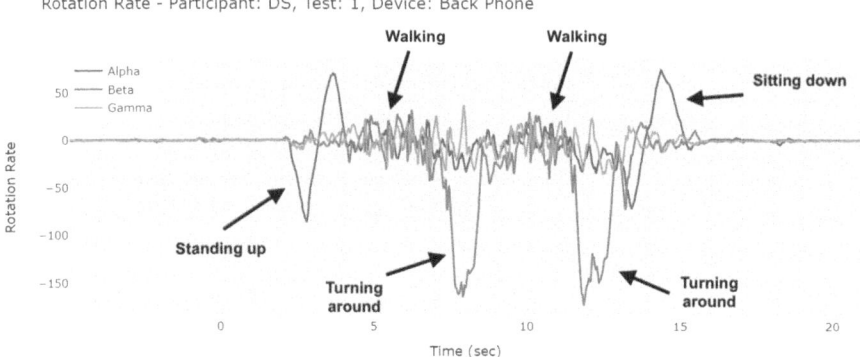

Fig. 3. Rotation rate signal from the phone placed on lower back during a Timed Up and Go test. The phases of the test are clearly visible on the signal.

We also present an example related to the signals captured with the mats placed on the floor. In Fig. 3 it is possible to observe the position of the feet during the walking phase of the test. This information can be used to analyze of the gait of the subject, including step length, step rate, and the center of pressure. In the picture, for example, one can extract the distance between the left and right feet, when both feet are on the floor (double support phase of the gait cycle). Gait analysis is not usually done in a TUG because of its complexity, but the use of technology allows to add this important aspect to the test (Fig. 4).

The data collection presented some challenges. Keeping all the involved sensors activated and streaming simultaneously turned out to be complex, especially

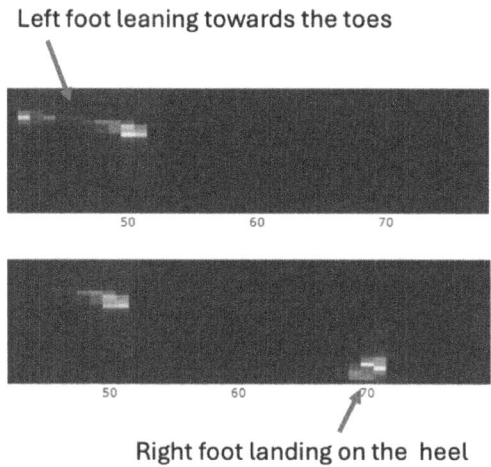

Fig. 4. Signals from one mat during the walking phase of the Timed Up and Go Test. The position of the feet is clearly visible during the gait cycle.

because some Bluetooth sensors disconnected during the tests. The software we employed did not implement automatic re-connection, which meant that, in some of tests, the data from some sensors may be missing. This was particularly true for the heart rate and running cadence sensors. Performing the tests required 3 researchers just to control all the equipment, which also introduced issues of communication and synchronization among them, as they had to agree when to start and stop the equipment. The effect was that some tests had to be repeated, especially on the first day of the data collection.

4   Conclusions

The advent of inexpensive sensor technology offers a promising alternative to conventional functional tests. These have the potential to provide reliable and objective data, and to augment the conventional mobility and functionality tests with measurements that go beyond simple distances and times, adding rich information such as precise gait analysis metrics. The study we are reporting on in this paper focuses on the creation of a publicly available dataset which combines a large number of different technologies used at the same time by our participants.

This allows researchers to harness an ensemble of cutting-edge sensors, including sensorized mats, sensorized shoes, smartphones, and smartwatches, and a camera-based technology which produces skeleton-like mappings of the body. We encourage other researchers to make use of the collected data to develop algorithms for segmentation of the tests and extraction of parameters, as well as to compare sensor configurations for real-world applications such as in home monitoring.

By making this dataset public, our research addresses a critical gap in the literature and lays the groundwork for innovative strategies to monitor and assess mobility, a key aspect of overall health and well-being across various populations. This could lead to personalized interventions and improved support for individuals with diverse health conditions and mobility challenges.

Future research should expand on these initial results, focusing on larger, more diverse participant groups, including individuals with specific health conditions or mobility impairments. Additionally, exploring the integration of these technologies into daily life could enable continuous monitoring and personalized interventions, potentially improving health outcomes and quality of life for a wider range of individuals.

Acknowledgements. This work was partially funded by the European Union - Next Generation EU, in the context of The National Recovery and Resilience Plan, Investment 1.5 Ecosystems of Innovation, Project Tuscany Health Ecosystem (THE), CUP: B83C22003930001, and by the Swedish Knowledge Foundation and the Internet of Things and People research center through the Synergy project Intelligent and Trustworthy IoT Systems.

References

1. Domínguez, J.J.G., et al.: Portable system for the functional assessment of older adults. In: 2020 IEEE International Symposium on Medical Measurements and Applications (MeMeA), pp. 1–6. IEEE (2020)
2. Dubois, A., Bihl, T., Bresciani, J.P.: Automating the timed up and go test using a depth camera. Sensors **18**(1), 14 (2017)
3. Goldberger, A.L., et al.: PhysioBank, PhysioToolkit, and PhysioNet: components of a new research resource for complex physiologic signals. Circulation **101**(23), e215–e220 (2000). http://circ.ahajournals.org/content/101/23/e215.full. https://doi.org/10.1161/01.CIR.101.23.e215. PMID: 1085218
4. Herman, T., Giladi, N., Hausdorff, J.M.: Properties of the 'timed up and go' test: more than meets the eye. Gerontology **57**(3), 203–210 (2011)
5. Kaeberlein, M., Rabinovitch, P.S., Martin, G.M.: Healthy aging: the ultimate preventive medicine. Science **350**(6265), 1191–1193 (2015)
6. Karas, M., Urbanek, J., Crainiceanu, C., Harezlak, J., Fadel, W.: Labeled raw accelerometry data captured during walking, stair climbing and driving (version 1.0. 0). PhysioNet (2021)
7. La Rosa, D., et al.: IoT smart shoe solution for neuromuscular disease monitoring. In: International Conference on Pervasive Computing Technologies for Healthcare, pp. 104–115. Springer (2022)
8. Matey-Sanz, M., González-Pérez, A., Casteleyn, S., Granell, C.: Instrumented timed up and go test using inertial sensors from consumer wearable devices. In: International Conference on Artificial Intelligence in Medicine, pp. 144–154. Springer (2022)
9. Michel, J.P., Sadana, R.: "healthy aging" concepts and measures. J. Am. Med. Dir. Assoc. **18**(6), 460–464 (2017)
10. Milosevic, M., Jovanov, E., Milenković, A.: Quantifying timed-up-and-go test: a smartphone implementation. In: 2013 IEEE International Conference on Body Sensor Networks, pp. 1–6. IEEE (2013)
11. Palermo, M., Lopes, J.M., André, J., Matias, A.C., Cerqueira, J., Santos, C.P.: A multi-camera and multimodal dataset for posture and gait analysis. Sci. Data **9**(1), 603 (2022)
12. Son, M., et al.: Evaluation of the turning characteristics according to the severity of Parkinson disease during the timed up and go test. Aging Clin. Exp. Res. **29**, 1191–1199 (2017)
13. Van Laerhoven, K., Hoelzemann, A., Pahmeier, I., Teti, A., Gabrys, L.: Validation of an open-source ambulatory assessment system in support of replicable activity studies. German J. Exerc. Sport Res. **52**(2), 262–272 (2022)

Objective Characterization of Timed Up and Go Test via Sensorized Mats

Hedda Eriksson[1], Malin Ramkull[1], Dario Salvi[1], Carl Magnus Olsson[1], Dario Ghezzi[2], Davide La Rosa[2], and Filippo Palumbo[2(✉)]

[1] Internet of Things and People Research Center, Computer Science and Media Technology (DVMT), Malmo University, Malmö, Sweden
`dario.salvi@mau.se`
[2] Institute of Information Science and Technologies "A. Faedo", National Research Council of Italy (ISTI-CNR), 56124 Pisa, Italy
`{dario.ghezzi,davide.larosa,filippo.palumbo}@isti.cnr.it`

Abstract. The Timed Up and Go (TUG) test is a widely recognized and standardized mobility test to measure basic mobility and balance capabilities. Despite the possibility to derive rich information about the patient, only the total time to complete the test is conventionally measured by a professional. This work examines the use of non-wearable sensors for the measurement of parameters of the test in an accurate and objective way. The study illustrates a system specifically designed for conducting the TUG test using a set of sensorized mats. The developed system is able to identify the following 4 phases of the test, with relative timestamps: TUG-time, Sit-to-Stand, Mid-Turning, and End-Turning-Stand-to-Sit. Additionally, meaningful parameters for gait assessment are also extracted: walking speed and stride length. Two experimental iterations were conducted to assess the reliability of the developed software. Both iterations involved two different groups of six healthy participants $(41.58 \pm 13.32$ yrs; 6 females, 6 males) performing various walking types. Our results demonstrate that sensorized mats can be used to segment the phases of the test reliably and can additionally be used to quantify gait parameters during the walk phase of the test.

Keywords: Timed Up and Go · Gait Analysis · Pressure Sensor · Sensorized Mat

1 Introduction

Walking is a fundamental human activity and by studying its characteristics, we can reveal significant information about an individual's physical health. In clinical terms, "gait" refers to the pattern of walking [8]. Gait analysis (GA) aims to identify meaningful parameters related to the measurement of walking activity [5]. Each parameter indicates a specific gait characteristic and can be used for various health assessments and to guide medical interventions [4].

© ICST Institute for Computer Sciences, Social Informatics and Telecommunications Engineering 2025
Published by Springer Nature Switzerland AG 2025. All Rights Reserved
H. Kondylakis and A. Triantafyllidis (Eds.): PervasiveHealth 2024, LNICST 612, pp. 179–189, 2025.
https://doi.org/10.1007/978-3-031-85575-7_11

In addition to gait analysis, other clinical tools exist for assessing posture [1], movement, and physical capacity, such as the Timed Up and Go (TUG) test [6]. The TUG test is a semi-subjective test frequently used in physical therapy to measure the ability to maintain balance while walking [9] and predict the probability of falls in older people [11].

Since these assessments require specialized personnel, there is a need for an automatic and inexpensive system for conducting such tests more frequently and autonomously. Recent technologies using sensors [7] allow for objective evaluation, making physical tests and gait characteristic measurements more efficient and effective, providing specialists with reliable information. One common approach is using sensorized mats, which can quantify pressure patterns under a foot over time.

The focus of this work is thus automatic identification of the phases of the TUG test through the use of sensorized mats. This allows the acquisition of rich, objective and reliable information about the patient being examined. Additionally, we aim at including gait analysis within the TUG test, which is, to the best of our knowledge, a scarcely explored area. Given its short duration, the TUG test is not typically used for objective gait analysis. However, guidelines related to the test suggest that clinicians should observe and annotate gait and balance during the test [6]. There are indications that gait-related parameters are, in fact, more sensitive to disease progression than the simple duration of the test [12,13].

Among the various approaches available for conducting the TUG test, we selected sensorized mats for this study due to their unique ability to provide detailed spatial and temporal pressure data across the foot during the entire test. Sensorized mats allow for the non-invasive, continuous monitoring of pressure distribution under the feet, which is crucial for accurately identifying the different phases of the TUG test, such as Sit-to-Stand and Mid-Turning. Additionally, they offer the advantage of being easy to use, requiring minimal setup, and not interfering with the subject's natural movement, making them ideal for both clinical and research environments. These characteristics make sensorized mats particularly effective for obtaining reliable and objective measurements of both TUG-time and gait parameters.

A relevant example of a sensorized system for gait analysis is the GAITRite system [3], which offers a pressure-sensitive walkway, measuring temporal and spatial gait parameters. Despite its ease of use and lack of required setup or calibration, the device is expensive. Another related study developed an algorithm for estimating gait parameters through a commercial sensorized mat [2]. This approach utilizes affordable commercial technology, making it more accessible for widespread use but with a lower spatial resolution. To be noted that none of these technologies have software developed specifically for conducting the TUG test.

There are gaps both in the literature and market concerning systems specifically designed to streamline and enhance analysis of the TUG test. For these reasons, we developed a system for conducting the TUG test using sensorized mats, improving reliability by objectively quantifying the time needed to complete the test versus the traditional semi-objective method, and incorporating additional gait parameters into the analysis.

The paper is structured as follows: Sect. 2 outlines the experimental setup, data collection and processing procedures, as well as parameter extraction methods and the validation techniques employed to assess the system's performance, in Sect. 3 we present and reflect on our results compared with our ground truth methods, as well as the evaluation of gait parameters which our system permits, and Sect. 4 concludes this paper with some final remarks.

2   Methods

2.1   Experimental Setup

The experimental setup consisted of two SensingTex[1] Fitness Mats embedding 2240 pressure as a matrix of 80×28, covering a sensing area of 1600×560 mm each arranged end-to-end to form a 3.2-meter walkway (see Fig. 1a). A chair, equipped with a SensingTex Seating Mat with a sensing area of 400×400 mm comprising 400 sensors in total (see Fig. 1b) was placed at the beginning of the walkway to accommodate the sit-to-stand and stand-to-sit transitions of the TUG test as shown in Fig. 1c. The mats capture pressure data at a sampling rate of 10 Hz.

2.2   Data Collection

Data collection was performed in two iterations. The first iteration involved six participants performing two types of walks: normal walk and slow walk. The second iteration included a new group of six participants who performed three walk types: normal walk, slow walk and abnormal walk. The walk types are defined as follows:

1. **Normal walk**: Participants are instructed to walk at their usual pace along the walkway. As they are all healthy and have no gait impairment, it is assumed that there is a coordinated sequence of movements enabling efficient and smooth movement from one location to another. This involves alternating weight-bearing steps with one foot while the other foot swings forward in a rhythmic manner, which is the description of a normal human walk.
2. **Slow walk**: Participants are directed to walk slowly, synchronized with a metronome set at 60 beats per minute (bpm), along the same walkway. This is done to simulate patients with reduced pace of their mobility.
3. **Abnormal walk**: Participants are instructed to mimic the gait pattern of individuals with walking impairments, such as those with back pain, reduced muscle and joint flexibility, a slightly stooped posture, and less fluid movement compared to younger individuals. This provides insight into abnormal locomotion.

---

[1] https://sensingtex.com.

Overall L: 1710 mm
Sensing L: 1600 mm

Overall W: 630 mm
Sensing W: 560 mm

(a) Sensor layout of the fitness mat.

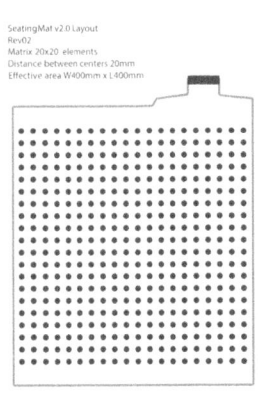

(b) Sensor layout of the seating mat.

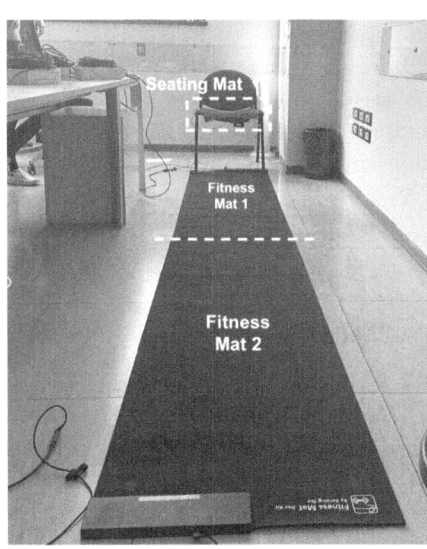

(c) The experimental setup at site.

Fig. 1. Overview of the sensor layouts and experimental setup.

In the second iteration, participants also wore a G-WALK[2] device by BTS Bioengineering to provide ground truth data. Video recordings were taken during each session to serve as an additional reference.

2.3   Parameter Extraction and Validation

The data processing pipeline consists of three subsystems: data collection, analysis algorithm, and parameter extraction algorithm. Each subsystem operates

---

[2] https://www.btsbioengineering.com/products/g-walk/.

independently, with the output of one serving as the input for the next (Fig. 2). The code, written in Python, utilizes the Streamlit[3] framework across all subsystems to develop web-based applications with user-friendly interfaces.

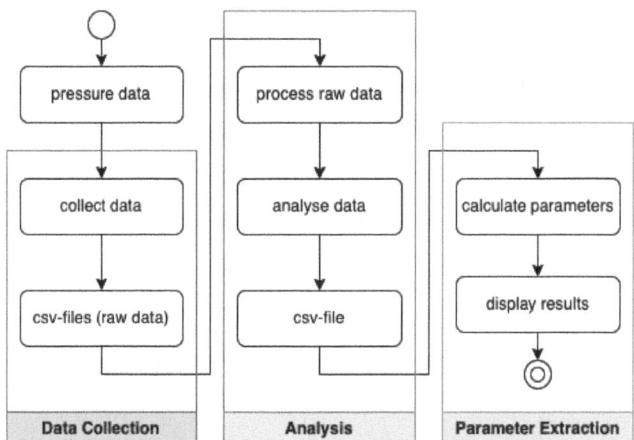

Fig. 2. Overview and flowchart of the system's events from test conduct to result analysis.

The collected data is stored in comma-separated-values (CSV) files, with each row containing readings from all sensors at a specific timestamp. The analysis algorithm processes the raw sensor data, ensuring the signals have constant sampling frequency, through resampling, and synchronization. It then employs a state machine to identify key events in the TUG test, such as transitions between sitting, standing, and walking phases (Fig. 3) and logs all the state transitions, or events, on a file.

In the initial state, when the individual is seated, a threshold on the seat mat total pressure triggers the transition to a standing position. Subsequent state transitions are tracked by monitoring the center of pressure (COP) coordinates against predefined thresholds illustrated in Fig. 4 and further referred to as A, B, and C.

During the forward and return gait states, the algorithm distinguishes between double and single stances by analyzing the distance in y-axis between the first and last recorded pressure values. Additionally, it determines the left or right placement of single stances by dividing the walkway at a horizontal axis at threshold C and the total pressure on each side of the walkway. The final state transition uses the same personalized threshold as the initial state transition, on the seat, in order to identify the end of the test.

Each state transition and gait phase is logged as an event. The analysis subsystem logs these events along with relevant parameters such as timestamps,

---
[3] https://streamlit.io.

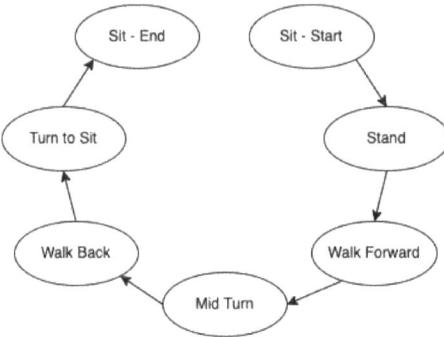

Fig. 3. The finite state machine used for the analysis of the TUG phases.

COP coordinates, total pressure distribution, and event placements (left or right foot) on a CSV file as an input for the next subsystem.

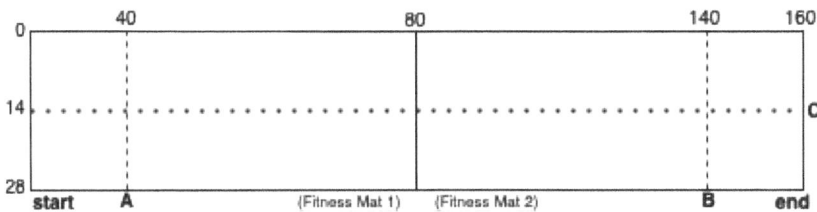

Fig. 4. Illustration of the predefined thresholds used on the sensing area matrix of the full walkway: A determines the start of forward gait and the end of return gait; B determines the end of forward gait and the start of return gait; C determines the placement of a single stance, either left or right, based on pressure distribution and direction of movement.

The parameter extraction algorithm identifies the phases of the TUG test (TUG-time, Sit-to-Stand time, Mid-Turning time, and End-Turning-Stand-to-Sit time) and gait parameters (walking speed and stride length) based on the logged events. Walking speed is determined by dividing the total distance covered during the forward and return gait phases by the total duration of those phases. Stride length is calculated by analyzing the distances between consecutive single-stance events. The subsystem also provides visual playback capabilities through heatmaps, as in Fig. 5.

The performance of the algorithms was validated using two ground truth methods: the measures produced by G-WALK and observations from video recordings. The accuracy of TUG parameters was assessed by comparing the system's output to the ground truth data. The mean error (ME), standard deviation (STD) were calculated to quantify the system's accuracy and consistency.

TUG Analysis Web Application

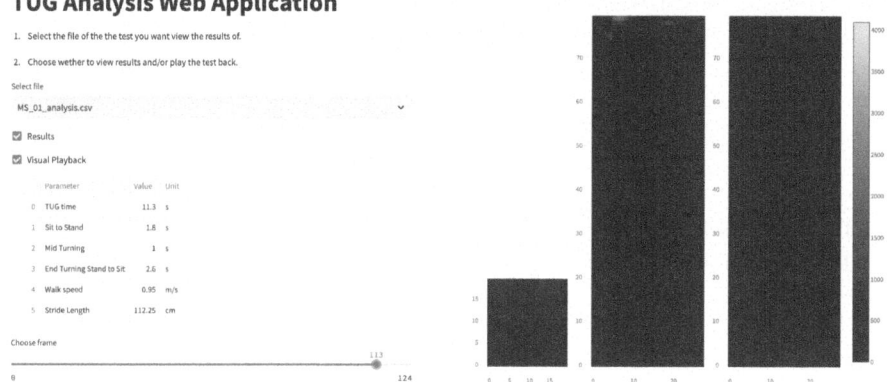

Fig. 5. The web application interface of the report model.

Bland-Altman analysis was also employed to evaluate the limits of agreement (LOA) between the two measurement methods.

3 Results and Discussion

3.1 Evaluation of the TUG Phases

The performance of the algorithms when identifying the TUG phases was evaluated using observations from video recordings. The results for TUG-time of normal and slow walks show errors below the Minimal Clinically Important Difference (MCID) threshold of 3.5 s for both normal and slow walks. The MCID represents the smallest change in a treatment outcome that is considered significant or meaningful to patients. The Bland-Altman Limits of Agreement (LOA) for normal walking were +2.00 s and −0.51 s, and for slow walking were +2.57 s and −0.13 s, indicating good agreement between the system's output and the ground truth. The system's performance was less accurate for abnormal walks however, highlighting the need for further refinement to accommodate diverse gait patterns. As our abnormal walk data was created by healthy volunteers simulating movement inhibitions, we were expecting this to be the worst case in terms of accuracy - possibly as a result of exaggerated abnormalities in the walking style.

The analysis of other TUG phases (Mid-Turning, Sit-to-Stand, and End-Turning-Stand-to-Sit) showed fair to good reliability, with the End-Turning-Stand-to-Sit parameter being the least reliable due to challenges in distinguishing it from the Stand-to-Sit phase. Table 1 summarizes the results for the TUG parameters. The mean absolute error (MAE) for all TUG parameters was below 1 s, indicating that, on average, the system's measurements were within 1 s of the ground truth. The mean error (ME) values were also relatively small, suggesting that the system did not consistently overestimate or underestimate the TUG

Table 1. Mean absolute error (MAE), mean error (ME), standard deviation (STD), and Bland-Altman limits of agreement (LOA) for TUG phases.

TUG Phases [s]	MAE (|GT-Ac|)	ME (GT-Ac)	STD (GT-Ac)	LOA (+)	LOA (−)
TUG-Time	0.71	0.59	0.67	1.90	−0.73
Sit-to-Stand	0.57	−0.44	0.63	0.80	−1.69
Mid-Turning	0.39	−0.12	0.54	0.94	−1.17
End-Turning-Stand-to-Sit	0.33	0.30	0.26	0.81	−0.22

parameters. The standard deviation (STD) values were generally low, indicating that the errors were relatively consistent across different trials. The Bland-Altman LOA were also relatively narrow, further supporting the system's reliability.

Table 2. Mean error (ME) and standard deviation (STD) of the error between G-WALK and the developed system for different TUG phases in different walking conditions.

TUG Phases [s]	Normal Walk (ME ± STD)	Slow Walk (ME ± STD)	Abnormal Walk (ME ± STD)
Sit-to-Stand	0.38 ± 0.66	−0.23 ± 0.94	−0.92 ± 1.72
Mid-Turning	0.35 ± 0.78	0.78 ± 2.03	−0.33 ± 1.11
End-Turning-Stand-to-Sit	1.05 ± 0.36	1.58 ± 0.62	1.73 ± 0.48

To provide a more comprehensive analysis, the TUG parameters were also evaluated separately for each walk type (normal, slow, and abnormal) using G-WALK as the ground truth. The results, presented in Table 2, reveal that the system's performance varied across different walking conditions. For normal and slow walks, the system generally performed well, with relatively low mean errors and standard deviations for most TUG parameters. However, the system's performance deteriorated for abnormal walks, particularly for the Sit-to-Stand and End-Turning-Stand-to-Sit parameters, which showed larger errors and higher variability. Furthermore, in Table 2, the Mid-turning phase for the slow walk shows relatively higher Mean Error (ME) and Standard Deviation (STD) compared to other phases. The relatively higher ME and STD observed in the slow walk for the Mid-turning phase can be partly attributed to the fact that participants were mimicking a slower pace rather than walking naturally. This act of mimicking could introduce inconsistencies and exaggerated movements, particularly during the Mid-turning phase, where precise coordination is required.

The variability in how participants executed the slower pace, combined with the subtler and more cautious movements, likely led to irregularities in sensor detection, resulting in greater measurement error. This highlights a limitation of the current system in accurately capturing movements that are not naturally performed, suggesting the need for further refinement to better accommodate varied gait patterns.

3.2 Evaluation of Gait Parameters

The system ability to calculate gait parameters was limited by its inability to consistently identify all phases of the gait cycle. While it could differentiate between double and single stances, it struggled to accurately detect heel strikes and toe-offs. This is mostly due to the low sampling frequency of 10 Hz which limits the ability to capture enough details of the movement of each foot. Sometimes only the heel strike is visible, other times only the tip of the foot is instead captured. Consequently, the calculated stride length exhibited high variability, especially during slow and abnormal walks. Table 3 summarizes the results for the gait parameters.

Table 3. Mean error (ME), standard deviation (STD), and Bland-Altman limits of agreement (LOA) for stride length in different walking conditions (in centimeters).

	ME (GT-Ac)	STD (GT-Ac)	LOA (+)	LOA (−)
Normal Walk	0.17	5.74	11.42	−11.09
Slow Walk	4.67	14.35	32.79	−23.46
Abnormal Walk	−22.00	18.86	14.96	−58.96
Total	−5.35	18.33	30.57	−41.28

The average walking speed calculated by the algorithm, for normal walking, was 0.93 m/s, which is within reasonable bounds when compared to reference values from the literature [10]. However, the high variability in stride length measurements, as evidenced by the wide Bland-Altman LOA and high standard deviation, suggesting the need for further refinement of the algorithm.

4 Conclusion

This paper sets out to address the need for algorithms relating to sensorized mats, to allow these to be used for TUG tests. The results from the system implementation and data collection of this study demonstrates the potential for using sensorized mats for objective characterization of the TUG test. The system developed was able to accurately measure TUG-time and other TUG parameters for normal and slow walks, with errors below the MCID threshold.

For abnormal walks, the system needs further research as performance was less accurate when trying to accommodate wider diversity of gait patterns. This would ideally be done in combination with data from participants with actual movement inhibitions rather than relying on simulated problems Furthermore, the estimation of gait parameters was limited by the system inability to consistently identify all phases of the gait cycle. This limitation could be addressed by increasing the sampling rate of the sensor data acquisition system or by incorporating additional sensor types, such as accelerometers.

Overall, the results of this study are promising and suggest that sensorized mats have the potential to be a valuable tool for objective gait analysis. With further refinement, the system developed in this research could be used to improve the accuracy and objectivity of clinical gait assessments.

Acknowledgements. This work was partially funded by the European Union - Next Generation EU, in the context of The National Recovery and Resilience Plan, Investment Partenariato Esteso PE8 *"Conseguenze e sfide dell'invecchiamento"* Project Age-IT, CUP: B83C22004800006, and by the Swedish Knowledge Foundation and the Internet of Things and People research center through the Synergy project Intelligent and Trustworthy IoT Systems.

References

1. Bacciu, D., et al.: A learning system for automatic berg balance scale score estimation. Eng. Appl. Artif. Intell. **66**, 60–74 (2017)
2. Bagarotti, R., Zini, E.M., Salvi, E., Sacchi, L., Quaglini, S., Lanzola, G.: An algorithm for estimating gait parameters through a commercial sensorized carpet. In: 2018 IEEE 4th International Forum on Research and Technology for Society and Industry (RTSI), pp. 1–6. IEEE (2018)
3. Bilney, B., Morris, M., Webster, K.: Concurrent related validity of the gaitrite walkway system for quantification of the spatial and temporal parameters of gait. Gait Posture **17**(1), 68–74 (2003)
4. Braun, B.J., et al.: Wearable technology in orthopedic trauma surgery-an AO trauma survey and review of current and future applications. Injury **53**(6), 1961–1965 (2022)
5. Chambers, H.G., Sutherland, D.H.: A practical guide to gait analysis. JAAOS-J. Am. Acad. Orthop. Surg. **10**(3), 222–231 (2002)
6. Giladi, N., Bloem, B.R., Hausdorff, J.M.: Chapter 36 - gait disturbances and falls. In: Schapira, A.H., et al. (eds.) Neurology and Clinical Neuroscience, pp. 455–470. Mosby, Philadelphia (2007). https://doi.org/10.1016/B978-0-323-03354-1.50040-7
7. Muro-de-la Herran, A., Garcia-Zapirain, B., Mendez-Zorrilla, A.: Gait analysis methods: an overview of wearable and non-wearable systems, highlighting clinical applications. Sensors **14**(2), 3362–3394 (2014)
8. Hulleck, A.A., Menoth Mohan, D., Abdallah, N., El Rich, M., Khalaf, K.: Present and future of gait assessment in clinical practice: towards the application of novel trends and technologies. Front. Med. Technol. **4**, 901331 (2022)

9. Mathias, S., Nayak, U., Isaacs, B.: Balance in elderly patients: the "get-up and go" test. Arch. Phys. Med. Rehabil. **67**(6), 387–389 (1986)
10. Murtagh, E.M., Mair, J.L., Aguiar, E., Tudor-Locke, C., Murphy, M.H.: Outdoor walking speeds of apparently healthy adults: a systematic review and meta-analysis. Sports Med. **51**(1), 125–141 (2021)
11. Shumway-Cook, A., Brauer, S., Woollacott, M.: Predicting the probability for falls in community-dwelling older adults using the timed up & go test. Phys. Ther. **80**(9), 896–903 (2000)
12. Soto-Varela, A., et al.: Modified timed up and go test for tendency to fall and balance assessment in elderly patients with gait instability. Front. Neurol. **11**, 543 (2020)
13. Zampieri, C., Salarian, A., Carlson-Kuhta, P., Aminian, K., Nutt, J.G., Horak, F.B.: The instrumented timed up and go test: potential outcome measure for disease modifying therapies in Parkinson's disease. J. Neurol. Neurosurg. Psychiatry **81**(2), 171–176 (2010)

A Flexible IMU-Based Unit for Validation Studies: A Step Counting Application

Alessandra Angelucci[1]([✉]) [ID], Lorenzo Barbieri[1] [ID], Sara Caramaschi[2] [ID], Clarysse A. Sarmiento[1] [ID], Virginia Sekules[1] [ID], and Andrea Aliverti[1] [ID]

[1] Dipartimento di Elettronica, Informazione e Bioingegneria, Politecnico di Milano, P.zza Leonardo da Vinci 32, 20133 Milan, Italy
alessandra.angelucci@polimi.it

[2] Internet of Things and People Research Center, Department of Computer Science and Media Technology, Malmö University, Nordenskiöldsgatan 1, 211 19 Malmö, Sweden

Abstract. Wearable step counting devices, such as smartwatches and activity trackers, have become ubiquitous, embedding sensors like Inertial Measurement Units (IMUs), barometers, and GPS systems to monitor physical activity. Despite their widespread use, these devices often restrict access to raw data, limiting their utility in research. This study introduces a customizable IMU-based unit, designed for flexible data acquisition and integration into a body sensor network (BSN), which can serve as a reference system for validating commercial smartwatches. The IMU-based unit transmits data via the ANT protocol and stores backups on an SD card to mitigate transmission data loss. Five volunteers participated in a protocol involving various conditions, such as resting, walking on a treadmill, walking outdoors, and climbing stairs. Preliminary results indicate that the IMU-based unit detects steps correctly accordingly to the typical waveforms reported in the literature The flexibility of the IMU-based unit allows for extensive post-processing and analysis, making it a valuable tool for validating commercial wearable devices and advancing research in physical activity monitoring. Future improvements include integrating multiple units and adopting Bluetooth Low Energy for enhanced data transmission and compatibility.

Keywords: Inertial Measurement Unit · step counting · wearable device · digital health

1 Introduction

1.1 Wearable Devices for Step Counting

Step counting devices, also known as pedometers or activity trackers, have gained significant popularity in recent years, as small wearable devices have become an integral part of many individuals' daily lives [1]. Wearables exist for different parts of the body, and the ones which embed step counting functions are generally watches (such as smartwatches and activity trackers) [2, 3], smartphones [4], foot-worn [5] and ankle-worn [6] devices, sensorized insoles [7, 8], smart glasses [9], smart rings [10], sensorized shirts [11], chest-worn bands [12], and earbuds [13].

© ICST Institute for Computer Sciences, Social Informatics and Telecommunications Engineering 2025
Published by Springer Nature Switzerland AG 2025. All Rights Reserved
H. Kondylakis and A. Triantafyllidis (Eds.): PervasiveHealth 2024, LNICST 612, pp. 190–200, 2025.
https://doi.org/10.1007/978-3-031-85575-7_12

Wearables embed different types of sensors, the most common of which are Inertial Measurement Units (IMUs), barometers, and GPS systems when they are used for step counting. IMUs are composed of accelerometers, gyroscopes, magnetometers, or a combination of those sensors. Miniaturized accelerometers can detect when a step is performed from the acceleration pattern [14]. In most circumstances, the accelerometer acts as the lead sensor while the gyroscope functions as the supplementary sensor. There are walking patterns, such as climbing stairs, where performance improves when gyroscopic data are used due to the oscillation of the body. Barometers can be useful in detecting steps while climbing stairs, due to the differences in elevation detectable from atmospheric pressures [15]. Additionally, GPS data can be fused with other sensor data to estimate the number of steps taken, distance and speed. All these sensors can be embedded in devices applied on different body locations, mostly on the wrist such as in the case of smartwatches and activity trackers.

Sensorized insoles can be based on several types of sensors, commonly capacitive or piezoresistive [16], and differ from the previously cited technology as they are directly applied under the foot, therefore they directly sense the pressures applied on the insole and can derive the number of steps. Another technology of interest is ankle force myography (FMG), which is recorded by using piezoresistive sensors surrounding the ankle to register the volumetric changes during muscle activities. Even during a low-speed walking, where accelerometer-based step counters encounter difficulties [6], the contraction and relaxation of the extensors and flexors causes different force distributions on the ankle-worn band, resulting in distinctive FMG patterns, and thus allowing to count the number of steps.

A limitation of commercial step counting wearable devices, and of wearable devices in general, is that users often have limited access to raw data, and platforms lack the flexibility needed for research purposes. Researchers require the ability to conduct simultaneous measurements from multiple devices and need the flexibility to customize acquisition parameters to suit their specific study needs. In fact, to do research effectively, a platform must be customizable in terms of number and type of devices to be acquired, sensors, sampling frequency, sensitivity, possibility to have a backup with no data loss, and choice between raw and processed data.

Furthermore, several devices currently available on the market, in particular smartwatches and activity trackers, do not have published validation data, therefore the accuracy and reliability of such devices must be assessed before using them. Some studies show how different smartwatches output different numbers of steps after the same walking activity is performed [17], thus raising doubts about the validity of some algorithms embedded in commercial smartwatches. Moore et al. [18] presented a scoping review on treadmill-based validation of step counting wearable technologies, in an attempt to provide a harmonized, empirically based set of best practices. As a recommendation on a given number of steps per day to take is being increasingly used both in individual and public health interventions, as in the case of the "10000 steps per day" recommendation from by the Centers for Disease Control and Prevention (CDC) [19], validation of wearables for step counting becomes critical.

1.2 Aim of the Work

This work presents two main aims. The first aim is to present a flexible IMU-based unit that allows to perform customizable acquisitions based on user's needs and that can be easily integrated into a body sensor network (BSN). This unit, thanks to the integration into the BSN, can be used in validation studies that employ wearable devices, either as a reference system (such as in the step counting application we present here) or as the device to be validated (such as the case of a 3-units configuration for respiratory measurements [20]). The second aim is to demonstrate that this IMU-based unit can be effectively used as a reference system in an experimental protocol to validate the step counting function of a commercial smartwatch.

2 Materials and Methods

2.1 Hardware

The hardware of the IMU-based unit is based on the MDBT50Q chip by Raytac, which embeds the nRF52840 microcontroller and a radiofrequency antenna. Two sensors are integrated in the printed circuit board (PCB), *i.e.*, the LSM6DSO 6-axis IMU and the LIS2MDL magnetometer, both by STMicroelectronics. Data from the sensors are sent to a smartphone app by means of the ANT protocol, which is further detailed in Sect. 2.2, and can also be saved on an on-board SD card. Figure 1 shows the IMU-based unit enclosed in a custom-made 3D-printed case designed to attach the unit to a person's shoe. Figure 1a, 1b, and 1c show the three dimensions of the device, and Fig. 1d how the device is worn on the shoe by means of an elastic strap.

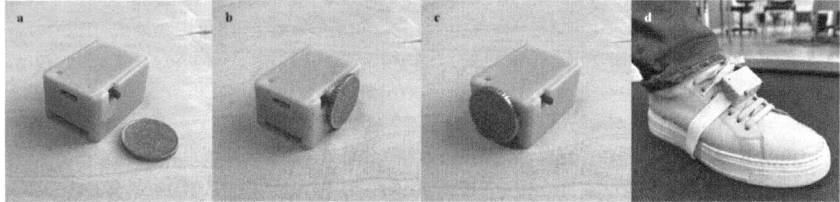

Fig. 1. Dimensions of the IMU-based device (a, b, c), and elastic strap to attach the device to the shoe (d).

2.2 ANT Network Topology

The ANT network topology implemented for this application is the star topology. The system is designed to simultaneously acquire a varying number of devices, but only one is used in this study. Each unit functions as a master node communicating through an independent channel to the smartphone with ANT USB2 stick acting as a slave. Additionally, a low frequency shared slave channel is used to control all the units.

The maximum data rate for sensor data is 180 Hz. In fact, the ANT USB2 stick supports up to 8 ANT channels and a combined message data rate of up to 190 Hz with 8-byte data payload in broadcast transmission. As 5 Hz of bandwidth are reserved for the control channel, 185 Hz are left for data transmission; we choose a maximum settable data rate of 180 Hz (BW_{total}) to facilitate computations when multiple units are used. To obtain the maximum bandwidth per unit (BW_{unit}), BW_{total} must be divided by the number of units n_{units} used in the acquisition, as in Eq. (1).

$$BW_{unit} = \frac{BW_{total}}{n_{units}} = \frac{180Hz}{n_{units}} \tag{1}$$

Furthermore, the maximum data rate (MDR) is influenced by the number of sensors used in the acquisition ($n_{sensors}$), as each sensor output occupies 6 bytes (1-byte LSB and 1-byte LSB for each axis). The formula is reported in Eq. (2).

$$MDR = \frac{BW_{unit}}{n_{sensors}} \tag{2}$$

2.3 Mobile Android Application

By means of a dedicated mobile Android application, the user can select the desired characteristics. Following user authentication and patient or participant selection, the user can set multiple parameters:

– Number of IMU-based units involved in the acquisition: at the present time, three units are available for selection.
– Sensors' data to collect: all combinations including accelerometer, gyroscope, and magnetometer are possible.
– Sensors' sensitivities: the user can select accelerometer and gyroscope sensitivities depending on the acquisition to be performed. Possible accelerometer sensitivities are ± 2 g, ± 4 g, ± 8 g and ± 16 g; possible gyroscope sensitivities are ± 125 dps, ± 250 dps, ± 500 dps and ± 1000 dps.
– Sampling frequency: the number of IMU-based units and sensors involved in the acquisition impacts the maximum selectable data rate, as it was explained in Sect. 2.2. The user must input the desired data rate output in Hz in the specific textbox. On-screen hints guide the user to a valid data rate selection.
– Backup file on the SD card: the user can choose whether to create a backup file on the SD card, and if so, select the file name.

2.4 Data Acquisition Protocol

5 healthy volunteers were enrolled in the protocol (3 men, mean age 24.2 ± 0.4 years, mean weight 66.8 ± 5.5 kg, mean height 172.4 ± 7.7 cm). The complete experimental setup consisted of three different devices: the Bangle.js 2 smartwatch from Espruino [21], the IMU-based unit presented in the previous sections, and the Polar H10 chest-worn strap [22]. In particular, the Bangle.js 2 smartwatch is an open, hackable smartwatch worn on the wrist which features several functions, including step counting and pulse

rate monitoring. The IMU-based unit attached to the shoe was used as a reference for the Bangle.js 2's step counting algorithm, while the Polar H10 chest-worn strap is equipped with an ECG sensor applied on the torso [23] and was used as a reference for the pulse rate monitored by the smartwatch. The IMU-based unit, in this protocol, sampled data at 100 Hz, used only the accelerometer with a sensitivity of $\pm$ 4 g, and simultaneously saved backup data on the SD card.

The complete protocol consisted of the following activities:

- Light activity, such as typing or working at the computer (5 min)
- Rest (3 min)
- Walking on a treadmill: baseline (2 min), walking at 3 km/h (3 min), walking at 4 km/h (3 min), walking at 5 km/h (3 min), recovery (3 min)
- Climbing up and down four flights of stairs three times
- Outdoor walking (1.03 km) with multiple 15-s stops where there are pedestrian crossings.

2.5 Signal Processing

Steps are computed by using a threshold-based algorithm. First, the global acceleration is computed using Eq. (3).

$$a_{global} = \sqrt{a_x^2 + a_y^2 + a_z^2} \qquad (3)$$

Then a_{global} is filtered using a 3 Hz low pass FIR filter to eliminate high-frequency noise and vibration not related to walking. After the FIR filter of order 300 is applied, a minimum distance between the peaks is selected to avoid overestimation of the number of peaks. The minimum distance between the peaks set by the algorithm changes depending on the walking speed, based on the work of Park et al. [24].

The acceleration threshold used to detect a step is then determined by adding two times the standard deviation of all collected global acceleration values to the mean global acceleration value after being filtered. Every time a peak is detected above this threshold, the algorithm detects a step. It must be noted that, in this case, only one IMU-based unit is used, therefore only one foot is monitored and to estimate the number of steps the obtained count must be multiplied by two.

3 Preliminary Results

3.1 Transmission Data Loss

Table 1 reports the data loss of the different phases of the protocol for each participant. Data loss is evaluated in terms of transmitted packets, but the lost samples could be retrieved from the SD card, thus making data loss virtually null during the research project. From the results in Table 1, it emerges that one participant had a systematically higher transmission data loss than the others, probably due to problems with the smartphone's ANT antenna. The results confirm that the SD card is a key feature of the system, which is overall reliable for flexible acquisitions both indoors and outdoors.

The higher data loss on during the acquisitions indoor on the treadmill can be attributed to by the high number of connected devices simultaneously present in the research laboratory and that might cause data transmission interference, while generally less connected devices are present outdoors.

Table 1. Transmission data loss of each acquisition, divided by participant.

Participant	Light activity	Rest	Treadmill	Stairs	Outdoor
1	7.40%	4.75%	15.04%	5.97%	8.4%
2	4.65%	5.02%	11.16%	8.45%	3.45%
3	25.5%	22.40%	27.90%	26.3%	27.6%
4	4.78%	5.00%	14.70%	9.58%	7.55%
5	6.63%	4.49%	9.85%	5.93%	2.86%

3.2 Examples of Step Counting Acquisitions Traces

Figure 2 shows three global acceleration traces, obtained from the same participant, during the three phases of walking on the treadmill (at 3 km/h in Fig. 2a, at 4 km/h in Fig. 2b, and at 3 km/h in Fig. 2c). The adaptive threshold is shown in each acquisition, and the number of steps that can be manually counted by looking at the signal is almost the same as the number of steps detected by the threshold-based algorithm. Furthermore, the possibility to have an adaptive threshold proved useful as in the three presented traces,

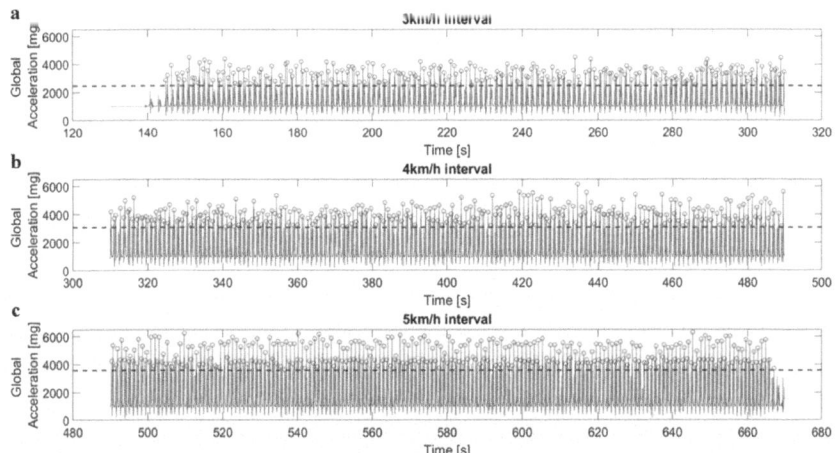

Fig. 2. Traces of global accelerations (blue line), identified steps (red dots), and thresholds determined by the algorithm for each trace (dotted line). (a) Walking on a treadmill at 3 km/h; (b) Walking on a treadmill at 4 km/h; (c) Walking on a treadmill at 5 km/h. (Color figure online)

all obtained from the same participant, the threshold is different, specifically higher as walking speed increases.

Figure 3 shows the number of steps detected by the Bangle.js smartwatch (Fig. 3a) and the values of acceleration detected by the IMU-based unit (Fig. 3b) during the outdoor acquisition of the same participant. The parts highlighted in yellow are in correspondence with pedestrian crossings, where the participant stopped for a few seconds. When no acceleration other than gravity is detected, *i.e.*, when the participant is still, also the count of steps stops until activity is resumed. It is however apparent how IMU data allow a more comprehensive understanding of the gait pattern and therefore of step counting.

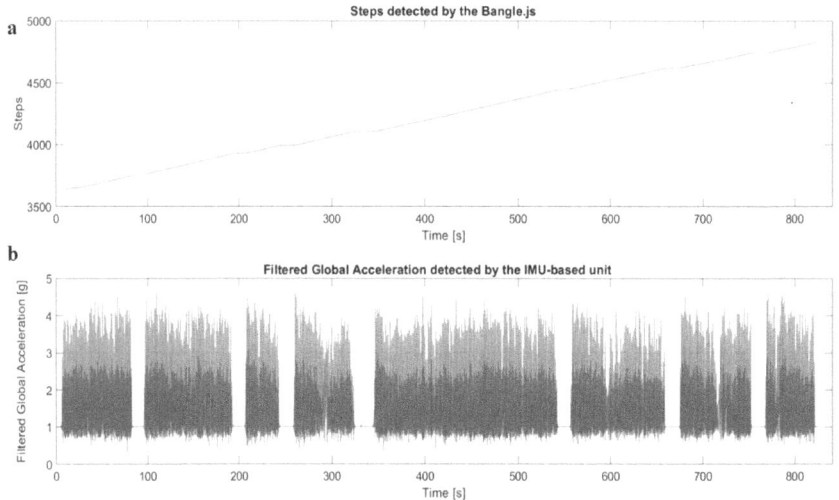

Fig. 3. Data obtained during the outdoor walking activity (a) Number of steps detected by the Bangle.js smartwatch; (b) Filtered global acceleration obtained from the IMU-based unit. The yellow areas highlight the moments when the participant stopped walking because of a pedestrian crossing. (Color figure online)

4   Discussion and Conclusions

This work describes the main characteristics of a flexible, custom-made IMU-based unit worn on the foot and used as a reference for step counting in an experimental protocol to validate a wrist-worn smartwatch. Positioning the unit on the foot allows not to detect artifacts due to arm and upper body movements, which is a major limitation of smartwatch-based step counting algorithms.

By means of a simple, threshold-based algorithm, the number of steps can be detected in a highly controlled situation such as walking on a treadmill. From the IMU-based unit, we are able to detect a signal with the typical waveforms reported in the literature [5]. One limitation of this work is that in more ecological conditions, such as walking outdoor or at an irregular pace, this algorithm is probably going to decrease its performance.

Furthermore, the number of enrolled participants is low, and it is therefore difficult to determine to what extent the signal processing strategy is robust even on a treadmill. Further tests are needed to assess the transmission data loss and the robustness of the threshold-based method. However, the flexibility of the designed IMU-based device allows to obtain raw accelerometer, and if needed gyroscope and magnetometer, data without data loss when the SD card is enabled, thus allowing researchers to perform further post-processing and analysis depending on the need.

The ANT protocol provides an easy strategy for integrating multiple units, but it has a limited bandwidth in the present configuration (broadcast transmission). This means that even with two IMU-based units instead of only one it would be no longer possible to collect data at 100 Hz from both, even if 100 Hz is a commonly used sampling frequency in motion analysis studies. As of today, the user sets the sampling frequency, and this value corresponds to the data transmission frequency too. One possible improvement consists in implementing the possibility of sampling data at a higher frequency, saving them into the SD card, and only send a subset of such data wirelessly. Furthermore, substituting the ANT protocol with BLE would allow to solve this problem, and to avoid the problem of supporting the ANT protocol in the first place, a feature that several smartphones do not have, including Apple smartphones. Using BLE, in combination with adequate app development in other programming languages such as Dart (*i.e.*, using Flutter, which is designed to work on all operating systems), would allow to install the app on almost all users' smartphones with no limitations.

Finally, the presented configuration uses only one IMU-based unit for step counting; however, the firmware and mobile application are designed with the purpose of integrating multiple devices in the BSN, either more IMU-based units, as it was discussed before, or other types of units. As mentioned in the Introduction, one of the main challenges of researchers is to be able to acquire exactly the combination of data needed for an experimentation, which varies from one experimental campaign to the other, and is a need that is not presently satisfied by commercial experimental platforms. The presented system enables the acquisition of various data combinations, including one setup with an IMU-based unit on the foot and another on the wrist. This configuration could be used to optimize step-counting algorithms on smartwatches in real-world settings, using foot-worn sensing as a reference. Another opportunity is to study the locomotor-respiratory coupling by acquiring raw data from two or three [25] chest-worn IMU-based units. In previous works, we have used different combinations of the following units: three IMU-based units [20, 25–28], a pulse oximeter [20, 27], a single-lead patch ECG [29], and an environmental monitor [30]. We plan to include in this platform other devices, including a wearable monitor of the partial pressure of transcutaneous carbon dioxide [31] and a module for electrodermal activity monitoring. This would enable much more complex analyses of multiple parameters and their interactions with each other during different activities and in various conditions.

Acknowledgements. We thank Prof. Dario Salvi of Malmö University for his support and guidance during this work.

Funding Information. This work was partly funded by the National Plan for National Recovery and Resilience Plan (NRRP) Complementary Investments (PNC, established with the decree-law 6 May 2021, n. 59, converted by law n. 101 of 2021) in the call for the funding of the Research Initiatives for Technologies and Innovative Trajectories in the health and care sectors (Directorial Decree n. 931 of 06–06-2022)–AdvaNced Technologies for Human-centrEd Medicine (ANTHEM) under Project PNC0000003. This work reflects only the authors' views and opinions, neither the Ministry for University and Research nor European Commission can be considered responsible for them.

References

1. Angelucci, A., Canali, S., Aliverti, A.: Digital technologies for step counting: between promises of reliability and risks of reductionism. Front Digit Health. **5** (2023)
2. Greco, M., et al.: Wearable health technology for preoperative risk assessment in elderly patients: the WELCOME study. Diagnostics **13** (2023). https://doi.org/10.3390/diagnostics13040630
3. Angelucci, A., et al.: Fitbit data to assess functional capacity in patients before elective surgery: pilot prospective observational study. J. Med. Internet Res. **25** (2023). https://doi.org/10.2196/42815
4. Qi, W., Su, H., Aliverti, A.: A smartphone-based adaptive recognition and real-time monitoring system for human activities. IEEE Trans. Hum. Mach. Syst. **50**, 414–423 (2020). https://doi.org/10.1109/THMS.2020.2984181
5. Anwary, A.R., Yu, H., Vassallo, M.: Optimal foot location for placing wearable IMU sensors and automatic feature extraction for gait analysis. IEEE Sens. J. **18**, 2555–2567 (2018). https://doi.org/10.1109/JSEN.2017.2786587
6. Jiang, X., Chu, K.H.T., Menon, C.: An easy-to-use wearable step counting device for slow walking using ankle force myography. In: 2017 IEEE International Conference on Systems, Man, and Cybernetics, SMC 2017. 2017-January, pp. 2219–2224 (2017). https://doi.org/10.1109/SMC.2017.8122950
7. Aliverti, A., Evangelisti, M., Angelucci, A.: Wearable tech for long-distance runners (2022). https://doi.org/10.1007/978-3-662-65064-6_10
8. Civeriati, V., et al.: A sensorized insole to estimate ground reaction forces and center of pressure during gait. In: 2024 IEEE International Workshop on Sport, Technology and Research (STAR), pp. 21–25 (2024). https://doi.org/10.1109/STAR62027.2024.10636002
9. Cristiano, A., Sanna, A., Trojaniello, D.: Validity of a smart-glasses-based step-count measure during simulated free-living conditions. Information **11**, 404 (2020). https://doi.org/10.3390/INFO11090404
10. Kristiansson, E., Fridolfsson, J., Arvidsson, D., Holmäng, A., Börjesson, M., Andersson-Hall, U.: Validation of Oura ring energy expenditure and steps in laboratory and free-living. BMC Med. Res. Methodol. **23** (2023). https://doi.org/10.1186/s12874-023-01868-x
11. Angelucci, A., et al.: Smart textiles and sensorized garments for physiological monitoring: a review of available solutions and techniques. Sensors (Switzerland) **21**, 1–23 (2021). https://doi.org/10.3390/s21030814
12. Angelucci, A., Kuller, D., Aliverti, A.: A home telemedicine system for continuous respiratory monitoring. IEEE J. Biomed. Health Inform. **25** (2021). https://doi.org/10.1109/JBHI.2020.3012621
13. Prakash, J., Yang, Z., Wei, Y.L., Choudhury, R.R.: STEAR: robust step counting from earables. In: Proceedings of the 1st International Workshop on Earable Computing, EarComp 2019, pp. 36–41. Association for Computing Machinery, Inc (2019). https://doi.org/10.1145/3345615.3361133

14. Angelucci, A., Aliverti, A.: Telemonitoring systems for respiratory patients: technological aspects. Pulmonology **26**, 221–232 (2020). https://doi.org/10.1016/j.pulmoe.2019.11.006
15. Massé, F., Gonzenbach, R.R., Arami, A., Paraschiv-Ionescu, A., Luft, A.R., Aminian, K.: Improving activity recognition using a wearable barometric pressure sensor in mobility-impaired stroke patients. J. Neuroeng. Rehabil. **12** (2015). https://doi.org/10.1186/s12984-015-0060-2
16. Chen, J.L., et al.: Plantar pressure-based insole gait monitoring techniques for diseases monitoring and analysis: a review (2022). https://doi.org/10.1002/admt.202100566
17. Montes, J., Tandy, R., Young, J., Lee, S.-P., Navalta, J.W.: Step count reliability and validity of five wearable technology devices while walking and jogging in both a free motion setting and on a treadmill. Int. J. Exerc. Sci. **13**, 410–426 (2020)
18. Moore, C.C., McCullough, A.K., Aguiar, E.J., Ducharme, S.W., Tudor-Locke, C.: Toward harmonized treadmill-based validation of step-counting wearable technologies: a scoping review (2020). https://doi.org/10.1123/jpah.2019-0205
19. Piercy, K.L., et al.: The physical activity guidelines for Americans. JAMA **320**, 2020–2028 (2018). https://doi.org/10.1001/JAMA.2018.14854
20. Angelucci, A., et al.: A wireless body sensor network for cardiorespiratory monitoring during cycling. In: 2023 IEEE International Workshop on Sport, Technology and Research (STAR), pp. 1–4 (2023). https://doi.org/10.1109/STAR58331.2023.10302438
21. Bangle.js 2 – Espruino. https://www.espruino.com/Bangle.js2. Accessed 28 June 2024
22. Schaffarczyk, M., Rogers, B., Reer, R., Gronwald, T.: Validity of the polar H10 sensor for heart rate variability analysis during resting state and incremental exercise in recreational men and women. Sensors **22** (2022). https://doi.org/10.3390/s22176536
23. Polar H10|Polar Global. https://www.polar.com/en/sensors/h10-heart-rate-sensor. Accessed 28 June 2024
24. Park, J., Ishikawa-Takata, K., Tanaka, S., Mekata, Y., Tabata, I.: Effects of walking speed and step frequency on estimation of physical activity using accelerometers. J. Physiol. Anthropol. **30**, 119–127 (2011). https://doi.org/10.2114/JPA2.30.119
25. Angelucci, A., Camuncoli, F., Galli, M., Aliverti, A.: A wearable system for respiratory signal filtering based on activity: a preliminary validation. In: 2022 IEEE International Workshop on Sport, Technology and Research, STAR 2022 - Proceedings (2022). https://doi.org/10.1109/STAR53492.2022.9860001
26. Angelucci, A., Aliverti, A.: An IMU-based wearable system for respiratory rate estimation in static and dynamic conditions. Cardiovasc Eng Technol. 1–13 (2023). https://doi.org/10.1007/S13239-023-00657-3/FIGURES/8
27. Angelucci, A., Bernasconi, S., D'Andrea, M., Contini, M., Gugliandolo, P., Agostoni, P., Aliverti, A.: Integration of a body sensor network of wearable devices for cardio-respiratory monitoring. In: 2023 45th Annual International Conference of the IEEE Engineering in Medicine & Biology Society (EMBC), pp. 1–4 (2023). https://doi.org/10.1109/EMBC40787.2023.10340495
28. Angelucci, A., Birettoni, F., Bufalari, A., Aliverti, A.: Validation of a wearable system for respiratory rate monitoring in dogs. IEEE Access. **12**, 80308–80316 (2024). https://doi.org/10.1109/ACCESS.2024.3408904
29. Angelucci, A., Villamar, O.W.P., Agostoni, P., Aliverti, A.: Design and evaluation of a wearable single-lead ECG for continuous monitoring. In: 2023 IEEE International Conference on Metrology for Extended Reality, Artificial Intelligence and Neural Engineering (MetroXRAINE), pp. 80–85 (2023). https://doi.org/10.1109/MetroXRAINE58569.2023.10405813

30. Bernasconi, S., Angelucci, A., Aliverti, A.: Evaluation of a new wearable device for indoor and outdoor environmental monitoring. In: 2024 IEEE International Workshop on Sport, Technology and Research (STAR), pp. 252–257 (2024). https://doi.org/10.1109/STAR62027.2024.10635952
31. Angelucci, A., et al.: A wearable device to monitor the partial pressure of transcutaneous carbon dioxide. IEEE Trans. Instrum. Meas.Instrum. Meas. **73**, 1–12 (2024). https://doi.org/10.1109/TIM.2024.3369136

Posters

Using Predictive Analysis and Wearables to Increase Physical Activity Among Individuals with Disabilities- SMART Design

Sangeetha Mohanraj[✉], Christen Mendonca, Laurie Malone, and Mohanraj Thirumalai

University of Alabama at Birmingham, Birmingham, AL 35244, USA
mohanraj@uab.edu

Abstract. Approximately half of individuals with disabilities in the United States lead inactive lifestyles despite the acknowledged health advantages of exercise. Barriers such as transportation issues, limited facility access, and a shortage of trained professionals hinder their engagement; thus, teleexercise via telehealth has emerged as a promising alternative, albeit lacking a universally effective modality. This study employs the Sequential Multiple Assignment Randomized Trial (SMART) methodology to determine the optimal sequence of tailored multimodal teleexercise interventions, utilizing predictive analytics and wearable sensor data to enhance adherence and evaluate feasibility and efficacy in a pilot trial commencing in Fall 2024.

Keywords: Predictive analysis · physical activity · disabilities · teleexercise · Sequential Multiple Assignment Randomized Trial (SMART) · multimodal intervention · wearable sensors · health coaching

1 Background

Approximately half of individuals with disabilities in the United States maintain a sedentary lifestyle despite overwhelming evidence showcasing the numerous health and quality of life benefits associated with physical activity [1–4]. Various factors hinder their participation in physical activities, such as challenges related to transportation, limited access to suitable facilities, and a shortage of skilled professionals who understand disability [5–9]. Teleexercise, which involves the remote delivery of exercise sessions through telehealth, has emerged as a feasible substitute for exercising in person at a nearby fitness facility [10]. Numerous tele-exercise modalities (asynchronous method, real-time exercise session in one-on-one or group setting, access to live or offline health coaches.) have been explored; however, no universally effective modality caters to the diverse needs of all individuals with disabilities.

© ICST Institute for Computer Sciences, Social Informatics and Telecommunications Engineering 2025
Published by Springer Nature Switzerland AG 2025. All Rights Reserved
H. Kondylakis and A. Triantafyllidis (Eds.): PervasiveHealth 2024, LNICST 612, pp. 203–205, 2025.
https://doi.org/10.1007/978-3-031-85575-7

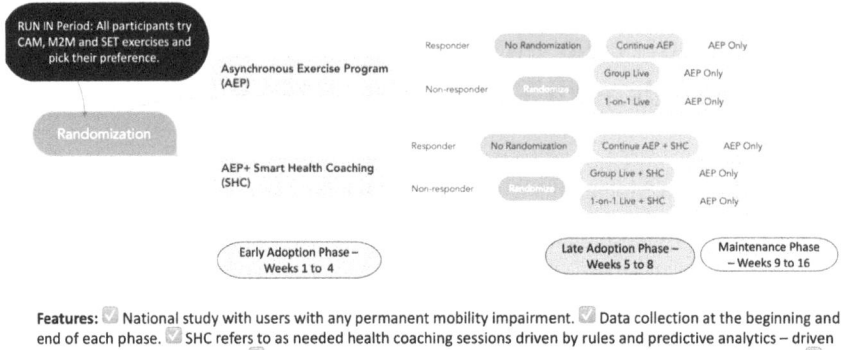

Features: ☑ National study with users with any permanent mobility impairment. ☑ Data collection at the beginning and end of each phase. ☑ SHC refers to as needed health coaching sessions driven by rules and predictive analytics – driven by data from all our prior-work. ☑ Accelerometry to objectively monitor physical activity levels (primary outcome). ☑ Fatigue as a secondary outcome. ☑ CAM – Complementary Alternative Medicine (Yoga/Pilates), M2M – Movement to Music, SET – Standard Exercise Training.

Fig. 1. Overview of SMART Design

2   Purpose

The primary aim of this research is to employ a novel experimental methodology called SMART (Sequential Multiple Assignment Randomized Trial) in order to ascertain the optimal strategy for organizing an optimal sequence of multimodal teleexercise tailored for individuals with disabilities (referred to as an adaptive intervention), in conjunction with predictive analytics on participant adherence within a structured series of physical activity interventions.

3   Methods

To address this need, a SMART (Sequential Multiple Assignment Randomized Trial) trial has been meticulously crafted to ascertain the effectiveness of an adaptive intervention that integrates asynchronous exercise videos, telehealth coaching, and one-on-one or group live exercise training sessions. The suggested multi-level intervention package (explained in Fig. 1) commences with the most cost-effective elements. Supplementary intervention components will gradually escalate if participants are deemed non-responsive to the intervention. By sequentially administering intervention components according to participant feedback, SMART enhances the likelihood of intervention success (e.g., boosting physical activity) with minimal resource utilization and lessening participant burden.

Predictive analytics is crucial in determining the ideal number of health coaching calls. At the same time, insights from patient-reported outcomes and data collected from wearable sensors aid in distinguishing between responders and non-responders to the initial treatment, thereby influencing the sequential randomization process. A comprehensive monitoring dashboard and automated messaging functionalities are implemented to enhance participant adherence to the intervention program.

4 Results

The primary focus of this study will center on evaluating the level of physical activity, while the secondary outcomes will delve into behavioral aspects, pain management, and fatigue levels. An initial pilot trial phase is slated to commence in the Fall of 2024 to test the efficacy and feasibility of this intervention approach.

5 Conclusion

Anticipated outcomes from this study are expected to pave the way for developing a groundbreaking adaptive teleexercise regimen tailored specifically for individuals with physical disabilities.

References

1. Rimmer, J.H., Chen, M.D., McCubbin, J.A., Drum, C., Peterson, J.: Exercise intervention research on persons with disabilities: what we know and where we need to go. Am. J. Phys. Med. Rehabil. **89**(3), 249–263 (2010). https://doi.org/10.1097/PHM.0b013e3181c9fa9d
2. Physical Activity Guidelines Advisory Committee report, 2008. To the Secretary of Health and Human Services. Part A: executive summary. Nutr. Rev. **67**(2), 114–20 (2009). https://doi.org/10.1111/j.1753-4887.2008.00136.x
3. Carroll, D.D., Courtney-Long, E.A., Stevens, A.C., et al.: Vital signs: disability and physical activity–United States, 2009–2012. MMWR Morb. Mortal. Wkly Rep. **63**(18), 407–413 (2014)
4. Hollis, N.D., Zhang, Q.C., Cyrus, A.C., Courtney-Long, E., Watson, K., Carroll, D.D.: Physical activity types among US adults with mobility disability, Behavioral Risk Factor Surveillance System, 2017. Disabil. Health J. **13**(3), 100888 (2020). https://doi.org/10.1016/j.dhjo.2020.100888
5. Martin Ginis, K.A., Ma, J.K., Latimer-Cheung, A.E., Rimmer, J.H.: A systematic review of review articles addressing factors related to physical activity participation among children and adults with physical disabilities. Health Psychol. Rev. **10**(4), 478–494 (2016). https://doi.org/10.1080/17437199.2016.1198240
6. Malone, L.A., Barfield, J., Brasher, J.D.: Perceived benefits and barriers to exercise among persons with physical disabilities or chronic health conditions within action or maintenance stages of exercise. Disabil. Health J. **5**(4), 254–260 (2012)
7. Rimmer, J.H., Padalabalanarayanan, S., Malone, L.A., Mehta, T.: Fitness facilities still lack accessibility for people with disabilities. Disabil. Health J. **10**(2), 214–221 (2017). https://doi.org/10.1016/j.dhjo.2016.12.011
8. Martin, J.J.: Benefits and barriers to physical activity for individuals with disabilities: a social-relational model of disability perspective. Disabil. Rehabil. **35**(24), 2030–2037 (2013)
9. Barfield, J., Malone, L.A.: Perceived exercise benefits and barriers among power wheelchair soccer players. J. Rehabil. Res. Dev. **50**(2) (2013)
10. Catalyst, N.: What is telehealth? NEJM Catalyst. **4**(1) (2018)

BeClean: Designing a Personalized Eco-Feedback Application to Promote Pro-Environmental Behavior

Pattiya Mahapasuthanon$^{(\boxtimes)}$ and Vivian Genaro Motti

George Mason University, 4400 University Drive, Fairfax, VA 22030, USA
pmahapas@gmu.edu, vmotti@gmu.edu

Abstract. Environmental health threats have created health problems globally. These problems can range from small skin irritations to premature deaths. To reduce such health threat exposure, persuasive technologies can be employed seeking to help citizens to reduce their carbon emission. Persuasive applications intended to promote pro-environmental behaviors have been rising along with research on climate change. However, persuasive techniques need to be adapted to users to engage them and increase their environmental awareness according to specific environmental concerns. In this paper, we present the design of BeClean–an interactive prototype that provides eco-feedback and contents tailored to users' environmental concerns and values. With appropriate persuasive techniques, we expected that BeClean users will reduce carbon emission in their daily activities; consequently reducing their exposure to environmental health threats.

Keywords: Sustainable Behavior · Persuasive Technology · Eco-Feedback

1   Introduction

Sustainability is defined by World Commission on Environment and Development as "meeting the needs of the present without compromising the ability of future generations to meet their own needs" [11]. Regarding environmental sustainability, the usage of technology to promote ecological awareness has shown large potential to persuade technology users towards adopting more sustainable behaviors [2]. Persuasive technologies or eco-feedback technologies that provide feedback based on users' behavior can be used to reduce their ecological footprint. These have been used to motivate people to achieve certain goals and to change their everyday behaviors.

Even though there is growing number of persuasive technologies implemented to promote sustainable behaviors, those have been designed to provide generic information and feedback to users. Existing research in persuasive applications do not take into consideration value differences among users [10]. In other words,

© ICST Institute for Computer Sciences, Social Informatics and Telecommunications Engineering 2025
Published by Springer Nature Switzerland AG 2025. All Rights Reserved
H. Kondylakis and A. Triantafyllidis (Eds.): PervasiveHealth 2024, LNICST 612, pp. 206–210, 2025.
https://doi.org/10.1007/978-3-031-85575-7

environmentally-motivated users likely use eco-feedback technologies as they tend to have higher environmental awareness. With varied environmental values, users are more receptive to different social influences as environmental concerns were proved to be related to culture. Therefore, persuasive technologies should employ different persuasive techniques which fit users' levels of environmental concerns and values.

This paper presents BeClean–an interactive prototype created as a persuasive mobile application. The application was designed to provide personalized information to users based on three environmental values including biospheric, altruistic, and egoistic. The design prototype was created to guide users through daily activities they can perform to reduce their own carbon footprint and live more sustainably. The design created was based on the Value-Belief-Norm (VBN) Theory [9] because values are the guiding principles for users' ways of living.

2   Related Work

Persuasive applications to promote pro-environmental behavior are designed to engage users in accomplish certain goals. These applications utilize several persuasive techniques to motivate users towards sustainable behaviors. Specifically, eco-feedback has been employed to provide the ability for users to track and compare their carbon emissions generated from their everyday activities. In this section, we explain existing eco-feedback technologies and how the environmental values affect the level of information accepted by users.

2.1   Eco-Feedback Technologies for Sustainable Behavior

Eco-feedback technologies provide feedback which allows users to understand their performance and progress towards specific goals [3]. For instance, persuasive applications can persuade users to manage their energy consumption. In the domain of sustainable behavior, researchers have been working on promoting sustainable behaviors via different technologies such as social robots [1], games [7], and mobile applications [5]. These were designed to provide one-size-fits-all information.

2.2   Environmental Values

Environmental values can be defined as beliefs. Values impact the attitudes and could lead users to selectively seek information that aligns with users' values. Environmental attitude directly influences users' pro-environmental behaviors [8]. These environmental values can be categorized into three values including egoistic, biospheric, and altruistic [9]. Biospheric (pro-environmental) attitude is a strong predictive factor of the willingness that a given user has to take environmental-friendly actions [9]. On the contrary, people with egoistic attitudes tend to voice their environmental health concerns on their own health benefits [8].

3   BeClean Application

We designed BeClean as an interactive mobile application comprising multiple features. Those features have been selected based on our extensive literature review and previous user studies. Figure 1 displays the main pages of BeClean. The application starts with the home page which displays the users' virtual pets as well as the vital sign which corresponds to the score from users' activities. For example, the health score will be in a high range when users continuously collect points from performing daily activities that contribute to environmental sustainability. Users can collect points from performing different activities (e.g. collecting trashes). Additionally, there is a leaderboard page which enables social comparison among users' connections and friends. The application also provides personalized information about ecological footprint using different modalities (e.g. video, text). In other words, the persuasive messages provided in this page will be adapted to users' environmental values. For example, users who have biospheric value will see recommendations about how to save the planet with their every day's actions. The source of information provided in the application is from established environmental impact website [6].

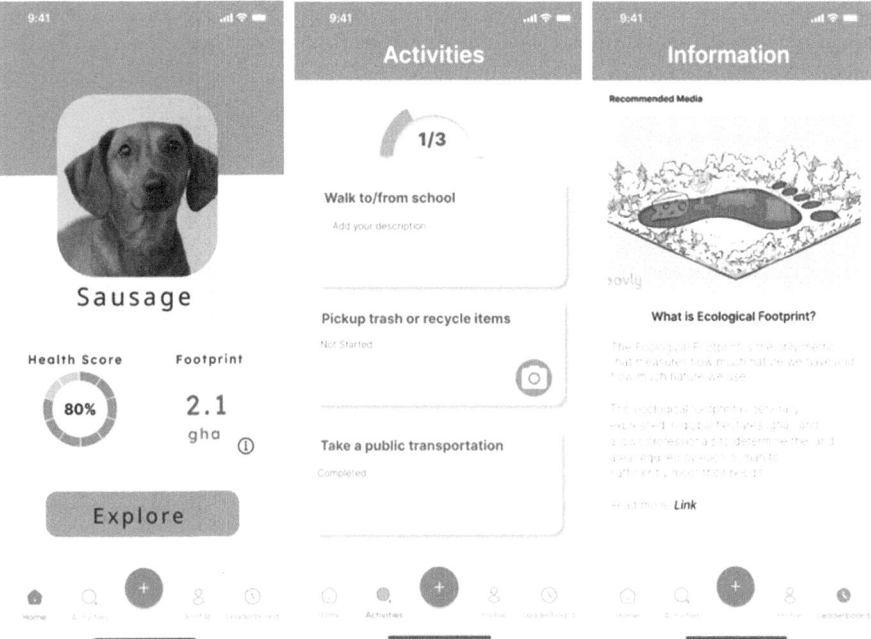

Fig. 1. BeClean application design demonstrating ecological footprint and to-do list for users to collect rewards

4   Expected Results

Based on the BeClean prototype we created, we are carrying out an online survey study to recruit participants from diverse backgrounds to evaluate the prototype. We expect that participants who have biospheric values will express a higher satisfaction with the app features overall. These biospheric participants are expected to download and use the application more than participants with egoistic and altruistic values. While, participants with egoistic and biospheric values will rank the to-do activity feature as their highest scores.

5   Conclusion

Overall, environmental values and concerns can be used to inform design decisions for persuasive applications. By accounting for environmental values, persuasive technologies which incorporate personalized eco-feedback can increase users' engagement as well as motivate users towards achieving more sustainable behaviors. The BeClean application was created to include features that are personalizable based on the users' environmental values. Our work is still in progress with the ongoing survey study to investigate the effects of environmental values on the usability and effectiveness of BeClean application.

References

1. Beheshtian, N., Moradi, S., Ahtinen, A., Väänanen, K., Kähkonen, K., Laine, M.: GreenLife: a persuasive social robot to enhance the sustainable behavior in shared living spaces. In: Proceedings of the 11th Nordic Conference on Human-Computer Interaction: Shaping Experiences, Shaping Society, pp. 1–12 (2020)
2. Dourish, P.: HCI and environmental sustainability: the politics of design and the design of politics. In: Proceedings of the 8th ACM Conference on Designing Interactive Systems, pp. 1–10 (2010)
3. Kollmuss, A., Agyeman, J.: Mind the gap: why do people act environmentally and what are the barriers to pro-environmental behavior? Environ. Educ. Res. **8**(3), 239–260 (2002)
4. Mahapasuthanon, P., Kalantari, N., Motti, V.G.: Evaluating an mHealth application: findings on visualizing transportation and air quality. In: Toeppe, K., Yan, H., Chu, S.K.W. (eds.) iConference 2021. LNCS, vol. 12645, pp. 301–312. Springer, Cham (2021). https://doi.org/10.1007/978-3-030-71292-1_24
5. Meurer, J., Lawo, D., Pakusch, C., Tolmie, P., Wulf, V.: Opportunities for sustainable mobility: re-thinking eco-feedback from a citizen's perspective. In: Proceedings of the 9th International Conference on Communities and Technologies-Transforming Communities, pp. 102–113 (2019)
6. Network, G.F.: Ecological footprint (2019)
7. Plichta, F., Mitschick, A., Klamka, K., Dachselt, R.: Growing green habits: unobtrusive gamified eco-feedback to motivate sustainable behavior. In: Proceedings of Mensch und Computer 2023, pp. 454–459 (2023)
8. Schultz, P.W.: Environmental attitudes and behaviors across cultures. Online Readings Psychol. Cult. **8**(1) (2002)

9. Stern, P.C., Dietz, T., Guagnano, G.A.: The new ecological paradigm in social-psychological context. Environ. Behav. **27**(6), 723–743 (1995)

10. Strengers, Y.A.: Designing eco-feedback systems for everyday life. In: Proceedings of the SIGCHI Conference on Human Factors in Computing Systems, pp. 2135–2144 (2011)

11. World Commission on Environment and Development: Our common future (1987). https://ideas.repec.org/b/oxp/obooks/9780192820808.html

Physical Activity, Physical Function and Quality of Life in Midlife Women

Oonagh M. Giggins[1]([⊠]) [ID], Suzanne Cullen-Smith[1] [ID],
Leen Broeckx[2] [ID], Romy Sels[3] [ID], Kim Helsen[2] [ID],
and Kris Cuppens[3] [ID]

[1] NetwellCASALA, Dundalk Institute of Technology, Dundalk, Ireland
oonagh.giggins@dkit.ie
[2] LiCalab Living and Care Lab, Thomas More University of Applied Sciences
Geel, Geel, Belgium
[3] Mobilab and Care, Thomas More University of Applied Sciences, Geel,
Belgium

Abstract. This cross-sectional observational study investigates the relationship between physical activity (PA) and physical function (PF), and menopause symptoms and quality of life (QoL) in a cohort of midlife women. Ten female volunteers (age: 56.7 ± 6.3 years, weight: 66.6 ± 7.1 kg, height: 163.8 ± 4.6 cm) took part in this investigation. Physical function was assessed in the laboratory, and the Menopause Rating Scale was used as a measure of QoL. Physical activity was quantified over 3-months using a wrist-worn PA monitor and average daily step counts were used to classify participants as; low active (n = 3), somewhat active (n = 4), or active (n = 3). The total MRS score (mean $\pm$ SD) was 22.5 ± 6. A strong negative correlation ($r_s = -0.8$, $p = 0.01$) was found between 6MWT distance and MRS scores and a moderate negative correlation was found between step count and MRS scores ($r_s = -0.56$, $p = 0.09$). However, overall, in the cohort studied PA levels were moderate. Midlife women tend to report low motivation for PA and experience barriers to PA engagement. Future work will seek to develop a digital health intervention for middle-aged, menopausal women to increase their PA and reduce their sedentary behavior.

Keywords: Women's Health · Midlife · Menopause · Physical Activity · Physical Function · Quality of Life

1 Introduction

Menopause is a normal part of the ageing process, characterized by the permanent cessation of menstrual periods and reproductive ability. During the menopause transition, women experience various physical, psychological, and social changes. Vasomotor symptoms, characterized by hot flushes and/or night sweats, are the main symptoms of menopause, with 40% of postmenopausal women in Europe reporting moderate-to-severe vasomotor symptoms [1]. Other psychosocial and physical complaints include weight gain, sleep disturbances, mood swings, anxiety, fatigue, joint

H. Kondylakis and A. Triantafyllidis (Eds.): PervasiveHealth 2024, LNICST 612, pp. 211–214, 2025.
https://doi.org/10.1007/978-3-031-85575-7

aches and pains, and sexual dysfunction. Many of these symptoms can be distressing and can negatively affect a woman's quality of life (QoL) [2, 3].

Physical activity (PA) may help attenuate the negative influence of menopause [4, 5]. However, despite the well-established benefits, most midlife women are not sufficiently active [5]. Physical activity is an important determinant of physical functioning (PF), which refers to the ability to perform basic and instrumental activities of daily living. In the Study of Women's Health across the Nation (SWAN), 29.6% of midlife women studied reported moderate functional limitations and 11.0% reported severe limitations [6]. However, women who maintain high or moderate PA during midlife showed significantly superior PF than those who maintain low PA [7].

2   Aim

This research sought to quantify PA and PF in midlife women and examine the relationship between PA and PF, and menopause symptoms and QoL in this cohort.

3   Methods

The protocol for this cross-sectional observational study was approved by the Ethics Committee in Dundalk Institute of Technology. All participants included in the study provided informed consent. Community-dwelling women, aged between 40 and 64 years of age took part and performed a series of PF tests in the laboratory, including measurement of handgrip strength, gait speed, and a six-minute walk test (6MWT). The Menopause Rating Scale (MRS) was used as a measurement of QoL. Following data collection in the laboratory, participants were provided with a Withings ScanWatch to wear to quantify PA for the following 3-months. Average steps count per day were used to categorize participants' PA levels; less than 5000 steps/day sedentary; 5000 to 7499 low active; 7500 to 9999 somewhat active; 10,000 to 12,499 active; and >12,500 highly active [8–10]. Because of the small sample size, Spearman correlation analysis was used to examine the association among studies variables.

4   Results

Ten female volunteers (age: 56.7 ± 6.3 years, weight: 66.6 ± 7.1 kg, height: 163.8 ± 4.6 cm) took part in the investigation. According to the WHO definition of menopause status, one participant was pre-menopausal, one peri-menopausal, and eight were classified post-menopausal. The prevalence of menopausal symptoms according to the MRS was high, but the severity of these symptoms was mild to moderate. The total MRS score (mean ± SD) was 22.5 ± 6. The most common symptom was sleep problems which was reported by all participants, followed by joint and muscular discomfort which was reported by 9/10 participants. Hot flushes and physical and mental exhaustion were also commonly reported (by 8/10 participants). The group mean (SD) for each of the PF measurements obtained in the laboratory and PA data collected during the 3-month periods are presented in Table 1. Average step counts per day obtained from the Withings Scanwatch classified participants as; low active (n = 3), somewhat active (n = 4), or active (n = 3). Results of the Spearman's rank correlation coefficient indicated that there was a strong negative correlation (r_s = −0.8, p = 0.01) between 6MWT distance and MRS scores. There was a moderate negative correlation between step count and MRS scores (r_s = −0.56, p = 0.09), while other correlations were weak.

Table 1 Group mean (SD) for PF measures obtained in the laboratory and PA data collected during 3-months. The relation between PF measures, PA and MRS scores are presented using Spearman's rank correlation coefficient (r_s)

	Grip Strength (Kg)	Gait speed (m/s)	6MWT (m)	Step Count
Mean (SD)	22.0 (4.3)	1.3 (0.1)	572.0 (80.3)	8159 (2131)
r_s	-0.28	0.14	-0.81	-0.56
p	0.43	0.70	0.01	0.09

5 Discussion

Women in midlife report a variety of symptoms associated with menopause, the most common being; sleep problems, joint and muscular discomfort, hot flushes and physical and mental exhaustion. The strong negative correlation between 6MWT distance and MRS scores, suggests that higher physical functioning improves the symptoms of menopause, thereby increasing QoL. In addition the negative correlation, albeit moderate between steps and MRS suggests that menopausal symptoms were experienced less by women who had higher levels of PA. This study provides evidence for the positive effects of PA in midlife women. However in the cohort studied, overall PA levels were moderate. Midlife women tend to report low motivation for PA and experience a number of barriers to PA engagement.

Digital health interventions may potentially encourage midlife women to increase PA. However, despite the development and evaluation of multiple technology-based interventions to promote PA, it remains unclear how to develop and design digital interventions that are both engaging and effective at changing PA behavior. In addition, there is a lack of digital interventions targeting an increase in PA levels specifically in menopausal women. Many digital intervention approaches are static and do not take into account the changing needs of the individual and their environment.

Recent progress in the field of digital health has enabled the development of interventions which provide responsive behavior change support in real-time. *Just-in-time adaptive interventions* (JITAI) holds enormous potential for promoting healthy behavior change. A JITAI leverages mobile and wireless technology and adapts "over time to an individual's changing status and contexts", with the goal to deliver support "at the moment and in the context that the person needs it most and is most likely to be receptive" [11]. JITAIs are designed to dynamically address the need of the user via the provision of the right amount or type of support needed at the right time [12].

Our future work seeks to develop a JITAI specifically targeting PA and sedentary behavior in middle-aged menopausal women. The developed intervention will apply deep learning and advanced analytics to the behavior and context related data gathered by the platform in order to optimize the intervention and achieve the best outcome. In addition to examining the feasibility of the approach, this proposed research will also examine the effectiveness of the developed adaptive intervention in promoting PA and reducing sedentary behavior in menopausal women.

References

1. Nappi, R.E., et al.: Global cross-sectional survey of women with vasomotor symptoms associated with menopause: prevalence and quality of life burden. Menopause **28**(8), 875–882 (2021). https://doi.org/10.1097/GME.0000000000001793
2. Avis, N.E., et al.: Change in health-related quality of life over the menopausal transition in a multiethnic cohort of middle-aged women. Menopause **16**(5), 860–869 (2009). https://doi.org/10.1097/gme.0b013e3181a3cdaf
3. Hess, R., et al.: The impact of menopause on health-related quality of life: results from the STRIDE longitudinal study. Qual. Life Res. **21**(3), 535–544 (2012). https://doi.org/10.1007/s11136-011-9959-7
4. Asikainen, T.-M., Kukkonen-Harjula, K., Miilunpalo, S.: Exercise for health for early postmenopausal women: a systematic review of randomised controlled trials. Sports Med. **34**, 753–778 (2004)
5. Wang, D., et al.: Healthy lifestyle during the midlife is prospectively associated with less subclinical carotid atherosclerosis: the study of women's health across the nation. J. Am. Heart Assoc. **7**(23), e010405 (2018)
6. Tseng, L.A., et al.: The association of menopause status with physical function: the Study of Women's Health Across the Nation. Menopause **19**(11), 1186–1192 (2012)
7. K. Pettee Gabriel, et al.: Physical activity trajectories during midlife and subsequent risk of physical functioning decline in late mid-life: The Study of Women's Health Across the Nation (SWAN). Prev Med (Baltim) **105**, 287–294 (2017). https://doi.org/10.1016/j.ypmed.2017.10.005.
8. Tudor-Locke, C., Bassett, D.R.: How many steps/day are enough? Preliminary pedometer indices for public health. Sports Med. **34**, 1–8 (2004)
9. Tudor-Locke, C., Johnson, W.D., Katzmarzyk, P.T.: Accelerometer-determined steps per day in US adults. Med. Sci. Sports Exerc. **41**(7), 1384–1391 (2009)
10. Tudor-Locke, C., Hatano, Y., Pangrazi, R.P., Kang, M.: Revisiting how many steps are enough?". Med. Sci. Sports Exerc. **40**(7), S537–S543 (2008)
11. Spruijt-Metz, D., et al.: Innovations in the use of interactive technology to support weight management. Curr. Obes. Rep. **4**(4), 510–519 (2015)
12. Nahum-Shani, I., et al.: Just-in-time adaptive interventions (JITAIs) in mobile health: key components and design principles for ongoing health behavior support. Ann. Behav. Med. **52**(6), 446–462 (2018). https://doi.org/10.1007/s12160-016-9830-8

Social Media and Its Impact on Orthorexia Nervosa. A Systematic Literature Review

Rron Lecaj[(✉)]

SMK College of Applied Sciences, Vilnius, Lithuania
rron.lecaj@smk.lt

1 Introduction

The present systematic literature review on social media and its impact on Orthorexia Nervosa (ON) was conducted for the purpose of better understanding the relationship between social media and the condition of ON. As communities evolve at the current fast paced manner, there is much room for the various developments in the human psyche. Most recently, a topic that has come into discussion has been that of Orthorexia Nervosa (ON) which is a condition mainly characterized by an obsessive need to eating healthy (Donini et al., 2022). Previous studies have linked it to obsessive-compulsive disorder (OCD) or Anorexia Nervosa (AN) (Koven & Abry, 2015; Barthels et al., 2016). However, ON is also comprised of other symptoms not found in other Eating and Feeding Disorders. Over the years, researchers have argued that ON's prominent indicator is that the anxiety in relation to food is correlated with quality as opposed to quantity (as is in AN, Bulimia Nervosa (BN), Binge-Eating Disorder (BED)) (Donini et al., 2022; Lopez-Gil et al., 2023). Other differences show that body image dissatisfaction and ON are not significantly correlated in some studies (Brytek-Matera et al., 2015). The latter means that the obsessive focus on healthy eating is not directly related to body image dissatisfaction as much as health satisfaction and perfectionism (Barnes & Caltabiano, 2016). Other factors that have been confirmed to have an influence on ON development are social media use (Scheiber et al., 2023), exercise (Hafstad et al., 2023), and discourses on social media platforms such as TikTok and Instagram (Santarosa et al., 2019) (Fig. 1).

In recent years, social media has become a pervasive part of daily life, influencing behaviors, attitudes, and perceptions with specific notations to healthy eating and eating habits. Platforms such as Instagram and TikTok allow for the rapid dissemination of information, including content related to health and nutrition (Greene et al., 2023). The visual and interactive nature of social media amplifies both positive and negative messages about eating habits (Santarosa et al., 2019). Therefore, the question is how are these relationships established and what the next steps are. This systematic literature review aims to examine the impact of social media on the development and reenforcement of ON symptoms.

H. Kondylakis and A. Triantafyllidis (Eds.): PervasiveHealth 2024, LNICST 612, pp. 215–219, 2025.
https://doi.org/10.1007/978-3-031-85575-7

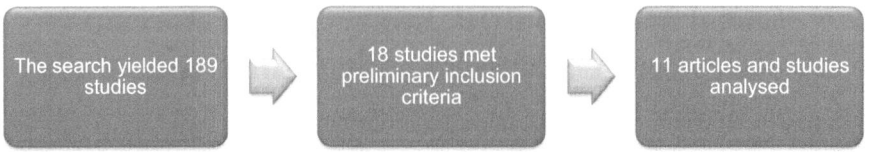

Fig. 1. Chart Display of Systematic Literature Review Process

2   Methods

A comprehensive search strategy was employed to identify relevant studies including databases such as EBSCO Host, Sage Journals Online, Taylor & Francis, and PubMed. The search terms used were "orthorexia nervosa", "social media", "impact", and "influence" alongside combinations. Owing to operators such as AND/OR, the search was refined and displayed studies specifically addressing the intersection of social media use and its impact on orthorexia nervosa. The review employed the review of literature within the references sections to maximise the coverage of relevant studies and research articles.

Inclusion criteria included: Published in the last ten years; peer reviewed articles; qualitative, quantitative and mixed-method studies; studies in the English language.

Exclusion criteria included: Studies indirectly looking into ON; Articles without empirical data (e.g., editorials, opinion pieces); Primarily non-English language publications.

Furthermore, the analysis employed several quality, accuracy, and consistency measures. To ensure the quality of the systematic literature review, studies were assessed using the PRISMA (Preferred Reporting Items for Systematic Reviews and Meta-Analyses) checklist. The checklist offered the means for a standardized approach to evaluate the rigor and reliability of the reviewed studies. The reviewer ensured that the databases were double-checked so as to ensure the accuracy and consistency of the studies extracted. Any discrepancies were resolved through discussion or consultation with a second unaffiliated reviewer (Fig. 2).

3   Results

The search yielded a total of 139 studies, out of which 18 made it through the preliminary inclusion criteria. Following a further systematic review of methodologies and samples, seven (7) studies were excluded for irrelevance to the discussion of the effects of social media on ON. Nine of the remaining studies were conducted in European countries such as Germany, Italy, the Netherlands, Turkey, Sweden, Russia, and the UK while one (1) study was conducted in Brazil, and another two (2) followed online discourse or ethnographic data collection and analyses. Out of these, 6 studies were quantitative (sample average: 1422), 3 were mixed-methods (quantitative and qualitative), and 3 were qualitative.

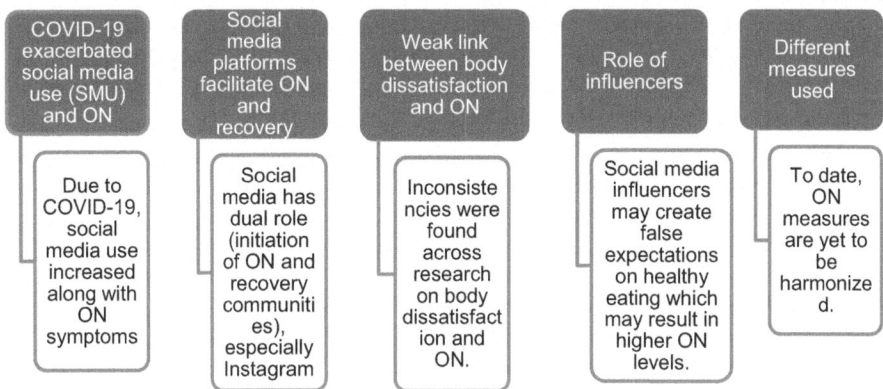

Fig. 2. Chart Display of Themes/Findings Extracted from the Systematic Literature Review

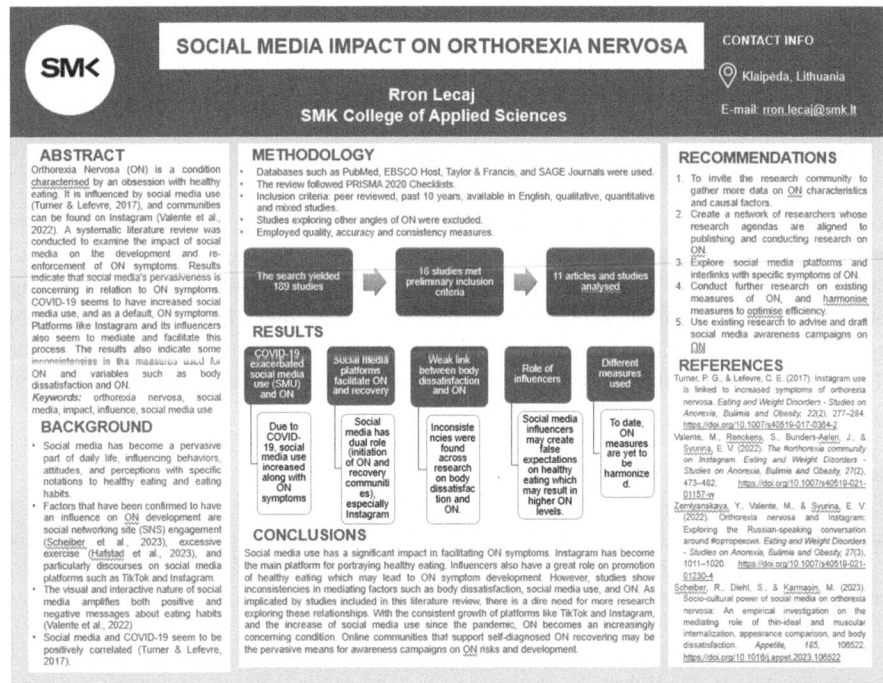

The reviewed literature highlighted and corroborate findings suggesting the positive correlation between social media use and higher tendencies for ON. Specifically, Instagram seems to be the platform which facilitates such trajectories with the use of hashtags, promotion of 'healthy eating' by influencers, and sense of community among self-identified ON victims. In part, some of the studies found that internalization of thin and muscular and body ideals as well as exposure to health and fitness content online as the main mediators. The influence social media has on the development and re-enforcement of ON symptoms seems to have been exacerbated by the COVID-19 pandemic and the induced and increased social media usage.

4   Conclusion

Social media use has a significant impact in facilitating ON symptoms as Instagram has become the main platform for portraying healthy eating. Influencers also have a great role on promotion of healthy eating which may lead to ON symptom development. However, studies show inconsistencies in mediating factors such as body dissatisfaction, social media use, and ON. As implicated by studies included in this literature review, there is a dire need for more research exploring these relationships. With the consistent growth of platforms like TikTok and Instagram, and the increase of social media use since the pandemic, ON becomes an increasingly concerning condition. Online communities that support self-diagnosed ON recovering may be the pervasive means for awareness campaigns on ON risks and development.

5   Recommendations for Future Research

To advance research on Orthorexia Nervosa (ON), the following recommendations are proposed: invite the research community to gather more data on ON characteristics and causal factors; create a network of researchers aligned with publishing and conducting research on ON; explore social media platforms and their links to specific ON symptoms; conduct further research on existing ON measures and harmonize them for efficiency; and use existing research to draft social media awareness campaigns on ON.

References

Asil, E., Yılmaz, M.V., Ayyıldız, F., Yalçın, T.: The effect of social media use on orthorexia nervosa: a sample from Turkey. Nutr. Hosp. (2023). https://doi.org/10.20960/nh.04217

Barnes, M.A., Caltabiano, M.L.: The interrelationship between orthorexia nervosa, perfectionism, body image and attachment style. Eat. Weight Disord. EWD **22**(1), 177–184 (2017). https://doi.org/10.1007/s40519-016-0280-x

Barthels, F., Meyer, F., Huber, T., Pietrowsky, R.: Orthorexic eating behaviour as a coping strategy in patients with anorexia nervosa. Eat. Weight Disord. - Stud. Anorexia Bulimia Obes. **22**(2), 269–276 (2017). https://doi.org/10.1007/s40519-016-0329-x

Brytek-Matera, A., Donini, L.M., Krupa, M., Poggiogalle, E., Hay, P.: Orthorexia nervosa and self-attitudinal aspects of body image in female and male university students. J. Eat. Disord. **3**(1), 2 (2015). https://doi.org/10.1186/s40337-015-0038-2

Cinquegrani, C., Brown, D.H.K.: 'Wellness' lifts us above the food Chaos': a narrative exploration of the experiences and conceptualisations of orthorexia nervosa through online social media forums. Qual. Res. Sport Exerc. Health **10**(5), 585–603 (2018). https://doi.org/10.1080/2159676X.2018.1464501

Donini, L.M., et al.: A consensus document on definition and diagnostic criteria for orthorexia nervosa. Eat. Weight Disord.: EWD **27**(8), 3695–3711 (2022). https://doi.org/10.1007/s40519-022-01512-5

Duarte, P., Silva, S.C.E., Sintra Pisco, A.M., De Campos, J.M.: Orthorexia nervosa: can healthy eating food trends impact food companies marketing strategies? J. Food Prod. Mark. **25**(7), 754–770 (2019). https://doi.org/10.1080/10454446.2019.1671931

Greene, A.K., Norling, H.N., Brownstone, L.M., Maloul, E.K., Roe, C., Moody, S.: Visions of recovery: a cross-diagnostic examination of eating disorder pro-recovery communities on TikTok. J. Eat. Disord.Disord. **11**(1), 109 (2023). https://doi.org/10.1186/s40337-023-00827-7

Håman, L., Barker-Ruchti, N., Patriksson, G., Lindgren, E.-C.: Orthorexia nervosa: an integrative literature review of a lifestyle syndrome. Int. J. Qual. Stud. Health Well Being **10**(1), 26799 (2015). https://doi.org/10.3402/qhw.v10.26799

Koven, N.S., Abry, A.W.: The clinical basis of orthorexia nervosa: emerging perspectives (2015)

López-Gil, J.F., Tárraga-López, P.J., Soledad Hershey, M., López-Bueno, R., Gutiérrez-Espinoza, H.: Neuropsychiatric Dis. Treat. **11**, 385–394 (2023). https://doi.org/10.2147/NDT.S61665

Soler-Marín, A., Fernández-Montero, A., Victoria-Montesinos, D.: Overall proportion of orthorexia nervosa symptoms: a systematic review and meta-analysis including 30 476 individuals from 18 countries. J. Glob. Health **13**, 04087 (2023). https://doi.org/10.7189/jogh.13.04087

Oliveira, M.F.D., Maglioni, A.B.R.R., Morais, B.A.B.D., Borges, L.R., Serafim, L.H.M., Ganen, A.D.P.: Relação entre comportamentos de risco para ortorexia nervosa, mídias sociais e dietas em estudantes de nutrição. Saúde e Pesquisa **14** (Supl. 1), 1–15 (2021). https://doi.org/10.17765/2176-9206.2021v14Supl.1.e9469

Opitz, M.-C., Newman, E., Sharpe, H.: Understanding perceived characteristics and causes of orthorexia nervosa in online communities—a Reddit analysis. Cyberpsychology: J. Psychosoc. Res. Cyberspace **16**(5) (2022). https://doi.org/10.5817/CP2022-5-6

Santarossa, S., Lacasse, J., Larocque, J., Woodruff, S.J.: #Orthorexia on Instagram: a descriptive study exploring the online conversation and community using the Netlytic software. Eat. Weight Disord. - Stud. Anorexia Bulimia Obes. **24**(2), 283–290 (2019). https://doi.org/10.1007/s40519-018-0594-y

Scheiber, R., Diehl, S., Karmasin, M.: Socio-cultural power of social media on orthorexia nervosa: an empirical investigation on the mediating role of thin-ideal and muscular internalization, appearance comparison, and body dissatisfaction. Appetite **185**, 106522 (2023). https://doi.org/10.1016/j.appet.2023.106522

Tarsitano, M.G., et al.: Symptoms of orthorexia nervosa are associated with time spent on social media: a web-based survey in an Italian population sample. Eur. Rev. Med. Pharm. Sci. **26**(24), 9327–9335 (2022). https://doi.org/10.26355/eurrev_202212_30683

Turner, P.G., Lefevre, C.E.: Instagram use is linked to increased symptoms of orthorexia nervosa. Eat. Weight Disord. - Stud. Anorexia, Bulimia Obes. **22**(2), 277–248 (2017). https://doi.org/10.1007/s40519-017-0364-2

Valente, M., Renckens, S., Bunders-Aelen, J., Syurina, E.V.: The #orthorexia community on Instagram. Eat. Weight Disord. - Stud. Anorexia Bulimia Obes. **27**(2), 473–482 (2022). https://doi.org/10.1007/s40519-021-01157-w

Zemlyanskaya, Y., Valente, M., Syurina, E.V.: Orthorexia nervosa and Instagram: exploring the Russian-speaking conversation around #орторексия. Eat. Weight Disord. - Stud. Anorexia Bulimia Obes. **27**(3), 1011–1020 (2022). https://doi.org/10.1007/s40519-021-01230-4

No One Teaches Me How to Do This: Clinical Research Coordinators Confront Challenges in Digital Clinical Trials

Jiyoon Han[1,2], Mangyeong Lee[1,2], Dongryul Oh[3], Jinseok Ahn[4], and Juhee Cho[1,2(✉)]

[1] SAIHST, Sungkyunkwan University, Seoul, South Korea
jcho@skku.edu
[2] Center for Clinical Epidemiology, Samsung Medical Center, Sungkyunkwan University School of Medicine, Seoul, South Korea
[3] Division of Hematology-Oncology, Department of Internal Medicine, Samsung Medical Center, Sungkyunkwan University School of Medicine, Seoul, South Korea
[4] Department of Radiation Oncology, Samsung Medical Center, Sungkyunkwan University School of Medicine, Seoul, South Korea

Abstract. Yet digital clinical trial is becoming more common, challenges in ensuring the clinical efficacy and safety of these trials persist. The quality of digital clinical trials depends on participant's competency, researcher's readiness, and supportive environments. While previous studies have examined the perspectives of nurses, physicians, and patients, the challenges faced by clinical research coordinators (CRCs) have been less addressed. This qualitative study, conducted at three university hospitals in South Korea from May to June 2024, aimed to identify barriers faced by CRCs in digital clinical trials and suggest requirements. Eight CRCs were interviewed using a semi-structured questionnaire, and thematic analysis was performed on the transcribed interviews. Key challenges identified included insufficient manuals, lack of environmental support, and inadequate manpower. CRCs emphasized outdated manuals, difficulties with unexpected technical issues, and lack of infrastructural support. They proposed updating manuals, improving internet connectivity, and increasing manpower. The findings of this study will provide valuable evidence for suggesting improvements and enhancing the current operations of digital clinical trials.

Keywords: Clinical research coordinator · Digital clinical trial · Challenges · Qualitative study

1 Introduction

Incorporating digital technologies into routine clinical practices and clinical trials became more common [1, 2]. However, challenges remain in ensuring the clinical efficacy and safety of digital clinical trials which utilize digital technology for conducting trials or deliver digital-based interventions [2]. The overall quality of digital

H. Kondylakis and A. Triantafyllidis (Eds.): PervasiveHealth 2024, LNICST 612, pp. 220–224, 2025.
https://doi.org/10.1007/978-3-031-85575-7

clinical trials depends on participant's competency, researcher's readiness, or facilitating environments in the context of digital technology usage [3]. Previous studies identified challenges or further requirements for quality assurance in digital clinical trial from the perspectives of nurses, physicians, and patients [4–7]. Although clinical research coordinators (CRCs) are responsible for most research activities of these trials, their challenges and requirements for ensuring quality of digital clinical trials were less addressed [8, 9]. Therefore, we conducted a qualitative study to identify what barriers CRCS faced during digital clinical trials, and to address key requirements to improve their workflows and the overall quality of clinical trials.

2   Materials and Methods

A qualitative study was conducted at three different university hospitals in South Korea from May to June 2024. Individuals responsible for the CRC role in their clinical trials and who agreed to participate in qualitative interviews were eligible for this study. This study was reviewed and approved by the Institutional Review Board (IRB No. SMC 2024–04-015), and all participants provided written informed consent.

In-depth or focus group interviews were conducted using a semi-structured questionnaire. Each interview lasted approximately 60 min. Prior to the interviews, participants were asked to complete a questionnaire on demographic characteristics such as age, gender, years of experience as a CRC, years of experience in digital clinical trial, and brief information of the clinical trials they coordinated. During the interviews, participants were asked about their experiences with digital clinical trials, the barriers and facilitators they encountered, and their suggestions for improvements. Every interview was audio-recorded, and confidentiality was maintained throughout the study.

All audio recordings were transcribed, and we performed a thematic analysis based on Braun and Clarke's method. With the verbatim transcription, two independent researchers generated initial codes, and defined themes that represented similar meanings across initial codes [10]. By examining each theme, final themes were identified including challenges posed to CRC and corresponding supports they requested.

3   Results

8 CRCs were recruited and included in the analysis. They were all female with an average age of 28.9 years. The average years of experience in digital clinical trials was 25.9 months. The most frequently used digital technology in the trial was smartphones (6 participants; 75%), followed by tablets, wearable devices, and other measuring devices. 75% of the CRCs had experience with digital clinical trials targeting cancer patients.

The identified challenges were mainly insufficient manuals for CRCs, lack of environmental support for conducting digital clinical trials, and lack of manpower (Table 1). CRC highlighted outdated manuals that fail to address real-world issues in

Table 1 Challenges and Requirements Clinical Research Coordinators Face While Conducting Digital Clinical Trials

Challenge	Requirements	Related Stakeholders
Insufficient manuals for CRCs	**Upgrading manuals**	
• Absence of action plan for addressing real-world issues, including technical and operational problems • Unexpected patient's request for technical issues on site • Coping with patient's negative attitude towards digital technology and trial participation	• Provide systematic education session or seminar on utilization of digital technology • Detailed instructions on the use of digital technology • Provide a FAQ page for prompt resolution on-site • Provide interpersonal strategies to address and improve patient compliance and reactions to digital technology use	SP[1], PI[2], TP[3]
• Technology provider's passive stance in the process of clinical trial	• Provide strategies for addressing patient reactions	TP[3]
• Additional assistance for patients with low digital literacy, especially the elderly, in utilizing digital technology	• Guidance for individuals with low digital literacy	SP[1], PI[2]
• Predominance of paper-based manuals, which is inefficient for information delivery	• Diversifying manual delivery through videos, simulations, and images	SP[1], PI[2]
Lack of environmental support	**Improving environmental support**	
• Poor internet connectivity for visitors(patient)	• Provision of portable Wi-Fi devices	SP[1], PI[2]
• Sharing empty rooms with multiple staff with no designated space	• Dedicated areas for patient management	
Lack of manpower	**Increasing manpower**	
• Delay of regular work tasks due to excessive patient technology inquiries	• Hiring additional staff to handle technical inquiries and assist patients • Reallocate task to enhance efficiency	SP[1], PI[2]
• Patient's request for face-to-face assistance in using digital technology	• Employ staff to assist patients with using digital technology	SP[1], PI[2]
• Inability to track patient's missing responses in real-time	• Employ continuous and periodic data monitoring staff	SP[1], PI[2]

digital clinical trial. They reported difficulties managing unexpected operational and technical problems, such as malfunctioning app/device or unintended data deletion. Also, handling patients with negative attitude toward digital technology and trial participation was challenging. They also noted the passive stance of technology providers as a problem. For the corresponding requirements, CRCs proposed upgrading manuals to detail the use of digital technology, provide strategies for addressing patient reactions, offer guidance for those with low digital literacy, and diversify manual delivery through videos, simulations, and images. Lack of environmental support was also highlighted by CRCs. Poor internet connectivity and inadequate space hindered their tasks. CRCs requested improvements such as portable Wi-Fi devices and dedicated areas for patient management. Lastly, lack of manpower involved in digital clinical trial was identified. Given the aspect of digital clinical trial, patients constantly inquire about technical issues. Also, patients with low digital literacy insist face-to-face assistance in problem-solving, resulting in CRC's burnout. They suggested hiring additional staff to improve their work conditions and enhance patient satisfaction.

SP[1]: Sponsor, PI[2]: Principal Investigator, TP[3]: Technology Provider.

4   Discussion and Conclusion

Identifying the barriers and requirements of CRCs in digital clinical trials is crucial to ensure the quality of trials, especially given their increasing prevalence. The findings of this study will provide valuable evidence for suggesting improvements and enhancing the current operations of digital clinical trials. We recommend that workflow and guidance for CRCs need to be tailored to digital clinical trials. In particular, decentralized or virtual clinical trials are emerging, which means that digital-based trial platforms will need to carry out most of the research activities performed by CRCs without their involvement. Thus, the current challenges of CRCs will be shifted to study participants interacting with the trial platform in virtual clinical trials, as their new barriers. Therefore, service vendors related to digital interventions or trial platforms should consider making their services more user and workflow-friendly in terms of digital health.

Acknowledgements. This research was supported by the Korea Health Industry Development Institute (KHIDI) grant and the National Research Foundation of Korea (NRF) grant (HI21C1787 and RS-2023-00212647).

References

1. De Brouwer, W., Patel, C.J., Manrai, A.K., Rodriguez-Chavez, I.R., Shah, N.R.: Empowering clinical research in a decentralized world. NPJ Digit. Med. **4**(1), 102 (2021)
2. Inan, O.T., et al.: Digitizing clinical trials. NPJ Digit. Med. **3**(1), 101 (2020)
3. Rosa, C., Marsch, L.A., Winstanley, E.L., Brunner, M., Campbell, A.N.: Using digital technologies in clinical trials: current and future applications. Contemp. Clin. Trials **100**, 106219 (2021)

4. Coert, R.M.H., et al.: Stakeholder perspectives on barriers and facilitators for the adoption of virtual clinical trials: qualitative study. J. Med. Internet Res. **23**(7), e26813 (2021)
5. McKenna, KC., et al.: Investigator experiences using mobile technologies in clinical research: qualitative descriptive study. JMIR mHealth uHealth **9**(2), e19242 (2021)
6. Safi, S., Thiessen, T., Schmailzl, K.J.: Acceptance and resistance of new digital technologies in medicine: qualitative study. JMIR research protocols **7**(12), e11072 (2018)
7. Meirte, J., et al.: Benefits and disadvantages of electronic patient-reported outcome measures: systematic review. JMIR Perioperative Med. **3**(1), e15588 (2020)
8. Mora, V., et al.: Clinical research coordinators: Key components of an efficient clinical trial unit. Contemp. Clin. Trials Commun. **32** (2023)
9. Davis, A.M., et al.: The invisible hand in clinical research: the study coordinator's critical role in human subjects protection. J. Law Med. Ethics **30**(3), 411–419 (2002)
10. Braun, V., Clarke, V.: Using thematic analysis in psychology. Qual. Res. Psychol. **3**(2), 77–101 (2006)

The User-Centred Design, and Evaluation of the MyGDM Prototype mHealth Tool: Poster

Jasmine R. Kirkwood[1]([✉]) [iD], Jane Dickson[2], Marryat Stevens[3],
Areti Manataki[4] [iD], Robert S. Lindsay[5] [iD], Deborah J. Wake[6] [iD],
and Rebecca M. Reynolds[1] [iD]

[1] Centre for Cardiovascular Science, University of Edinburgh, Edinburgh EH16 4TJ, UK
J.R.Kirkwood@sms.ed.ac.uk
[2] University of Dundee Medical School, Dundee DD1 9SY, UK
[3] My Way Digital Health, Dundee G2 4SQ, UK
[4] School of Computer Science, University of St Andrews, St Andrews KY16 9SX, UK
[5] School of Cardiovascular and Metabolic Health, The University of Glasgow, Glasgow G12 8TA, UK
[6] Usher Institute, The University of Edinburgh, Edinburgh EH16 4TJ, UK

Abstract. Gestational diabetes mellitus (GDM), is diabetes at the that is first recognised during pregnancy. It has increasing clinical issue affecting up to 10% of women in pregnancy. We have designed a user-centred prototype mHealth app for GDM care (MyGDM) using includes a clinical dashboard linked with a patient-facing app, that allows automatic transfer of blood glucose data, visualisations, education, culturally inclusive meals ideas and languages, and ability to request a call. We have designed and evaluated MyGDM through: ethnographic observations and 11 semi-structured interviews (6 healthcare professionals and 5 women with GDM) followed by an iterative design through three focus groups with 31 participants (17 healthcare professionals and 14 researchers); 13 questionnaires with women with GDM. From the focus groups, participants were pleased with the user-experience and could see how it would be beneficial in their clinics. During the questionnaires, 100% of women with GDM said that the MyGDM app would fit into their lifestyle and would have helped them manage their GDM. Additionally, 61.54% (8/13) and 69.23% (9/13) of women with GDM responded with likely or very likely to have used the educational resources and the 'request a call' function respectively. In summary, end-users were positive toward the MyGDM prototype mHealth tool, and future work includes piloting in a clinical setting.

Keywords: Gestational Diabetes Mellitus · mhealth · User-Centred Design

© ICST Institute for Computer Sciences, Social Informatics and Telecommunications Engineering 2025
Published by Springer Nature Switzerland AG 2025. All Rights Reserved
H. Kondylakis and A. Triantafyllidis (Eds.): PervasiveHealth 2024, LNICST 612, pp. 225–226, 2025.
https://doi.org/10.1007/978-3-031-85575-7

1 Poster

The proposed poster to present the work on MyGDM prototype is shown in Fig. 1.

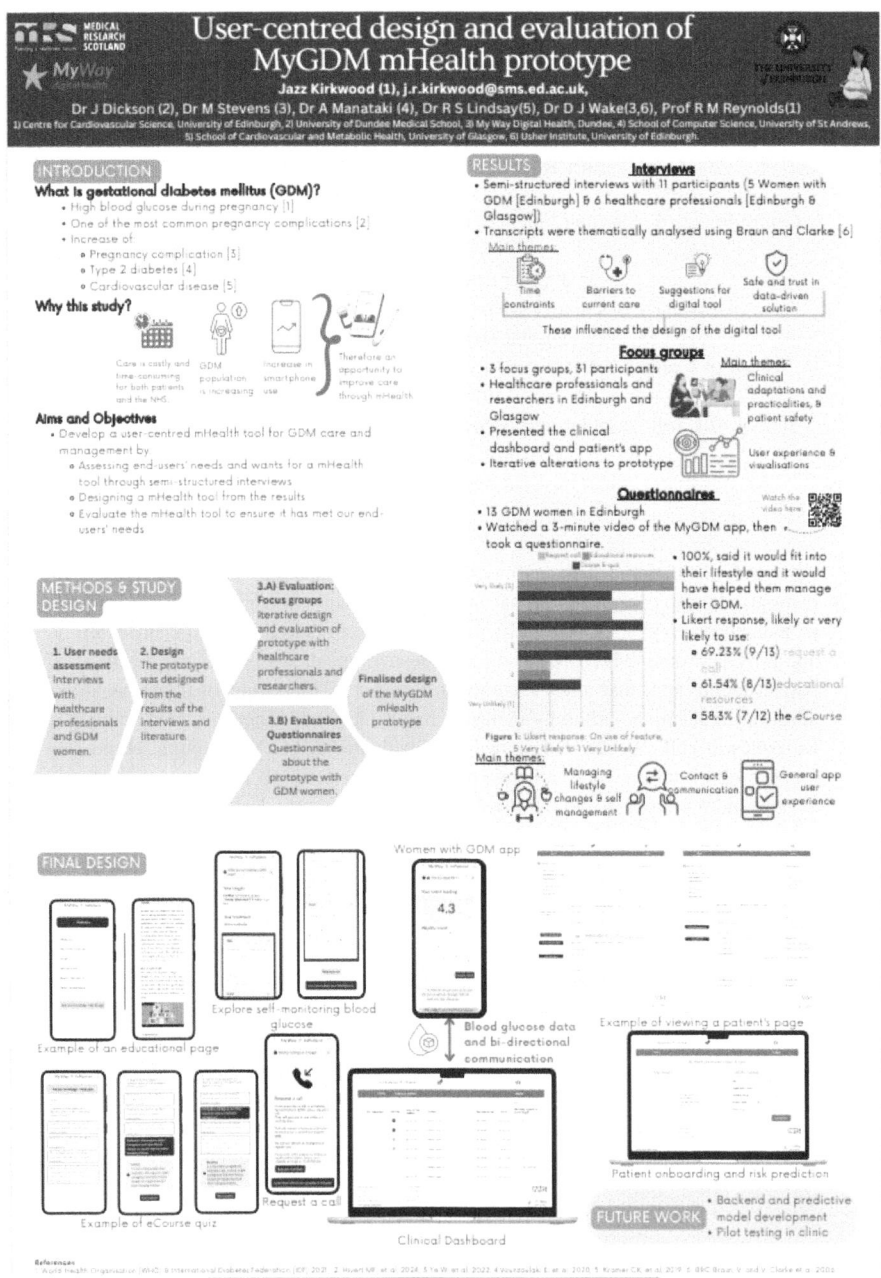

Fig. 1. Preposed poster to present the MyGDM prototype at EAI Pervasive Health conference 2024

Unveiling Inequalities in Mobile Health Utilization across Different Implementation Phases: Analyzing Factors Associated with Access, Adoption, Adherence, and Maintenance

Seongwoo Yang[1,2], Myoung Jin Cha[1], Mangyeong Lee[2,3], and Juhee Cho[2,3(✉)]

[1] Department of Digital Health, Samsung Advanced Institute for Health Sciences and Technology, Sungkyunkwan University, Seoul, Korea
[2] Center for Clinical Epidemiology, Samsung Medical Center, Seoul, Korea
jcho@skku.edu
[3] Department of Clinical Research Design and Evaluation, Samsung Advanced Institute for Health Sciences and Technology, Sungkyunkwan University, Seoul, Korea

Background. Despite increased downloads and utilization of various mobile health (mHealth) apps emphasizing the significance of technology-based remote monitoring and diagnosis for further progress [1], a major barrier to patient care in the use of mHealth interventions is attrition [2]. In addition, many mHealth studies struggle with high participant dropout rates due to the fundamental challenge of maintaining participant engagement [3]. For instance, similar to other extensive mHealth investigations, the prominent MyHeart Counts study led by Stanford University encountered significant dropout rates; the average app engagement lasted only 4.1 days [4]. In addition to this, other previous studies have found that as many as 80% of participants in mHealth interventions may only minimally engage with the service, defined as logging in fewer than twice, and only a small percentage of users consistently use the intervention over the long term [5, 6]. Although clinical trials often report retention rates of 70% or higher, these trials are typically short-term, some lasting fewer than two months, and may not reflect real-world use [7]. Besides, an observational study of app usage in a large real-world cohort discovered that only 2% had maintained continuous usage which would likely lead to improved clinical outcomes [8]. These low retention rates may indicate the minimal benefit of mHealth. In addition, some people could not be able to access or adopt mHealth to manage their health, which varies significantly by country and target population, resulting in unequal opportunities for health [9, 10]. Therefore, scrutinization of factors related to low retention rates of mHealth apps or interventions in real-world settings and barriers that prevent people from accessing and adopting mHealth is a crucial precondition for better clinical or behavioral outcomes. The main purpose of the study is to identify factors related to inequalities in the use of mobile health in each phase by conducting a systematic review of previously published articles.

© ICST Institute for Computer Sciences, Social Informatics and Telecommunications Engineering 2025
Published by Springer Nature Switzerland AG 2025. All Rights Reserved
H. Kondylakis and A. Triantafyllidis (Eds.): PervasiveHealth 2024, LNICST 612, pp. 227–231, 2025.
https://doi.org/10.1007/978-3-031-85575-7

Keywords: mobile health · inequalities · implementation · adoption · digital health

1   Methods

Databases searched included PubMed, Web of Science, Medline, and ProQuest. Inequality indicators for mHealth utilization were identified and measures of effect were collected. Inclusion and exclusion criteria for study selection are described in Table 1. The primary outcomes were mHealth utilization by implementation phase: access, adoption, adherence, and maintenance. Meta-analyses were performed on factors identified in three or more articles.

Table 1. Inclusion and exclusion criteria for study selection

Inclusion	Exclusion
Define mobile health specifically	Reviews, commentaries, opinions, clinical trial protocols, or app development papers
Have inequality indicators related to mobile health	No user engagement
Include participants using smartphones, mHealth applications, wearables	Engage face-to-face or other digital tools such as computers or websites
	No peer-reviewed articles
	Not written in English

2   Results

For the systematic review, a total of 62 and 37 out of 1,170 articles were finally included in qualitative and quantitative synthesis, respectively (Fig. 1). More than half studies (61.3%) were conducted in North America, especially in the United States (59.7%). Most included studies were observational studies (75.8%), including cross-sectional (37.1%), prospective (12,9%), and retrospective (25.8%) studies. While the qualitative and observational studies tended to meet the most criteria for quality assessment using the MMAT [11], the RCTs were less likely to meet the criteria.

All included studies were then classified into four implementation phases: access (37.1%), adoption (75.8%), adherence (14.5%), and maintenance (3.2%), which were also considered as the outcome. In addition, inequality indicators were collected from the included studies, and these were classified by levels of influence (individual, interpersonal, community, and societal) and domains of influence (biological, behavioral, physical/built environment, digital/mobile environment, sociocultural environment, and health care system). Based on these principles, a visual framework that represents all extracted inequality indicators in mHealth utilization was constructed. From this framework, it was found that a myriad number of inequality indicators are involved across the implementation phases, especially at the access and adoption phases. To summarize, genetic factors and education level were consistently associated with mHealth utilization across the phases. In addition, comorbidities and mentally or physically impaired health conditions were related to access to mHealth. The behavioral and sociocultural domains had many factors related to access, adoption, and adherence to mHealth. The digital/mobile domains also had a sheer number of factors associated with mHealth utilization, such as digital literacy/numeracy, frequency of smartphones, using the Internet for health issues, readiness to use mHealth and awareness about mHealth. Besides, the healthcare system and physical environment domains were related to access and adoption of mHealth.

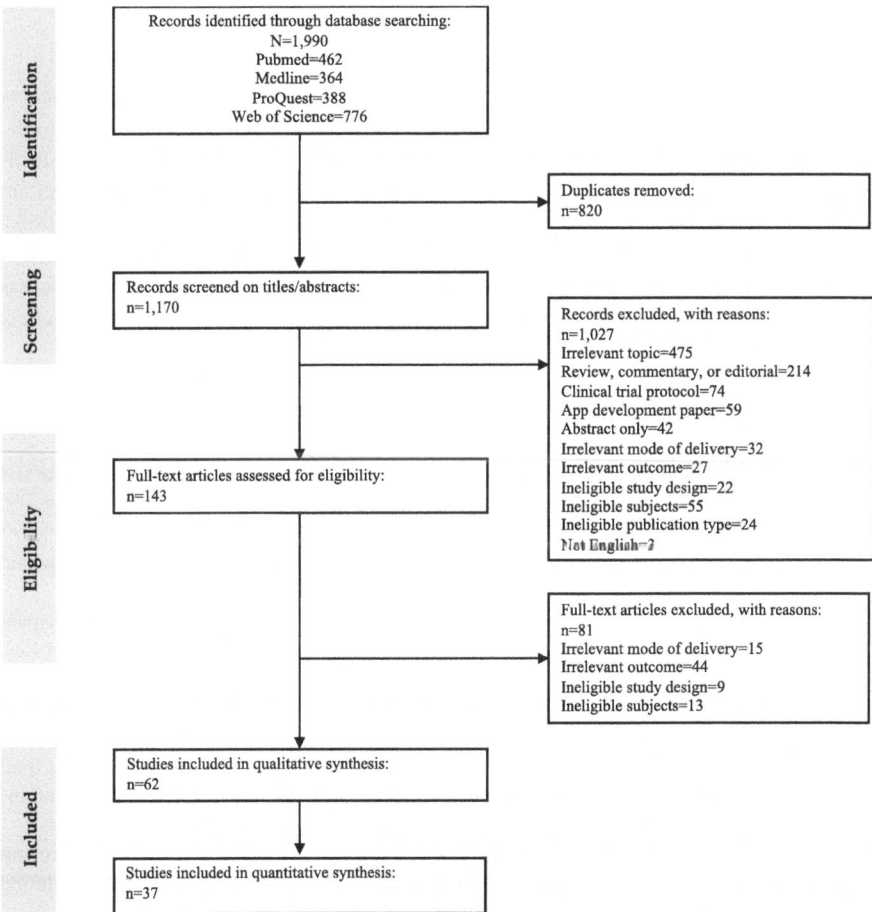

Fig. 1. Preferred Reporting Items for Systematic Reviews and Meta-Analyses flow diagram representing the selection of studies in the systematic review

Meta-analyses were conducted only for the access and adoption phases, due to the criteria, which required at least three articles for each inequality indicator. At the access phase, while the increase in age was negatively associated with mHealth utilization (OR = 0.96; 95% CI = 0.95, 0.97), a higher level of education had a positive association with mHealth utilization (OR = 2.08; 95% CI = 1.25, 3.46). At the adoption phase, older people compared to those younger (OR = 0.20; 95% CI = 0.06, 0.73), higher income (OR = 1.93; 95% CI = 1.16, 3.21), more comorbidities (OR = 1.50; 95% CI = 1.35, 1.67), and more physical activity (OR = 1.92; 95% CI = 1.29, 2.87) are statistically significant for the association with mHealth utilization. However, the results were less likely to be reliable because of the heterogeneity in most meta-analyses.

3 Conclusions

In conclusion, the multifaceted nature of mHealth adoption and utilization underscores the need for tailored interventions addressing specific demographic and socioeconomic barriers. Enhancing DHL, improving accessibility and affordability of mHealth technologies, and building trust through user-centered design and clear communication are essential strategies to promote equitable and effective use of mHealth applications. These findings provide a robust foundation for developing policies and programs that can drive the broader adoption and more effective use of mHealth technologies across diverse populations, aligning with broader trends in digital health policy and practice.

References

1. Almalki, M., Giannicchi, A.: Health apps for combating COVID-19: descriptive review and taxonomy. JMIR Mhealth Uhealth 9(3), e24322 (2021)
2. Meyerowitz-Katz, G., Ravi, S., Arnolda, L., Feng, X., Maberly, G., Astell-Burt, T.: Rates of attrition and dropout in app-based interventions for chronic disease: systematic review and meta-analysis. J. Med. Internet Res. 22(9), e20283 (2020)
3. Amagai, S., Pila, S., Kaat, A.J., Nowinski, C.J., Gershon, R.C.: Challenges in participant engagement and retention using mobile health apps: literature review. J. Med. Internet Res. 24(4), e35120 (2022)
4. Hershman, S.G., et al.: Physical activity, sleep and cardiovascular health data for 50,000 individuals from the MyHeart Counts Study. Sci. Data 6(1), 24 (2019)
5. Fleming, T., Bavin, L., Lucassen, M., Stasiak, K., Hopkins, S., Merry, S.: Beyond the trial: systematic review of real-world uptake and engagement with digital self-help interventions for depression, low mood, or anxiety. J. Med. Internet Res. 20(6), e199 (2018)
6. Pfammatter, A.F., Mitsos, A., Wang, S., Hood, S.H., Spring, B.: Evaluating and improving recruitment and retention in an mHealth clinical trial: an example of iterating methods during a trial. Mhealth 3 (2017)
7. Wang, Y., Xue, H., Huang, Y., Huang, L., Zhang, D.: A systematic review of application and effectiveness of mHealth interventions for obesity and diabetes treatment and self-management. Adv. Nutr. 8(3), 449–462 (2017)
8. Helander, E., Kaipainen, K., Korhonen, I., Wansink, B.: Factors related to sustained use of a free mobile app for dietary self-monitoring with photography and peer feedback: retrospective cohort study. J. Med. Internet Res. 16(4), e3084 (2014)

9. Alam, M.Z., Hoque, M.R., Hu, W., Barua, Z.: Factors influencing the adoption of mHealth services in a developing country: a patient-centric study. Int. J. Inf. Manage. **50**, 128–143 (2020)
10. Cajita, M.I., Hodgson, N.A., Lam, K.W., Yoo, S., Han, H.-R.: Facilitators of and barriers to mHealth adoption in older adults with heart failure. CIN: Comput. Inform. Nurs. **36**(8), 376–382 (2018)
11. Pluye, P., Gagnon, M.-P., Griffiths, F., Johnson-Lafleur, J.: A scoring system for appraising mixed methods research, and concomitantly appraising qualitative, quantitative and mixed methods primary studies in mixed studies reviews. Int. J. Nurs. Stud. **46**(4), 529–546 (2009)

Diagnostic Hysteroscopy Electronic Health Record System

Alexandros Theodosiou[1,2(✉)], Constantinos Pattichis[1],
Vasilis Tanos[4], and Andreas Panayides[2,3]

[1] Department of Computer Science, University of Cyprus, Nicosia, Cyprus
{alexandros.theodosiou,pattichi}@ucy.ac.cy
[2] 3AE Health Ltd, Nicosia, Cyprus
a.panayides@3ahealth.com
[3] CYENS CoE, Nicosia, Cyprus
[4] Aretaieion Iatrikon Kentron Limited, Nicosia, Cyprus
v.tanos@aretaeio.com

Abstract. Introduction: Hysteroscopy is the most frequently performed procedure in gynecology, essential for diagnosing and treating menstrual abnormalities, infertility, suspected endometrial cancer, and congenital uterine anomalies. Diagnostic hysteroscopy lacks a standardized protocol for reporting findings, resulting in inconsistent documentation practices among doctors and hospitals. In Cyprus, but also in a significant percentage of public and private clinics internationally, health records remain paper-based, which hampers efforts to standardize and share health data globally. This situation is untenable in an era where global health data standards are becoming increasingly important for secondary use, cross-system and cross-border communication.

Current Systems: Existing systems for diagnostic hysteroscopy allow for image capture through hysteroscopes. However, the equipment used, is not typically connected to Electronic Health Records (EHR) systems, especially in smaller clinics. The latter introduces a manual process, where healthcare professionals transfer these images and/or videos via external storage equipment (i.e., USB drives) to their personal computers for creating clinical reports. This process is inefficient and prone to errors, highlighting the need for a more streamlined and standardized approach.

Proposed System: We developed a fully customizable add-on module to our Electronic Health Record system but also for any 3rd party EHR solution, that revolutionizes the current processes. The proposed module connects directly to hysteroscopes, capturing medical images and medical video operated via a user-friendly interface and/or voice commands, and then stores them in a database, linked to the patient's profile, thus eliminating the need for additional transfers and hardware. It standardizes the report structure for all users (e.g., doctors), thus allowing for automated clinical report generation, which can be further customized to conform to health insurance organizations' requirements. Importantly, it enables the introduction of additional software as a service (SaaS) AI guidance module(s) based on images/ video during hysteroscopy procedures, while it supports 2nd opinion provision via real-time and/or on demand medical video streaming [9]. Moreover, the resulting system benefits from the Health Level 7 (HL7) Clinical Document Architecture (CDA) certification inherited

H. Kondylakis and A. Triantafyllidis (Eds.): PervasiveHealth 2024, LNICST 612, pp. 232–238, 2025.
https://doi.org/10.1007/978-3-031-85575-7

from our EHR system, ensuring that it adheres to global health data standards, facilitating international data sharing, interoperability, and aligning and reinforcing the European Health Data Space (EHDS) regulation.

Conclusion: This work demonstrates that simple healthcare procedures often overlooked by technology vendors can greatly benefit from novel, customizable interventions. Our EHR system not only makes hysteroscopic data globally accessible but also provides a powerful tool for capturing data to train AI models, ensuring that critical health data is standardized, shareable, and usable on a global scale.

Keywords: Gynecology · Hysteroscopy · Diagnostic Hysteroscopy ·
Electronic Health Record (EHR) · Health Data Standardization · AI-guidance ·
Image Capture · CDA HL7 Certification · Health Data Interchange · Global
Health Data

1 Introduction

1.1 Gynecology

Gynecology is a specialized field in medicine focusing on the health and diseases of the female reproductive system, including the uterus, ovaries, fallopian tubes, and breasts. This branch of medicine encompasses a wide range of conditions and treatments, from routine health checks and preventive care to complex surgical procedures [4, 5]. Gynecologists manage reproductive health, diagnose and treat disorders such as endometriosis, fibroids, polycystic ovary syndrome (PCOS), and cancers of the reproductive organs. They also provide essential services related to pregnancy, childbirth, and menopause, ensuring comprehensive care throughout a woman's life [6, 7].

1.2 Health IT and Gynecology

Health Information Technology (Health IT) in gynecology involves the application of advanced information processing techniques, including both hardware and software, to manage healthcare information effectively [2]. This integration of Health IT in gynecology has revolutionized the way patient data is stored, retrieved, and utilized. It has facilitated the digitization of gynecological records, enabling better data management and accessibility. Health IT supports various functions such as electronic health records (EHRs), telemedicine, and decision support systems [3]. These technologies enhance the quality of care by improving diagnostic accuracy, treatment planning, and patient monitoring. Moreover, the use of big data and artificial intelligence in gynecology aids in predictive analytics and personalized medicine, ultimately leading to better patient outcomes.

1.3 Health IT in Cyprus

In Cyprus, the implementation of Health Information Technology (Health IT) faces significant challenges, especially within the field of gynecology. The current healthcare infrastructure relies heavily on paper-based records, impeding the standardization and efficient sharing of health data. This lack of digitization presents obstacles to aligning with global health data standards, which are increasingly critical in the modern healthcare landscape. At the same time, existing systems in Cypriot hospitals for diagnostic hysteroscopy are outdated and inefficient. While hysteroscopes can capture images, the process requires manual transfer of these images via USB to personal computers, followed by report creation using text editors. This manual approach is time-consuming and prone to errors, leading to inconsistent documentation practices among healthcare providers.

These challenges highlight the urgent need for more streamlined and standardized Health IT solutions to improve the efficiency, accuracy, and standardization of medical documentation and data management in Cyprus.

2 Current EHR Systems and Hysteroscopy

2.1 Existing Procedures

In Cypriot hospitals, the current systems for conducting and documenting diagnostic hysteroscopies are largely antiquated and inefficient. These systems enable the capture of images via hysteroscopes, which are essential for visualizing the uterine cavity. However, the process for handling these images is cumbersome and somewhat outdated. After capturing the images, doctors are required to manually transfer them from the hysteroscope to their personal computers. Once the images are transferred, reports must be generated manually using text editors. This process involves inserting the captured images into a report format and adding descriptive text to document the findings. The latter process is typically repeated based on different health insurance organizations' requirements.

2.2 Challenges and Motivation

The existing approach to handling diagnostic hysteroscopy data presents several significant problems. Firstly, the manual transfer of images and report creation is a time-consuming process. It requires multiple steps, each of which adds to the overall time taken to complete the procedure and document the findings. Secondly, manual processes are inherently prone to human error. Mistakes can occur during the transfer of images, the input of data, and the creation of reports, leading to inconsistencies and inaccuracies in medical documentation. Importantly, there is no support for video files, posing significant security and privacy concerns to accompanying video files.

Additionally, there is a lack of standardized protocol for reporting hysteroscopy findings, resulting in varied documentation practices among doctors and hospitals. This lack of uniformity makes it difficult to compare data across different institutions and hinders collaborative efforts. The reliance on paper-based health records further complicates the situation. Paper records are difficult to manage, prone to physical degradation, and do not support easy sharing or integration with digital health systems. Lastly, the absence of adherence to global health data standards in the current systems limits the ability to share and utilize health data at an international scale. This is increasingly untenable in an era where interoperability and global data exchange are crucial for advancing research via the secondary use of health data towards improving patient care.

Clearly, there is a pressing need for an advanced, efficient, and standardized approach to diagnostic hysteroscopy documentation. Addressing these issues can significantly enhance the quality of care, streamline workflows, and facilitate the integration of Cypriot health data into the global healthcare ecosystem.

3 Proposed Hysteroscopy Solution

Our cutting-edge Electronic Health Record system integrates advanced Health Information Technology (Health IT) to revolutionize the management and documentation of medical procedures. Designed with a user-friendly interface, it facilitates seamless data capture, storage, and analysis, transforming how healthcare providers manage patient information and conduct diagnostic procedures (Fig. 1).

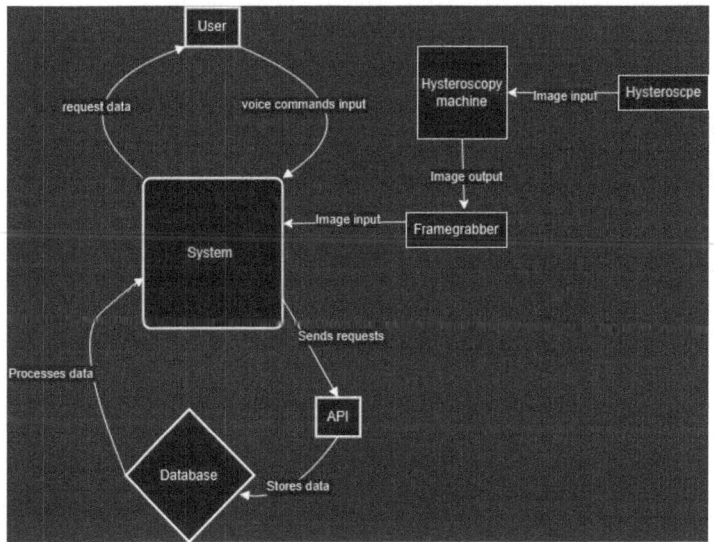

Fig. 1. System diagram

3.1   EHR Components and Features

General Characteristics
Our EHR system provides several significant improvements over existing systems. The direct integration and data capture feature of our EHR system connects directly to medical devices such as hysteroscopes, ultrasound machines, cameras and other video equipment, allowing for real-time image and video data capture. This eliminates the need for manual transfers, thus reducing the risk of data loss and errors while speeding

up enhancing the healthcare professional experience of interacting with a (single) EHR system. This is achieved by using frame grabbers to get the video output from the medical devices and channel it to our system. This allows us to directly manipulate the data from medical devices as we want and store them directly in our system's database.

The system automates the generation of medical reports, standardizing the report structure across all users. This ensures consistency and accuracy in documentation, which is crucial for maintaining high standards of patient care.

Our EHR provides sophisticated data visualization tools that help healthcare providers quickly interpret and analyze patient data. This includes interactive dashboards that display vital statistics, patient demographics, and treatment outcomes, making it easier to track patient progress and make informed decisions.

Incorporating support for plug and play artificial intelligence modules ranging from predictive analytics such as Intensive Care Unit (ICU) Sepsis prediction, to medical image segmentation and disease classification. This enhances diagnostic accuracy and supports personalized treatment plans.

The system supports International Patient Summary (IPS) and has Clinical Document Architecture certification for Health Level 7 (HL7) standards, ensuring compliance with global health data standards. This facilitates international data sharing and interoperability, which is critical for collaborative research and global health initiatives.

Our EHR system ensures that patient data is secure, with access controls and encryption. It also supports remote access, allowing healthcare providers to access patient information from anywhere, ensuring continuous care.

Unique Hysteroscopy Module Characteristics

The hysteroscopy module within our EHR system addresses several key issues. It addresses the lack of standardization in reporting hysteroscopy findings by automating the report generation process. This ensures that all findings are documented in a consistent format, making it easier to compare and share data.

The module directly connects to hysteroscopes, capturing images in real-time and storing them in a centralized database. This eliminates the need for manual image transfers and reduces the risk of data loss or mismanagement.

The system not only captures images but also records videos during hysteroscopic procedures. This provides a more comprehensive view of the procedure, aiding in better diagnosis and treatment planning. Furthermore, by embedding in our solution video processing software such as FFMPEG, we allow the user to perform various video-related processes (i.e., compression, resizing, temporal down sampling, etc.). Importantly, we establish the necessary pillars for 2nd opinion provision via real-time and on-demand video streaming of the hysteroscopic procedure, widening the healthcare professional's clinical options, for the benefit of the patient. At the same time, via the setup of a video streaming server, adopting a radiology departments' -like data sharing philosophy, the video recordings can be shared securely, respecting the patient's privacy.

The hysteroscopy module supports voice commands, allowing doctors to capture images and videos without manual intervention. This eliminates delays associated with manual image capture, ensuring high-quality images and videos, and reduces the risk of errors due to interruptions in the procedure. To use voice recognition as well as vocal feedback from the computer to the doctor we used HTML5 Web Speech API that allows us to implement the features we want in almost any browser.

By integrating the hysteroscopy module with the EHR, we streamline the entire workflow from image capture to report generation. This reduces the time taken to document findings and allows healthcare providers to focus more on patient care.

Future modules target AI-driven tools that will assist the medical expert in identifying abnormalities and suggesting possible diagnoses [8]. This will aid doctors in making more accurate, informed and timely decisions during diagnostic hysteroscopies.

With CDA certification, the hysteroscopy module ensures that all data is standardized and can be easily shared with other healthcare institutions globally. This promotes collaborative research and improves the overall quality of care.

By capturing detailed and standardized data, the module provides valuable resources for training new healthcare providers and conducting research. This data can be used to train AI models, further enhancing diagnostic tools and techniques.

4   Conclusion

Our EHR system shows how using advanced technology in healthcare can greatly improve efficiency, accuracy, and data management. One example of this is the hysteroscopy module, which highlights the advantages of automating and standardizing medical procedures. By doing so, it guarantees that important health information can be easily accessed and utilized worldwide. This system doesn't just enhance patient care but also serves as a strong foundation for medical research and AI advancement.

Acknowledgment. This project has received funding from the European Union's Horizon Widening participation and spreading excellence program under the HORIZON-WIDERA-2022-ACCESS-04-01 - Excellence Hubs call with grant agreement no. 101087483.

References

1. Proposal for a Regulation of the European parliament and the council on the European Parliament and the Council on the European Health Data Space, COM (2022) 197. https://eur-lex.europa.eu/legal-content/EN/TXT/?uri=CELEX%3A52022PC0197&fbclid=IwZXh0%5b%E2%80%A6%5dnPQtH5RnOxTwONrhMN8-NJQ1n0Qe0weJo_aem_bizZ1kk8jXdIg6iC8H4HPQ. Accessed Jul 2024
2. N.A.: The History of Healthcare Technology and the Evolution of HER (2018). The History of Healthcare Technology and the Evolution of EHR–baytechIT
3. DelVecchio, A., Wallask, S.: Health IT (health information technology). What is Health IT (health information technology)?—Definition from TechTarget
4. N.A.: Diagnostic Hysteroscopy. Diagnostic Hysteroscopy—Baylor Medicine (bcm.edu)
5. Moore, J.F., Carugno, J.: Hysteroscopy In: StatPearls [Internet]. Treasure Island (FL): StatPearls Publishing (2022). Hysteroscopy - StatPearls - NCBI Bookshelf (nih.gov)
6. Britannica, T. Editors of Encyclopaedia, "Obstetrics and Gynecology"

7. Encyclopedia Britannica (2018). Obstetrics and gynecology—Women's Health, Pregnancy Care & Delivery—Britannica
8. Panayides, A.S., et al.: AI in medical imaging informatics: current challenges and future directions. IEEE J. Biomed. Health Inform. **24**(7), 1837–1857 (2020). https://doi.org/10.1109/JBHI.2020.2991043
9. Antoniou, Z.C., et al.: Real-time adaptation to time-varying constraints for medical video communications. IEEE J. Biomed. Health Inform. **22**(4), 1177–1188 (2018). https://doi.org/10.1109/JBHI.2017.2726180

Improving Personalized Medicine via AI-Based Precision Tracheostomy

Evropi Toulkeridou[1], Panagiota Kosmidou[2], Kristis Vevis[2],
Zinonas Antoniou[3], Loizos Kallinos[3], Ioanna Valiandi[1],
and Andreas Panayides[1,3(✉)]

[1] Videomics FRG, CYENS Center of Excellence, Nicosia, Cyprus
`a.panayides@cyens.org.cy`
[2] German Oncology Center (GOC), Limassol, Cyprus
[3] R&D Department, 3aHealth, Nicosia, Cyprus

Abstract. Tracheostomy is a medical procedure frequently used to secure patients' airways. Typically, healthcare providers measure the patients' neck diameters and tracheas using 3D-CT in order to select specific sizes of tracheostomy tubes. Further, specific decisions before and/or during the procedure may also depend on collected and evaluated data regarding the clinical condition or unique characteristics of the patients. To this day, healthcare providers rely on their intuitive judgment based on previous relevant experience, with no systematic metrics unequivocally guiding their decisions, since no research exists in the literature that investigates patterns in these data. On the other hand, artificial intelligence (AI)-based methods have proved to be powerful tools used in medical care. However, although Deep Learning (DL) techniques have already shown excellent performance in image processing and diagnosis, their combination with the analysis of data informing the clinical condition and unique characteristics of patients remains unexplored, especially in the ENT (i.e., ear, nose, throat) surgical practice. Herein, we will combine these analyses to reveal patterns that previous statistical methods failed to identify. Our model will incorporate both convolutional neural networks for the automated measurement of 3D-CT scans and automated natural language processing of DL to extract clinically relevant information. We aim to create a tool with high diagnostic accuracy comparable to that of experienced healthcare providers. Our study will provide an implementation of AI-based systems that will be able to assist physicians in handling big data and improving diagnostic efficiency, as well as in clinical decision making in cases of high complexity or uncertainty.

Keywords: Tracheostomy · Artificial Intelligence · Deep Learning

1 Introduction

Tracheostomy is one of the most frequently performed procedures in ENT (i.e., ear, nose, throat) surgical practice [1]. Tracheostomy patient care requires some of the highest financial expenditures compared to other diagnostic or procedural groups. It is common for patients with acute respiratory failure and may be required in an emergency setting to bypass an obstructed airway. More commonly, it facilitates mechanical

H. Kondylakis and A. Triantafyllidis (Eds.): PervasiveHealth 2024, LNICST 612, pp. 239–246, 2025.
https://doi.org/10.1007/978-3-031-85575-7

ventilation, helps wean patients from a ventilator, or allows for more efficient management [2]. The procedure of tracheostomy consists of several steps, during which the healthcare provider is expected to choose various parameters of the process and act according to the patient's unique characteristics. The number of parameters along with the frequency of tracheostomy and the patient's characteristics result in a huge amount of data, which can be analyzed and reveal patterns.

This multitude of parameters than may be considered for the customization of the tracheostomy procedure to individual patients offers a great choice to the practitioners; at the same time, however, it presents them with a formidable challenge. According to the National Confidential Enquiry into Patient Outcome and Death (NCEPOD), tracheostomy-related complications were experienced by 24% of patients in Intensive Care Unit (ICU) and 31% of ward patients [3]. Therefore, efforts to optimize tracheostomy practice may favorably affect both the quality of care and the resources expended in delivering this care of secretions, among other reasons.

To this day, healthcare providers rely on their intuitive judgment and relevant experience with previous medical cases to make estimates, as no systematic metrics unequivocally guide their decisions. To our knowledge, there is no research in the literature that investigates patterns in these data [4].

Artificial Intelligent (AI) methods have proved to be powerful tools in the medical care community in recent years. The creation of complex network architectures that process mathematical functions with millions of parameters has enabled machines to analyze and interpret intricate data with high accuracy [5]. From image processing to analysis of electronic health data, Machine Learning (ML) and Deep Learning (DL) techniques have demonstrated incredible performance. ML in healthcare has rapidly evolved, offering groundbreaking advancements in diagnostics, treatment planning, patient monitoring, and operational efficiency. DL on the other hand has notably enhanced computer vision. The advent of convolutional neural networks (CNNs) has greatly improved AI's ability to classify images, detect objects, and determine their locations, surpassing the results achieved with traditional machine-learning techniques. Recent initiatives to apply DL to medical image classification have revealed its enormous potential. These applications have shown significant progress in supporting diagnostic decisions, predicting prognoses, and managing hospital triage, underscoring AI's transformative role in healthcare [6].

Our study is aiming to combine these ML and DL methods to automatically predict the tracheostomy parameters and identify hidden patterns in the clinical data.

2   Methodology

2.1   Data Collection

A total of 50 patients will be included in the study. As a first step, their demographic and health data will be obtained before the procedure. Moreover, a 3D-CT will be conducted and analyzed using DL methods as described in the next section. The results of the image analysis will include measurements of the diameter of the abscess in all 3 axes of the CT and the nearest distance from the abscess to the inlet of the trachea. An example of tracheostomy tube is shown in Fig. 1. After the tracheostomy, the characteristics of the tube used in the procedure as well as data of the complications and after-surgical health indicators will complete each patient's medical record. Several clinical characteristics that will be used are shown in Table 1.

Table 1. Clinical characteristics of the 50 patients with tracheostomy.

Characteristics	N%
Gender	**Male, Female**
Age, years	**>18**
Smoking	**Yes/No**
Alcohol	**Yes/No**
BMI	
Height	
Neck circumference	
Heart Disease	
WBC	
Lympocytes	
Neutrophils	
CRP	
Hematocrit	
Tube length	
Outer/Inner Diameter	
Cuff Diameter	
Reasons for Tracheostomy	
Outcomes	
Capnography	

The project requires two different but connected tasks, one for the image and one of the total data analyses. After all data are collected, they will be split and used as training and testing sets in both tasks.

2.2   Image Processing

A segmentation task involves outlining an exact boundary around histologic structures to extract detailed morphological features accurately. Segmentation is generally challenging, especially when the structures have various possible appearances. As a result, a single comprehensive classifier or model may struggle to capture the entire range of visual cues and features needed to identify a specific histologic structure. Due to the variation of the patients' tracheas, we will use an already established CNN architecture which has already shown high performance in segmentation tasks, that of U-Net (Fig. 2).

The U-Net architecture, first introduced by Ronneberger et al. in 2015 [7], has gained popularity for its ability to produce high-quality segmentation results with

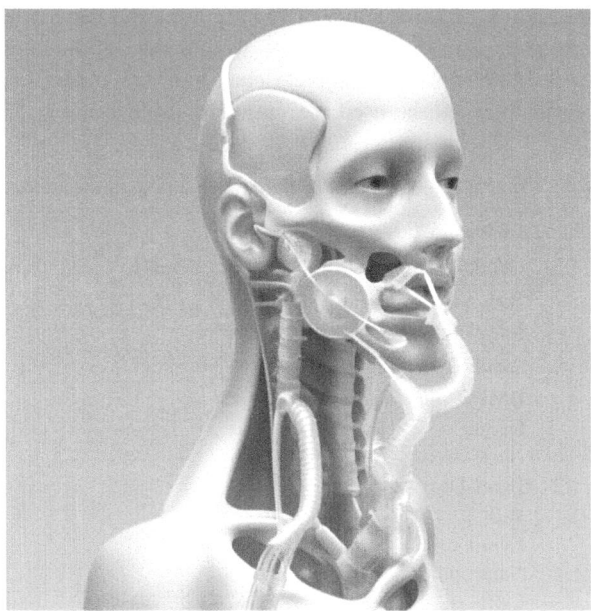

Fig. 1. AI-Generated image of tracheostomy tube. The characteristics of the optimal tube are connected with the unique characteristics of the patient.

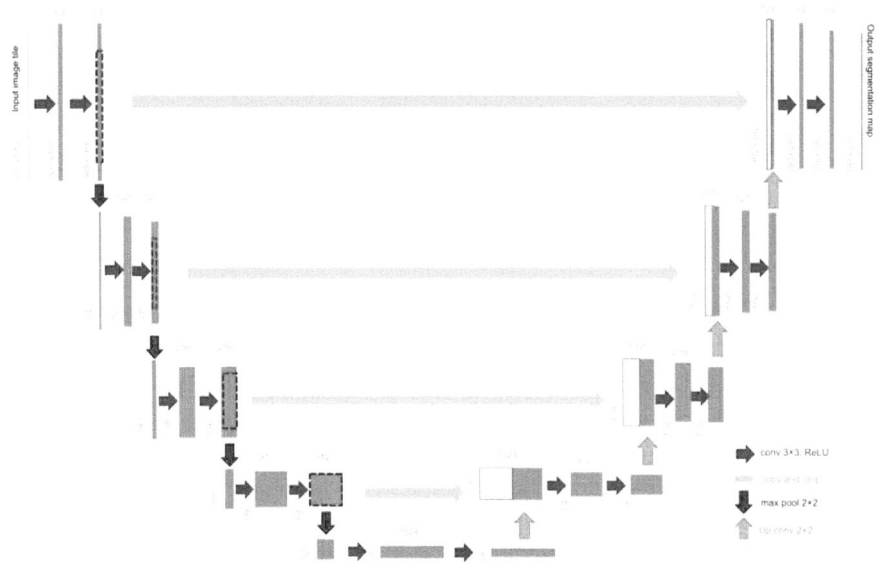

Fig. 2. U-Net architecture as presented in Ronneberger et al. in 2015 [7]. The introduced architecture was first applied in 2D images. In our study, a 3D implementation will be used.

relatively few training images. Its design facilitates the capture of both local and global features, making it highly effective for precise segmentation tasks.

The contracting path is the first half of the U-Net, resembling a traditional CNN. It consists of repeated application of two 3 × 3 convolutions (unpadded) followed by a rectified linear unit (ReLU) and a 2 × 2 max pooling operation with stride 2 for downsampling. At each downsampling step, the number of feature channels is doubled. The purpose of the contracting path is to capture context by progressively reducing the spatial dimensions of the input image while increasing the number of feature maps.

Located at the bottom of the U shape, the bottleneck consists of two 3 × 3 convolutions followed by ReLU activation. It serves as a bridge between the contracting and expanding paths, capturing high-level abstract features.

The expanding path is the second half of the U-Net. It consists of an upsampling of the feature map followed by a 2 × 2 convolution ("up-convolution") that halves the number of feature channels. A concatenation with the correspondingly cropped feature map from the contracting path is followed by two 3 × 3 convolutions and ReLU. This step is repeated multiple times, progressively increasing the spatial dimensions and decreasing the number of feature channels. The purpose of the expanding path is to enable precise localization by combining the high-level abstract features from the bottleneck with the detailed information from the contracting path.

At the end of the expanding path, a 1 × 1 convolution is used to map each feature vector to the desired number of classes, usually one for each class in the segmentation task. This results in a segmented output image with the same spatial dimensions as the input image.

The automated segmentation of the 3D-CT using 3D U-Net [8] will enable the automated measurement of the abscess and the distance from the abscess to the inlet of the trachea. Since the CNN performance is highly connected to the quality and characteristics of the data, tuning the hyperparameters and use several variations of the architecture is a necessary process. The U-Net architecture will act as a starting point, but we aim to create a data-oriented architecture for the specific project.

2.3   Clinical Data Analysis

As a next step, the results of the automated image process in addition to the clinical data will be used for the training and testing of k-Nearest Neighbors method [9, 10].

k-Nearest Neighbors (k-NN) is a valuable tool for analyzing clinical data, offering simplicity, flexibility, and intuitive predictions. Its effectiveness in disease classification, treatment outcome prediction, and patient risk stratification makes it a valuable asset in the realm of healthcare analytics. However, careful consideration of the algorithm's parameters and preprocessing steps is essential to ensure accurate and reliable results.

k-NN is an instance-based or lazy learning algorithm, meaning it does not explicitly learn a model during training. Instead, it stores the entire training dataset and makes predictions based on the stored data.

To determine the "closeness" or similarity between data points, k-NN relies on distance metrics. Commonly used distance metrics include Euclidean distance, Manhattan distance, and Minkowski distance [9].

The parameter k represents the number of nearest neighbors to consider when making a prediction. The choice of k significantly impacts the algorithm's performance. A smaller k may lead to noisy predictions, while a larger k can smooth out predictions but may ignore local variations.

As all ML methods, k-NN requires adjustment to the specific data. Moreover, we aim to explore more ML algorithms for data analysis.

3 Discussion

DL models are increasingly used for predictive analytics based on prior observations. Various DL algorithms can analyze large datasets, transforming complex and heterogeneous data into actionable clinical insights. Applications of DL in medicine include cancer diagnosis, prognostic predictions, integration of clinical and genomic data, clinical trial design, and the analysis of readmission and mortality data. In the context of infectious diseases, DL aids in diagnosis, severity prediction, and determination of the most appropriate antimicrobial treatments [11–13]. Nowadays, high diagnostic performance DL models are becoming increasingly available for clinical practice regarding lesion detection and prediction. Moreover, DL models have been widely used in medical imaging, as their accuracy is human levelled. Additionally, ML and DL algorithms have revealed patterns in clinical data and improved the decision-making in pharmaceutical data. However, in the case of tracheostomy, the only study using ML techniques to date (i.e., the state-of-the-art) focuses merely on the decision whether to perform tracheostomy or not (based on preliminary data), without specifying about other related factors (e.g., size or type of tracheostomy, etc.) [14–16]. In our study, a DL model will be developed to predict the optional parameters of tracheostomy of patients based on clinical and CT data, demonstrating potential clinical utility [17].

The k-NN algorithm, one of the oldest and simplest ML algorithms, is renowned for its accuracy in data mining and pattern classification. It assumes that instances in a dataset will be close to other instances with similar characteristics, basing classification on the similarity with nearest neighbors. The algorithm prioritizes relative distances between instances over their absolute positions, making it suitable for large, multidimensional datasets, especially when prior knowledge of data distribution is absent. Additionally, k-NN requires no off-line training, enhancing time efficiency. It is widely used in fields such as transportation, information security, and medicine [18].

Significant factors will be identified and used for classification. For our DL model, factors will be chosen for their ease of implementation and interpretability, helping clinicians decide the parameters of tracheostomy.

As CNNs and k-means clustering are different methods used for different data structures, more than one performance criteria are needed [19]. The most well-established and commonly used estimator for the results of CNN algorithms are the Dice coefficient and F1 scores. Additionally, to evaluate the k-means performance, Adjusted Rand Index (ARI) will be used. After the accuracy and performance of the used algorithms reaches its top value, the results of both will be combined to predict the factors of the tracheostomy procedure. The developed algorithms will be refined throughout the project duration as more data, as well as clinical feedback from the pilot studies, become available [20].

4   Conclusion

This study presents an AI framework designed to extract clinically relevant information from patient data to predict tracheostomy parameters. This framework has the potential to enhance patient care by streamlining the tracheostomy process. As clinical workflows become more sophisticated, these AI systems could serve as valuable diagnostic aids for physicians, particularly in situations involving diagnostic uncertainty or complexity. By augmenting physician reasoning, these frameworks can provide significant support.

Acknowledgments. The project Improving Personalized Medicine via AI-based Precision Tracheostomy – PRECIOUS, ENTERPRISES/0223/Sub-Call1/0263 is co-financed by the European Regional Development Fund and the Republic of Cyprus through the Research and Innovation Foundation.

References

1. Freeman, B.D.: Tracheostomy update: when and how. Crit. Care Clin. **33**(2), 311–322 (2017). https://doi.org/10.1016/j.ccc.2016.12.007. PMID: 28284297
2. Sheshadri, A., et al.: Pulmonary function testing in patients with tracheostomies: feasibility and technical considerations. Lung **199**(3), 307–310 (2021). https://doi.org/10.1007/s00408-021-00441
3. Wilkinson, K., Freeth, H., Martin, I.: Are we 'on the right trach?' The national confidential enquiry into patient outcome and death examines tracheostomy care. J. Laryngol. Otol. **129** (3), 212–216 (2015). https://doi.org/10.1017/S00222151150001588
4. Growson, M.G., et al.: A contemporary review of machine learning in otolaryngology – head and neck surgery. Laryngoscope **130**, 45–51 (2020)
5. Liang, H., et al.: Evaluation and accurate diagnoses of pediatric diseases using artificial intelligence. Nat. Med. **25**, 433–438 (2019). https://doi.org/10.1038/s41591-018-0335-9
6. Janowczyk, A., Madabhushi, A.: Deep learning for digital pathology image analysis: a comprehensive tutorial with selected use cases. J. Pathol. Inform. **7**, 29 (2016)
7. Ronneberger, O., Fischer, P., Brox, T.: U-Net: convolutional networks for biomedical image segmentation. In: Navab, N., Hornegger, J., Wells, W., Frangi, A. (eds.) Medical Image Computing and Computer-Assisted Intervention, vol. 9351 MICCAI (2015)
8. Çiçek, Ö., Abdulkadir, A., Lienkamp, S. S., Brox, T., Ronneberger, O: 3D U-Net: learning dense volumetric segmentation from sparse annotation. In: Ourselin, S., Joskowicz, L., Sabuncu, M., Unal, G., Wells, W. (eds.) Medical Image Computing and Computer-Assisted Intervention, vol. 9901, MICCAI (2016)
9. Fix, E., Hodges, J.L.: Discriminatory analysis. Nonparametric discrimination: consistency properties (PDF) (Report). USAF School of Aviation Medicine, Randolph Field, Texas. Archived (PDF) from the original on September 26, 2020 (1951)

10. Cover, T.M., Hart, P.E.: Nearest neighbor pattern classification (PDF). IEEE Trans. Inf. Theory. **13**(1), 21–27 (1967). CiteSeerX 10.1.1.68.2616. https://doi.org/10.1109/TIT.1967. 1053964. S2CID 5246200

11. Balkenende, L., Teuwen, J., Mann, R.M.: Application of deep learning in breast cancer imaging. Semin. Nucl. Med. **52**(5), 584–596 (2022). https://doi.org/10.1053/j.semnuclmed. 2022.02.003

12. Zeng, C., Gu, L., Liu, Z., Zhao, S.: Review of deep learning approaches for the segmentation of multiple sclerosis lesions on brain MRI. Front. Neuroinformatics **14**, 1662–5196 (2020). https://doi.org/10.3389/fninf.2020.610967

13. Kijowski, R., et al.: Deep learning for lesion detection, progression, and prediction of musculoskeletal disease. **52**(6), 1607–1619 (2020). https://doi.org/10.1002/jmri.27001.

14. Esteva, A., et al.: Dermatologist-level classification of skin cancer with deep neural networks. Nature **542**, 115–118 (2017)

15. Mayo, R.C., Leung, J.: Artificial intelligence and deep learning -radiology's next frontier? Clin. Imaging **49**, 87–88 (2018). https://doi.org/10.1016/j.clinimag.2017.11.007

16. Mahmood, R., et al.: Automated treatment planning in radiation therapy using generative adversial networks. Proc. Mach. Learn. Res. **85**, 1–15 (2018)

17. Chen, S.-L., Chin, S.-C., Ho, C.-Y.: Deep learning artificial intelligence to predict the need for tracheostomy in patients of deep neck infection based on clinical and computed tomography findings— preliminary data and a pilot study. Diagnostics **2022**, 12 (1943). https://doi.org/10.3390/diagnostics1208194

18. Zhang, Z.: Introduction to machine learning: k-nearest neighbors. Annal. Transl. Med. **4**(11), 218 (2012)

19. Emmert-Streib, F., et.al: An introductory review of deep learning for prediction models with big data. Front. Artif. Intell. **3**, 2624–8212 (2020). https://doi.org/10.3389/frai.2020.00004

20. Hubert, L., Arabie, P.: Comparing partitions. J. Classif. **2**(1), 193–218 (1985)

Author Index

© ICST Institute for Computer Sciences, Social Informatics and Telecommunications Engineering 2025
Published by Springer Nature Switzerland AG 2025. All Rights Reserved
H. Kondylakis and A. Triantafyllidis (Eds.): PervasiveHealth 2024, LNICST 612, pp. 247–249, 2025.
https://doi.org/10.1007/978-3-031-85575-7

The manufacturer's authorised representative in the EU is Springer

Nature Customer Service Centre GmbH, Europaplatz 3, 69115 Heidelberg,

Germany. If you have any concerns regarding our products, please

contact ProductSafety@springernature.com

Printed and bound by CPI Group (UK) Ltd, Croydon, CR0 4YY
27/04/2026

02097586-0004